Men's Health Concerns

SOURCEBOOK

Fifth Edition

Health Reference Series

Fifth Edition

Men's Health Concerns

SOURCEBOOK

Basic Consumer Health Information about Trends and Issues in Men's Health, Including Information about Gender-Specific Health Differences, the Leading Causes of Death in Men, Reproductive and Sexual Concerns, Male-Linked Genetic Disorders, Mental Health Concerns, Alcohol and Drug Abuse, and Other Concerns of Special Significance to Men

Along with Information about the Screenings, Vaccinations, and Self-Examinations Recommended for Men, Guidelines for Nutrition, Physical Activity, Weight Control, and Other Lifestyle Choices That Affect Wellness, a Glossary of Related Terms, and a Directory of Resources for Further Help and Information

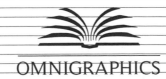

OMNIGRAPHICS

615 Griswold, Ste. 901, Detroit, MI 48226

Bibliographic Note
Because this page cannot legibly accommodate all the copyright notices, the Bibliographic
Note portion of the Preface constitutes an extension of the copyright notice.

* * *

Health Reference Series
Keith Jones, *Managing Editor*
***

OMNIGRAPHICS
A PART OF RELEVANT INFORMATION
***

Copyright © 2017 Omnigraphics
ISBN 978-0-7808-1482-0
E-ISBN 978-0-7808-1481-3

Library of Congress Cataloging-in-Publication Data

Names: Omnigraphics, Inc., issuing body.

Title: Men's health concerns sourcebook: basic consumer health information about
trends and issues in men's health, including information about gender-specific
health differences, the leading causes of death in men, reproductive and sexual
concerns, male-linked genetic disorders, mental health concerns, alcohol and drug
abuse, and other concerns of special significance to men; along with information
about the screenings, vaccinations, and self-examinations recommended for men,
guidelines for nutrition, physical activity, weight control, and other lifestyle
choices that affect wellness, a glossary of related terms, and a directory of
resources for further help and information.

Description: Fifth edition. | Detroit, MI: Omnigraphics, [2016] | Includes
bibliographical references and index.

Identifiers: LCCN 2016032535 (print) | LCCN 2016033061 (ebook) | ISBN
9780780814820 (hardcover: alk. paper) | ISBN 9780780814813 (ebook) | ISBN
9780780814813 (eBook)

Subjects: LCSH: Men--Health and hygiene--Popular works.

Classification: LCC RA776.5 .M457 2016 (print) | LCC RA776.5 (ebook) | DDC
613/.0423--dc23

LC record available at https://lccn.loc.gov/2016032535

Table of Contents

Preface xiii

Part I: Men's Health Basics

Chapter 1—Gender-Specific Health Differences........................... 3

    Section 1.1—Differences in Men's and
                    Women's Health: An Overview 4

    Section 1.2—Why Women Live Longer
                    than Men.. 7

    Section 1.3—Alcohol Use and Risks to
                    Men's Health.................................. 10

    Section 1.4—Gender Differences in Heart
                    Disease 14

    Section 1.5—Gender Differences in
                    Substance Abuse........................... 17

    Section 1.6—PTSD Study: Men versus
                    Women... 21

Chapter 2—Self-Examinations Recommended for Men 25

    Section 2.1—Breast Self-Examination................ 26

    Section 2.2—Oral Cancer Self-Examination....... 28

    Section 2.3—Skin Cancer Self-Examination 30

    Section 2.4—Testicular Self-Examination.......... 33

Chapter 3—Recommended Screening Tests for Men.................. 35

    Section 3.1—Screening Tests for Men:
           What You Need and When............. 36

    Section 3.2—Abdominal Aortic Aneurysm
           Screening... 39

    Section 3.3—Blood Pressure Screening.............. 41

    Section 3.4—Cholesterol Screening..................... 44

    Section 3.5—Colorectal Cancer Screening.......... 47

    Section 3.6—Osteoporosis Screening 52

    Section 3.7—Prostate Cancer Screening............. 53

Chapter 4—Vaccinations for Men.. 57

    Section 4.1—Recommended Vaccinations
           for Adults....................................... 58

    Section 4.2—Human Papillomavirus
           Vaccination..................................... 61

    Section 4.3—Seasonal Influenza Vaccination..... 63

Chapter 5—Managing Common Disease Risk Factors............... 67

    Section 5.1—Preventing High Blood
           Pressure 68

    Section 5.2—Preventing High Cholesterol.......... 70

    Section 5.3—Ensuring Adequate Sleep............... 72

    Section 5.4—Managing Stress............................. 75

Chapter 6—Aim for a Healthy Weight 81

    Section 6.1—Assessing Your Weight and
           Health Risk 82

    Section 6.2—About Body Mass Index (BMI)....... 84

    Section 6.3—Health Risks of Overweight
           and Obesity 88

    Section 6.4—Tips for Healthy Weight Loss 92

    Section 6.5—Choosing a Safe and Successful
           Weight-Loss Program..................... 97

Chapter 7—Nutrition Tips for Men 103

    Section 7.1—Healthy Eating for Men 104

Section 7.2—Nutrition Tips for Building
Strength and Increasing
Muscle Mass 106

Chapter 8—Physical Activity: Key to a Healthy Life 111

Section 8.1—How Much Physical Activity
Do Adults Need? 112

Section 8.2—The Benefits of Physical
Activity 115

Part II: Leading Causes of Death in Men

Chapter 9—Mortality in the United States 121

Section 9.1—Causes of Death: A
Statistical Overview 122

Section 9.2—Cancer among Men: Some
Statistics..................................... 124

Chapter 10—Alzheimer Disease 127

Chapter 11—Chronic Liver Disease 133

Section 11.1—Viral Hepatitis 134

Section 11.2—Cirrhosis................................... 140

Chapter 12—Chronic Obstructive Pulmonary
Disease (COPD) 149

Chapter 13—Colorectal Cancer.. 161

Chapter 14—Diabetes.. 165

Chapter 15—Heart Disease... 169

Section 15.1—Congestive Heart Failure 170

Section 15.2—Coronary Artery Disease 179

Section 15.3—Heart Attack 189

Section 15.4—Taking Aspirin to Prevent
Heart Attacks............................. 199

Chapter 16—HIV and AIDS... 203

Chapter 17—Homicide 211

Chapter 18—Influenza and Pneumonia 215

    Section 18.1—Influenza 216

    Section 18.2—Pneumonia 219

Chapter 19—Chronic Kidney Disease 223

Chapter 20—Liver Cancer.. 229

Chapter 21—Lung Cancer.. 239

Chapter 22—Motor Vehicle Accidents...................................... 245

    Section 22.1—Aggressive Driving 246

    Section 22.2—Distracted Driving.................... 248

    Section 22.3—Drowsy Driving........................ 254

    Section 22.4—Impaired Driving 257

    Section 22.5—Older Drivers 261

Chapter 23—Other Accidents and Injuries 265

    Section 23.1—Falls... 266

    Section 23.2—Fire-Related Injuries 269

    Section 23.3—Occupational Injuries 275

    Section 23.4—Poisoning................................. 280

    Section 23.5—Water-Related Accidents.......... 284

Chapter 24—Penile Cancer.. 291

Chapter 25—Prostate Cancer 301

Chapter 26—Testicular Cancer.. 315

Chapter 27—Stroke 325

Chapter 28—Suicide 335

Part III: Sexual and Reproductive Concerns

Chapter 29—Kidney and Urological Disorders......................... 343

    Section 29.1—Kidney Stones 344

    Section 29.2—Urinary Incontinence in
              Men... 351

Chapter 30—Penile Concerns 363

    Section 30.1—Circumcision 364

    Section 30.2—Balanitis 367

    Section 30.3—Penile Intraepithelial
                    Neoplasia (Erythroplasia
                    of Queyrat) 370

    Section 30.4—Penile Trauma 372

    Section 30.5—Peyronie Disease...................... 374

    Section 30.6—Phimosis and Paraphimosis..... 381

Chapter 31—Disorders of the Scrotum and Testicles............... 385

    Section 31.1—Epididymitis............................. 386

    Section 31.2—Hydrocele................................ 390

    Section 31.3—Inguinal Hernia 393

    Section 31.4—Spermatocele............................ 401

    Section 31.5—Testicular Torsion 403

    Section 31.6—Perineal Injury in Males 407

    Section 31.7—Undescended Testicle............... 414

    Section 31.8—Varicocele 416

Chapter 32—Noncancerous Prostate Disorders....................... 421

    Section 32.1—Benign Prostatic
                    Hyperplasia.............................. 422

    Section 32.2—Prostatitis................................ 428

Chapter 33—Sexual Dysfunction... 439

Chapter 34—Male Infertility.. 449

Chapter 35—Vasectomy and Vasectomy Reversal 453

Chapter 36—Nonsurgical Contraception 459

    Section 36.1—Birth Control Methods:
                    How Well Do They Work? 460

    Section 36.2—Condoms.................................. 462

    Section 36.3—Withdrawal 464

Chapter 37—Safer Sex Guidelines 467

Chapter 38—Sexually Transmitted Diseases 471

    Section 38.1—What Are Sexually
                   Transmitted Diseases? 472

    Section 38.2—Chlamydia 475

    Section 38.3—Genital Herpes 480

    Section 38.4—Gonorrhea 485

    Section 38.5—Hepatitis B 488

    Section 38.6—Human Papillomavirus 490

    Section 38.7—Pubic Lice (Crabs).................... 494

    Section 38.8—Scabies.................................... 498

    Section 38.9—Syphilis................................... 501

    Section 38.10—Trichomoniasis...................... 507

Part IV: Other Medical Issues of Concern to Men

Chapter 39—Male-Linked Genetic Disorders 513

    Section 39.1—Color Vision Deficiency............. 514

    Section 39.2—Fragile X Syndrome................. 521

    Section 39.3—Hemophilia.............................. 526

    Section 39.4—Klinefelter Syndrome 535

    Section 39.5—Muscular Dystrophy 543

Chapter 40—Breast Concerns in Men 553

    Section 40.1—Breast Cancer in Men.............. 554

    Section 40.2—Gynecomastia.......................... 563

Chapter 41—Osteoporosis in Men 565

Chapter 42—Sleep Apnea in Men... 573

Chapter 43—Male Pattern Baldness 583

Chapter 44—Mental Health Concerns in Men.......................... 587

    Section 44.1—Depression............................... 588

    Section 44.2—Posttraumatic Stress
                   Disorder...................................... 593

    Section 44.3—Schizophrenia.......................... 600

Chapter 45—Alcohol, Tobacco, and Drug Use in Men.............. 611

    Section 45.1—Alcohol: Frequently Asked
                 Questions.................................. 612

    Section 45.2—Smoking: Harmful Effects
                 and Benefits of Quitting........... 617

    Section 45.3—Quitting Smoking 625

    Section 45.4—Smokeless Tobacco................... 628

    Section 45.5—Drugs: What You Should
                 Know.. 630

    Section 45.6—Anabolic Steroid Use 633

Chapter 46—Violence Against Men... 637

    Section 46.1—Myths and Realities of
                 Domestic Abuse Against
                 Men.. 638

    Section 46.2—Sexual Assault of Men.............. 641

Chapter 47—A Guy's Guide to Body Image 645

Chapter 48—Body Dysmorphic Disorder 651

Chapter 49—Male Menopause 655

Part V: Additional Help and Information

Chapter 50—Glossary of Men's Health Terms......................... 661

Chapter 51—Directory of Resources That Provide
                 Information about Men's Health......................... 669

Index... 677

Preface

About This Book

The life expectancy gap between men and women has narrowed in recent years, but men still face many health disadvantages. Men are more likely than women to smoke and drink, engage in risky behaviors, and put off checkups and regular preventative care. Men also face a number of disorders unique to their gender, including prostate cancer, penile and testicular disorders, low testosterone, and sex-linked genetic disorders.

Men's Health Concerns Sourcebook, Fifth Edition, discusses health issues that disproportionally affect men. It explains how men can help protect themselves and preserve their health with self-examinations, vaccinations, screening tests, and lifestyle choices. It provides facts about the specific diseases and injuries that comprise the list of leading causes of death in men and explains how men can avoid them or lessen their impact. Detailed information about sexual and reproductive concerns, prostate disorders, substance use, mental health concerns, and other disorders affecting men is included. Lifestyle choices, nutrition and physical activity for men are also covered. A glossary of related terms and a list of resources provide further help and information.

How to Use This Book

This book is divided into parts and chapters. Parts focus on broad areas of interest. Chapters are devoted to single topics within a part.

Part I: Men's Health Basics provides fundamental information about differences in men's and women's health, screening tests, self-examinations, and vaccinations that are recommended for men. It offers suggestions for managing common disease risk factors, including tips on weight management, nutrition, and physical activity.

Part II: Leading Causes of Death in Men describes the factors that contribute most significantly to men's mortality, including heart disease, cancer, diabetes, Alzheimer disease, liver and kidney disease, chronic obstructive pulmonary disease, and other respiratory illnesses. It discusses common injuries and accidents frequently associated with fatalities in men, including motor vehicle accidents, falls, occupational injuries, homicide, and suicide.

Part III: Sexual and Reproductive Concerns provides information about conditions that affect male reproductive organs, including urological disorders, prostate disorders, disorders of the scrotum and testicles, circumcision, and penile concerns. It offers suggestions for dealing with sexual dysfunction and male infertility. It includes facts about birth control methods, sexually transmitted diseases, and safer sex practices.

Part IV: Other Medical Issues of Concern to Men discusses male linked genetic disorders, including color vision deficiency, hemophilia, and muscular dystrophy. It examines physical and mental health concerns with gender differences in their expression or incidence rates. In addition, men's issues related to disorders traditionally associated with women, such as body image and body dysmorphic disorder, breast cancer, and osteoporosis, are also addressed.

Part V: Additional Help and Information includes a glossary of terms related to men's health and a directory of resources offering additional help and support.

Bibliographic Note

This volume contains documents and excerpts from publications issued by the following U.S. government agencies: Agency for Healthcare Research and Quality (AHRQ); Bureau of Labor Statistics (BLS); Centers for Disease Control and Prevention (CDC); *Eunice Kennedy Shriver* National Institute of Child Health and Human Development (NICHD); Genetics Home Reference (GHR); National Cancer Institute (NCI); National Eye Institute (NEI); National Heart, Lung, and Blood Institute (NHLBI); National Institute of Arthritis and Musculoskeletal and Skin Diseases (NIAMS); National Institute of Dental and Craniofacial Research (NIDCR); National Institute of Diabetes and Digestive and Kidney Diseases (NIDDK); National Institute of Mental Health (NIMH); National Institute on Aging (NIA); National Institute on Drug Abuse (NIDA); National Institutes of Health (NIH); Office of Disease Prevention and Health Promotion (ODPHP); Office of Population Affairs (OPA); Office on Women's Health (OWH); Substance Abuse and Mental Health Services Administration (SAMHSA); U.S. Department of Agriculture (USDA); U.S. Department of Veterans Affairs (VA); U.S. Fire Administration (USFA); and U.S. Food and Drug Administration (FDA).

In addition, this volume contains copyrighted documents from the following organization: The Nemours Foundation

It may also contain original material produced by Omnigraphics and reviewed by medical consultants.

About the Health Reference Series

The *Health Reference Series* is designed to provide basic medical information for patients, families, caregivers, and the general public. Each volume takes a particular topic and provides comprehensive coverage. This is especially important for people who may be dealing with a newly diagnosed disease or a chronic disorder in themselves or in a family member. People looking for preventive guidance, information about disease warning signs, medical statistics, and risk factors for health problems will also find answers to their questions in the *Health Reference Series*. The *Series*, however, is not intended to serve as a tool for diagnosing illness, in prescribing treatments, or as a substitute for the physician/patient relationship. All people concerned about medical symptoms or the possibility of disease are encouraged to seek professional care from an appropriate health care provider.

A Note about Spelling and Style

Health Reference Series editors use *Stedman's Medical Dictionary* as an authority for questions related to the spelling of medical terms and the *Chicago Manual of Style* for questions related to grammatical structures, punctuation, and other editorial concerns. Consistent adherence is not always possible, however, because the individual volumes within the *Series* include many documents from a wide variety of different producers, and the editor's primary goal is to present material from each source as accurately as is possible. This sometimes means that information in different chapters or sections may follow other guidelines and alternate spelling authorities.

Medical Review

Omnigraphics contracts with a team of qualified, senior medical professionals who serve as medical consultants for the *Health Reference Series*. As necessary, medical consultants review reprinted and originally written material for currency and accuracy. Citations including the phrase, "Reviewed (month, year)" indicate material reviewed by this team. Medical consultation services are provided to the *Health Reference Series* editors by:

Dr. Vijayalakshmi, MBBS, DGO, MD
Dr. Senthil Selvan, MBBS, DCH, MD
Dr. K. Sivanandham, MBBS, DCH, MS (Research), PhD

Our Advisory Board

We would like to thank the following board members for providing initial guidance on the development of this series:

- Dr. Lynda Baker, Associate Professor of Library and Information Science, Wayne State University, Detroit, MI

- Nancy Bulgarelli, William Beaumont Hospital Library, Royal Oak, MI

- Karen Imarisio, Bloomfield Township Public Library, Bloomfield Township, MI

- Karen Morgan, Mardigian Library, University of Michigan-Dearborn, Dearborn, MI

- Rosemary Orlando, St. Clair Shores Public Library, St. Clair Shores, MI

Health Reference Series *Update Policy*

The inaugural book in the *Health Reference Series* was the first edition of *Cancer Sourcebook* published in 1989. Since then, the *Series* has been enthusiastically received by librarians and in the medical community. In order to maintain the standard of providing high-quality health information for the layperson the editorial staff at Omnigraphics felt it was necessary to implement a policy of updating volumes when warranted.

Medical researchers have been making tremendous strides, and it is the purpose of the *Health Reference Series* to stay current with the most recent advances. Each decision to update a volume is made on an individual basis. Some of the considerations include how much new information is available and the feedback we receive from people who use the books. If there is a topic you would like to see added to the update list, or an area of medical concern you feel has not been adequately addressed, please write to:

Managing Editor
Health Reference Series
Omnigraphics
615 Griswold, Ste. 901
Detroit, MI 48226

Part One

Men's Health Basics

Part One

Chapter 1

Gender-Specific Health Differences

Chapter Contents

Section 1.1—Differences in Men's and Women's
       Health: An Overview 4

Section 1.2—Why Women Live Longer than Men 7

Section 1.3—Alcohol Use and Risks to Men's Health 10

Section 1.4—Gender Differences in Heart Disease.................... 14

Section 1.5—Gender Differences in Substance Abuse............... 17

Section 1.6—PTSD Study: Men versus Women 21

Section 1.1

Differences in Men's and Women's Health: An Overview

This section includes text excerpted from "Sex and Gender," *NIH News in Health*, National Institutes of Health (NIH), May 2016

Sex and Gender

How Being Male or Female Can Affect Your Health

Are you male or female? The answer to this seemingly simple question can have a major impact on your health. While both sexes are similar in many ways, researchers have found that sex and social factors can make a difference when it comes to your risk for disease, how well you respond to medications, and how often you seek medical care. That's why scientists are taking a closer look at the links between sex, gender, and health.

Many people use the words sex and gender interchangeably, but they're distinct concepts to scientists.

Defining Differences: Sex is biological. It's based on your genetic makeup. Males have one X and one Y chromosome in every cell of the body. Females have two X chromosomes in every cell. These cells make up all your tissues and organs, including your skin, heart, stomach, muscles, and brain.

Gender is a social or cultural concept. It refers to the roles, behaviors, and identities that society assigns to girls and boys, women and men, and gender-diverse people. Gender is determined by how we see ourselves and each other, and how we act and interact with others. There's a lot of diversity in how individuals and groups understand, experience, and express gender. Because gender influences our behaviors and relationships, it can also affect health.

Influences on Health: "Sex and gender play a role in how health and disease affect individuals. There was a time when we studied men and applied those findings to women, but we've learned that there

4

are distinct biological differences between women and men," explains Dr. Janine Austin Clayton, who heads research on women's health at NIH. "Women and men have different hormones, different organs, and different cultural influences—all of which can lead to differences in health."

As scientists learn more about the biology of males and females, they're uncovering the influences of both sex and gender in many areas of health.

For instance, women and men can have different symptoms during a heart attack. For both men and women, the most common heart attack symptom is chest pain or discomfort. But women are more likely than men to have shortness of breath, nausea and vomiting, fatigue, and pain in the back, shoulders, and jaw. Knowing about such differences can lead to better diagnoses and outcomes.

Men and women also tend to have different responses to pain. NIH-funded researchers recently learned that different cells in male and female mice drive pain processing.

"Without studying both sexes, we wouldn't know if we're taking steps in the right direction toward appropriate clinical treatment for men and women," Clayton says. "Our differences also affect how we respond to medications, as well as which diseases and conditions we may be prone to and how those diseases progress in our bodies." For example, women metabolize nicotine faster than men, so nicotine replacement therapies can be less effective in women.

Attention to Addiction: Scientists are finding that addiction to nicotine and other drugs is influenced by sex as well. "When it comes to addiction, differences in sex and gender can be found across the board," says Dr. Sherry McKee, lead researcher at an NIH-funded center at Yale University that studies treatments for tobacco dependence. "There are different reasons men and women pick up a drug and keep using a drug, and in how they respond to treatment and experience relapse. Sex also influences disease risk in addiction. For example, women who smoke are more susceptible to lung and heart disease than men who smoke."

One NIH-funded research team has detected some of these differences in the brain. In a recent study, 16 people who smoke—8 men and 8 women—underwent brain scans while smoking to create "movies" of how smoking affects dopamine, the chemical messenger that triggers feelings of pleasure in the brain.

These brain movies showed that smoking alters dopamine in the brain at different rates and in different locations in males and females.

Dopamine release in nicotine-dependent men occurred quickly in a brain area that reinforces the effect of nicotine and other drugs. Women also had a rapid response, but in a different brain region—the part associated with habit formation. "We were able to pinpoint a different brain response between male and female smokers, a finding that could be useful in developing sex-specific treatments to help smokers quit," says lead study researcher Dr. Kelly Cosgrove, a brain-imaging expert at Yale University.

Finding better ways to help men and women quit smoking is important for everyone's health. More than 16 million Americans have diseases caused by smoking. It's the leading cause of preventable death in the U.S.

Autoimmune Disorders: Scientists have found sex influences in autoimmune disorders as well. About 80% of those affected are women. But autoimmune conditions in men are often more severe. For instance, more women than men get multiple sclerosis (MS), a disease in which the body's immune system attacks the brain and spinal cord. But men seem more likely to get a progressive form of MS that gradually worsens and is more challenging to treat.

"Not only are women more susceptible to MS, but women also have many more considerations in the management of the disease, especially since it often begins during child-bearing years," says Dr. Ellen Mowry, a specialist who studies MS at Johns Hopkins University.

"There are a lot of unanswered questions when it comes to the study of sex differences in MS and other autoimmune disorders," Mowry explains. "Researchers can learn a lot by studying women and men separately and together, considering possible risk or predictive factors that may differ based on sex or gender, and working collaboratively with other scientists to improve the likelihood of detecting these factors."

Section 1.2

Why Women Live Longer than Men

"Why Women Live Longer than Men," © 2017 Omnigraphics.
Reviewed August 2016.

According to statistics compiled by the United Nations, women typically live 4.5 years longer than men worldwide. In 2013 the global average life expectancy for women was 71 years compared to 66.5 for men. This pattern has been observed in every country in the world, and it has held true the entire time that reliable birth and death records have existed.

Although social and lifestyle factors are believed to play a role in adult mortality rates, evidence suggests that biological and genetic factors are also involved. Significantly, studies have found gender-related differences in life expectancy among other primates—female gorillas, chimpanzees, and orangutans consistently outlive males of their species as well. By studying the various factors that may account for increased female longevity, scientists hope that they will identify ways to help both men and women live longer, healthier lives.

Biological Factors

Biologists have put forth a number of theories to explain why women live longer than men. Some of the major genetic and biological factors they believe may contribute to increased female longevity include the following:

- **Women carry two X chromosomes, while men have one X and one Y chromosome.**

  This biological difference means that men are more vulnerable to genetic mutations that can cause life-threatening health conditions. Whereas women may avoid the expression of genetic diseases by relying on a normal gene on the other X chromosome, men lack a second copy of the defective gene.

- **Women's bodies tend to be smaller in size than men's bodies.**

Since larger people have more cells in their bodies, they may have a greater tendency to develop harmful cellular mutations. In addition, larger bodies use more energy, which creates wear and tear on organs and tissues and may increase the rate of long-term damage.

- **Women's immune system function declines at a slower rate than men's.**

All people's immune function gradually declines with age. But blood samples of healthy people have shown that the normal loss of white blood cells—which help protect the body from infection—occurs faster in men than in women. As a result, women may enjoy protection from illness to a more advanced age.

- **The male hormone testosterone may increase disease risk later in life.**

Testosterone, which is secreted by the testicles, is the hormone primarily responsible for the development of male sex traits, such as deep voices and hairy chests. Although testosterone contributes to male strength and virility, it may also increase men's risk of developing cardiovascular disease and cancer later in life. A modern analysis of records from nineteenth-century Korea revealed that eunuchs (men whose testicles are removed before puberty, and thus have significantly lower lifetime exposure to testosterone) lived an average of 20 years longer than typical Korean men and were far more likely to reach their hundredth birthday.

- **The female hormone estrogen may decrease disease risk later in life.**

Estrogen, which is produced in the ovaries, is the hormone primarily responsible for female sex traits, such as breast development and menstruation. In contrast to testosterone, estrogen appears to protect against disease. Estrogen has antioxidant properties, meaning that it helps eliminate harmful chemicals that may cause cell damage. Studies have shown that when the ovaries are removed from female animals, the animals experience an increase in disease risk and a decrease in longevity.

- **Women develop heart disease a decade later than men.**

Heart disease is the leading cause of death for both men and women in the United States. But partly due to the protective effects of estrogen, which helps control cholesterol and prevent plaque formation in the arteries, women tend to develop heart disease ten years later than men. In fact, women's risk of heart disease only begins to increase after menopause, when the production of estrogen declines. In addition, more than four times as many men as women smoke worldwide, and smoking is a major contributor to heart disease. Another theory to explain the delayed onset of cardiovascular illness in women is that women's heart rate tends to increase during the second half of the menstrual cycle. Some researchers claim that this increase offers the same health benefits as moderate exercise.

Lifestyle Factors

In addition to biological differences between men and women, studies have also suggested that sociological and lifestyle factors may contribute to women's longer lifespan. Some of the main factors that are believed to influence mortality rates include the following:

- **Men are more prone to risk-taking behavior.**

  According to the U.S. Centers for Disease Control and Prevention (CDC), unintentional injuries are the third-leading cause of death for American men. For women, on the other hand, unintentional injuries rank sixth. Scientists point out that the frontal lobe of the brain develops more slowly in males than in females. Since this part of the brain is involved in calculating risks and behaving responsibly, men are more likely to exhibit dangerous or risky behavior than women of the same age. As a result, studies show that men are less likely to wear seatbelts and more likely to drive aggressively and be involved in motor vehicle accidents.

- **Women have stronger social networks.**

  Men are often socialized to hide their emotions and keep their concerns bottled up inside. For women, however, it is more culturally acceptable to express emotions and confide in friends or family members about sources of worry or stress. Studies have shown that strong social connections can decrease a person's risk of dying by 50%. Men can experience the protective nature of social ties by getting married—studies have also shown that married men tend to be healthier and live longer than single men.

- **Women take better care of their health.**

  Another contributing factor to women's longevity is that they tend to take better care of their health. Men often ignore or deny symptoms of illness and avoid seeking medical attention. In fact, studies have shown that men are 24% less likely than women to have visited a doctor within the past year.

References

1. Bergland, Christopher. "Why Do Women Live Longer Than Men?" *Psychology Today,* July 8, 2015.

2. Innes, Emma. "Women Live Longer Than Men Because Their Immune Systems Age More Slowly" MailOnline, May15, 2013.

3. Levine, Hallie. "5 Reasons Women Live Longer Than Men" Health.com, October 13, 2014.

4. Zeilinger, Julie. "The Real Reason Women Live Longer Than Men?" *Huffington Post,* August 3, 2013.

Section 1.3

Alcohol Use and Risks to Men's Health

This section contains text excerpted from the following sources: Text beginning with the heading "Alcohol Use and Your Health" is excerpted from "Fact Sheets—Alcohol Use and Your Health," Centers for Disease Control and Prevention (CDC), June 29, 2016; Text beginning with the heading "Excessive Alcohol Use and Risks to Men's Health" is excerpted from "Fact Sheets—Excessive Alcohol Use and Risks to Men's Health," Centers for Disease Control and Prevention (CDC), March 7, 2016.

Alcohol Use and Your Health

Drinking too much can harm your health. Excessive alcohol use led to approximately 88,000 deaths and 2.5 million years of potential life lost (YPLL) each year in the United States from 2006–2010, shortening the lives of those who died by an average of 30 years. Further, excessive drinking was responsible for 1 in 10 deaths among working-age adults aged 20–64 years. The economic costs of excessive alcohol consumption in 2010 were estimated at $249 billion, or $2.05 a drink.

What Is a "Drink"?

In the United States, a standard drink contains 0.6 ounces (14.0 grams or 1.2 tablespoons) of pure alcohol. Generally, this amount of pure alcohol is found in

- 12-ounces of beer (5% alcohol content).

- 8-ounces of malt liquor (7% alcohol content).

- 5-ounces of wine (12% alcohol content).

- 1.5-ounces of 80-proof (40% alcohol content) distilled spirits or liquor (e.g., gin, rum, vodka, whiskey).

What Is Excessive Drinking?

Excessive drinking includes binge drinking, heavy drinking, and any drinking by pregnant women or people younger than age 21.

Binge drinking, the most common form of excessive drinking, is defined as consuming

- For women, 4 or more drinks during a single occasion.

- For men, 5 or more drinks during a single occasion.

Heavy drinking is defined as consuming

- For women, 8 or more drinks per week.

- For men, 15 or more drinks per week.

Most people who drink excessively are not alcoholics or alcohol dependent.

What Is Moderate Drinking?

The *Dietary Guidelines for Americans* defines moderate drinking as up to 1 drink per day for women and up to 2 drinks per day for men. In addition, the *Dietary Guidelines* do not recommend that individuals who do not drink alcohol start drinking for any reason.

However, there are some people who should **not** drink any alcohol, including those who are:

- Younger than age 21.

- Driving, planning to drive, or participating in other activities requiring skill, coordination, and alertness.

- Taking certain prescription or over-the-counter medications that can interact with alcohol.

- Suffering from certain medical conditions.

- Recovering from alcoholism or are unable to control the amount they drink.

By adhering to the *Dietary Guidelines*, you can reduce the risk of harm to yourself or others.

Short-Term Health Risks

Excessive alcohol use has immediate effects that increase the risk of many harmful health conditions. These are most often the result of binge drinking and include the following:

- Injuries, such as motor vehicle crashes, falls, drownings, and burns.

- Violence, including homicide, suicide, sexual assault, and intimate partner violence.

- Alcohol poisoning, a medical emergency that results from high blood alcohol levels.

- Risky sexual behaviors, including unprotected sex or sex with multiple partners. These behaviors can result in unintended pregnancy or sexually transmitted diseases, including HIV.

Long-Term Health Risks

Over time, excessive alcohol use can lead to the development of chronic diseases and other serious problems including:

- High blood pressure, heart disease, stroke, liver disease, and digestive problems.

- Cancer of the breast, mouth, throat, esophagus, liver, and colon.

- Learning and memory problems, including dementia and poor school performance.

- Mental health problems, including depression and anxiety.
- Social problems, including lost productivity, family problems, and unemployment.
- Alcohol dependence, or alcoholism.

By not drinking too much, you can reduce the risk of these short- and long-term health risks.

Excessive Alcohol Use and Risks to Men's Health

Men are more likely than women to drink excessively. Excessive drinking is associated with significant increases in short-term risks to health and safety, and the risk increases as the amount of drinking increases. Men are also more likely than women to take other risks (e.g., drive fast or without a safety belt), when combined with excessive drinking, further increasing their risk of injury or death.

Drinking Levels among Men

- Approximately 58% of adult men report drinking alcohol in the last 30 days.
- Approximately 23% of adult men report binge drinking 5 times a month, averaging 8 drinks per binge.
- Men are almost two times more likely to binge drink than women.
- Most (90%) people who binge drink are not alcoholics or alcohol dependent.
- About 4.5% of men and 2.5% of women met the diagnostic criteria for alcohol dependence in the past year.

Injuries and Deaths as a Result of Excessive Alcohol Use

Men consistently have higher rates of alcohol-related deaths and hospitalizations than women.

Among drivers in fatal motor-vehicle traffic crashes, men are almost twice as likely as women to have been intoxicated (i.e., a blood alcohol concentration of 0.08% or greater).

Excessive alcohol consumption increases aggression and, as a result, can increase the risk of physically assaulting another person.

Men are more likely than women to commit suicide, and more likely to have been drinking prior to committing suicide.

Reproductive Health and Sexual Function

Excessive alcohol use can interfere with testicular function and male hormone production resulting in impotence, infertility, and reduction of male secondary sex characteristics such as facial and chest hair.

Excessive alcohol use is commonly involved in sexual assault. Also, alcohol use by men increases the chances of engaging in risky sexual activity including unprotected sex, sex with multiple partners, or sex with a partner at risk for sexually transmitted diseases.

Cancer

Alcohol consumption increases the risk of cancer of the mouth, throat, esophagus, liver, and colon in men.

There are a number of health conditions affected by excessive alcohol use that affect both men and women.

Section 1.4

Gender Differences in Heart Disease

This section contains text excerpted from the following sources: Text beginning with the heading "Facts about Heart Disease" is excerpted from "Know the Facts about Heart Disease," Centers for Disease Control and Prevention (CDC), March 2010. Reviewed August 2016; Text beginning with the heading "Facts on Men and Heart Disease" is excerpted from "Men and Heart Disease Fact Sheet," Centers for Disease Control and Prevention (CDC), June 16, 2016.

Facts about Heart Disease

What Is Heart Disease?

Heart disease is the leading cause of death in the United States. More than 600,000 Americans die of heart disease each year. That's one in every four deaths in this country.

The term "heart disease" refers to several types of heart conditions. The most common type is coronary artery disease, which can cause heart attack. Other kinds of heart disease may involve the valves in the heart, or the heart may not pump well and cause heart failure. Some people are born with heart disease.

Are You at Risk?

Anyone, including children, can develop heart disease. It occurs when a substance called plaque builds up in your arteries. When this happens, your arteries can narrow over time, reducing blood flow to the heart.

Smoking, eating an unhealthy diet, and not getting enough exercise all increase your risk for having heart disease.

Having high cholesterol, high blood pressure, or diabetes also can increase your risk for heart disease. Ask your doctor about preventing or treating these medical conditions.

What Are the Signs and Symptoms?

The symptoms vary depending on the type of heart disease. For many people, chest discomfort or a heart attack is the first sign.

Someone having a heart attack may experience several symptoms, including:

- Chest pain or discomfort that doesn't go away after a few minutes.

- Pain or discomfort in the jaw, neck, or back.

- Weakness, light-headedness, nausea (feeling sick to your stomach), or a cold sweat.

- Pain or discomfort in the arms or shoulder.

- Shortness of breath.

If you think that you or someone you know is having a heart attack, call 9-1-1 immediately.

How Is Heart Disease Diagnosed?

Your doctor can perform several tests to diagnose heart disease, including chest X-rays, coronary angiograms, electrocardiograms (ECG or EKG), and exercise stress tests. Ask your doctor about what tests may be right for you.

Can It Be Prevented?

You can take several steps to reduce your risk for heart disease:

- Don't smoke.

- Maintain a healthy weight.

- Eat a healthy diet.

- Exercise regularly.

- Prevent or treat your other health conditions, especially high blood pressure, high cholesterol, and diabetes.

How Is It Treated?

If you have heart disease, lifestyle changes, like those just listed, can help lower your risk for complications. Your doctor also may prescribe medication to treat the disease. Talk with your doctor about the best ways to reduce your heart disease risk.

Facts on Men and Heart Disease

- Heart disease is the leading cause of death for men in the United States, killing 321,000 men in 2013—that's **1 in every 4** male deaths.

- Heart disease is the **leading cause** of death for men of most racial/ethnic groups in the United States, including African Americans, American Indians or Alaska Natives, Hispanics, and whites. For Asian American or Pacific Islander men, heart disease is second only to cancer.

- About 8.5% of all white men, 7.9% of black men, and 6.3% of Mexican American men have coronary heart disease.

- **Half** of the men who die suddenly of coronary heart disease have **no previous symptoms**. Even if you have no symptoms, you may still be at risk for heart disease.

- **Between 70% and 89%** of sudden cardiac events occur in men.

Risk Factors

High blood pressure, high LDL cholesterol, and smoking are key risk factors for heart disease. About **half of Americans** (49%) have at least one of these three risk factors.

Several other medical conditions and lifestyle choices can also put people at a higher risk for heart disease, including:

- diabetes

- overweight and obesity

- poor diet

- physical inactivity

- Excessive alcohol use

Section 1.5

Gender Differences in Substance Abuse

This section includes text excerpted from "Gender Differences in Primary Substance of Abuse across Age Groups," Substance Abuse and Mental Health Services Administration (SAMHSA), April 3, 2014.

National data consistently show that gender is an important factor to consider when examining patterns of substance abuse, such as overall prevalence rates and substances of choice. For example, males are more likely than females to report marijuana and alcohol use, whereas females are more likely than males to report nonmedical use of prescription drugs. Also, differences in substance abuse patterns among men and women vary by age. Data from the 2011 National Survey on Drug Use and Health show that men aged 18 or older have almost twice the rate of substance dependence as adult women, but among youths aged 12 to 17, the rate of substance dependence for both genders is the same (6.9 percent). Knowledge of how gender can interact with age and patterns of substance abuse may be useful to those responsible for the design of outreach, prevention, and treatment programs.

The Treatment Episode Data Set (TEDS) collects data on admissions to substance abuse treatment facilities across the United States and can be used to examine differences in primary substance of abuse among males and females by age. TEDS collects information on up to three substances of abuse that led to the treatment episode. The main substance abused by the client is known as the "primary substance of abuse." For each admission, data on primary substance of abuse are reported at the time of treatment entry. The analyses in this report are based on TEDS data for 2011.

TEDS is a census of all admissions to treatment facilities reported to the Substance Abuse and Mental Health Services Administration (SAMHSA) by State substance abuse agencies. Because TEDS involves actual counts rather than estimates, statistical significance and confidence intervals are not applicable. The differences mentioned in the text of this report have Cohen's h effect size ≥ 0.20, indicating that they are considered to be meaningful

Overview and Demographic Characteristics

In 2011, about 609,000 of the 1.84 million admissions to substance abuse treatment were female (33.1 percent), and 1.23 million were male (66.9 percent). No meaningful gender differences were found by race/ ethnicity. Specifically, the majority of female and male admissions (66.4 and 58.2 percent, respectively) were non-Hispanic White. The percentages of female and male admissions that were non-Hispanic Black and Hispanic were similar.

Gender Profiles

No appreciable gender differences were found by primary substances of abuse overall (Figure 1.1). Alcohol was the most commonly reported primary substance of abuse by female (33.3 percent) and male (42.3 percent) admissions. Among females, alcohol was followed by heroin (15.3 percent), marijuana (14.6 percent), and prescription pain relievers (13.8 percent); among males, the next most frequently reported substances were marijuana (19.9 percent), heroin (15.0 percent), and prescription pain relievers (7.8 percent).

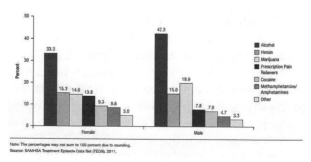

Figure 1.1. *Substance Abuse Treatment Admissions Aged 12 or Older, by Gender and Primary Substance*

18

Differences in Primary Substance of Abuse

Analyses by gender and age were conducted for the six most commonly reported primary substances of abuse: alcohol, marijuana, heroin, prescription pain relievers, cocaine, and methamphetamine/amphetamines. Four of these substances (the exceptions were cocaine and heroin) showed meaningful gender difference (Cohen's h ≥ .20) in at least one age group.

Alcohol and Marijuana

Compared with their male counterparts, a larger proportion of female admissions aged 12 to 17 reported alcohol as their primary substance of abuse (21.7 vs. 10.5 percent). This pattern changed among adult admissions. Among admissions aged 25 to 34, a smaller proportion of female admissions than male admissions reported alcohol as their primary substance of abuse (25.9 vs. 36.5 percent). Marijuana was reported as the primary substance of abuse less frequently by females than males among admissions aged 12 to 17 (60.8 vs. 80.7 percent) and 18 to 24 (22.1 vs. 33.4 percent). There was no variation by gender in primary marijuana abuse among admissions aged 25 or older.

Methamphetamine / Amphetamines

The proportions of female and male admissions reporting methamphetamine/amphetamines as their primary substance of abuse were similar across all age groups with the exception of those aged 18 to 24. Specifically, among admissions aged 18 to 24, 8.9 percent of female admissions reported primary methamphetamine/amphetamine abuse compared with 3.7 percent of male admissions.

Prescription Pain Relievers

The highest proportions of primary abuse of prescription pain relievers (e.g., oxycodone) were found among admissions aged 18 to 24 and 25 to 34. In the 25 to 34 age group, 19.0 percent of female admissions and 12.2 percent of male admissions reported prescription pain relievers as their primary substance of abuse. In terms of the effect size, however, the differences between male and female admissions in these age groups were negligible. The only meaningful difference by effect size between males and females was observed among admissions aged 65 or older. Within the 65 or older age group, the proportion of female admissions reporting primary abuse of prescription pain relievers was nearly 3 times that of their male counterparts (7.2 vs. 2.8 percent).

Discussion

This report highlights important differences in primary substance of abuse between males and females admitted to substance abuse treatment. These differences were found at various stages of life, from adolescence through older adulthood, particularly for abuse of alcohol, marijuana, methamphetamine/amphetamines, and prescription pain relievers. Although this report does not explain the potential reasons for these differences, it brings awareness to the fact that they exist. This may help inform the design of prevention, outreach, and treatment services for specific gender and age groups across multiple settings, including primary care. For example, other research shows that compared with men, women have been found to initiate use of methamphetamine at younger ages and have a greater vulnerability to methamphetamine dependence due to physiological factors. This research, coupled with the findings in this report, might suggest that age-appropriate methamphetamine prevention and outreach efforts directed towards adolescents and young women in particular may be important in areas with moderate to high rates of methamphetamine use.

Additionally, the findings related to differences in the abuse of prescription pain relievers between older adult males and females may warrant further investigation particularly in the context of older adults receiving medications in general medical settings. Further research is needed to understand who would benefit from programs that target particular gender and age groups compared with gender-specific programs and standard treatment.

Section 1.6

PTSD Study: Men versus Women

This section includes text excerpted from "PTSD Study: Men versus Women," U.S. Department of Veterans Affairs (VA), April 18, 2013. Reviewed August 2016.

"In the general population, women are twice as likely as men to develop posttraumatic stress disorder," noted Dr. Sonja Batten, VA's Deputy Chief Consultant for Specialty Mental Health. "But among recent returnees seeking care at VA, PTSD rates among men and women are the same. Statistics such as these suggest the need to better understand the role of gender in PTSD, particularly as it may impact our Veterans seeking care."

Researchers at the Department of Veterans Affairs are now taking some initial steps toward understanding this complex subject. To that end, Dr. Sabra Inslicht, a staff psychologist at the San Francisco VA Medical Center and an assistant professor of psychiatry at the University of California, San Francisco recently led a VA study that took a closer look at how men and women learn to fear. Her work was published in the October 2012 issue of the Journal of Psychiatric Research.

Men Are from Mars; Women Are from Venus

"If we can learn more about potential gender differences in the process of fear learning," Inslicht said, "it may help us develop more targeted treatments that are geared more precisely to the unique needs of men and women."

For their study, Inslicht and her team recruited 18 men and 13 women who had been diagnosed with PTSD. These participants were all shown various images on a computer screen. Electrodes were attached to their palms so researchers could measure participants' physiological response to each image.

After certain images appeared, the test subject received a small electrical shock. Gradually, the test subject came to associate these particular images with something unpleasant.

"They learned to anticipate the impending shock," Inslicht said. "They learned the danger cues. We call this 'fear conditioning.'"

Researchers carefully monitored test subjects' skin conductive responses—that is, how sweaty their palms got—to measure the body's stress reaction to the image on the screen.

"We discovered that women responded more strongly to the visual cues than men when they saw a particular image that they knew was going to be followed by an electric shock," Inslicht explained. "This suggests that women conditioned more robustly than men. In our future work, we'd like to get a better understanding as to why these differences may occur."

Fight or Flight

"To some extent, learning to fear is important for survival," the researcher said. "When we are threatened by something dangerous, we tend to react with a stress response or 'fight-or-flight' response. It helps keep us safe by mobilizing our bodies to either fight or flee a threat, thus enabling us to protect ourselves from harm in dangerous situations."

Inslicht said this 'fight or flight' response, however, can sometimes persist even in non-threatening situations.

"For example," she said, "if you witnessed a suicide bombing while on patrol in a crowded marketplace in Afghanistan, you might develop a fear of crowded places. While you're on patrol and in potential danger, a heightened level of vigilance can be protective. However, if that response persists even after returning home and to a safe place, it can become problematic.

"When you're unable to turn it off in safe situations, the stress becomes prolonged," she continued. "This can cause wear and tear on both the mind and the body. When this heightened reactivity starts to negatively impact your daily life, we begin to worry about posttraumatic stress."

But if fear conditioning does, in fact, occur differently in men and women, then might not the process known as 'fear extinction' also be affected by gender differences?

"Fear extinction happens," Inslicht said, "when you are gradually exposed to the previously learned danger cues, such as crowds, and you gradually come to realize that the cue will not be followed by a stressful or potentially traumatic event. This results in the diminishing of the fear response. Since extinction learning is believed to be important for recovery from PTSD, a deeper understanding of this process could alter our strategy for how we treat PTSD in men and women."

Much More to Learn

Inslicht said her small study leaves a number of questions unanswered, and that more in-depth research is needed.

"For example, all our study participants had PTSD," she said, "so we couldn't arrive at any conclusions regarding whether women, as a general rule, condition more strongly than men do, or whether this difference is found only among women who have already developed PTSD."

"Finally, we did not examine what may drive the gender differences that we found," the researcher noted. "For example, there may be biological differences such as particular hormones and neuropeptides that may mediate these effects."

Inslicht said the research community is only just beginning to understand fear learning and extinction mechanisms and their relationship to PTSD.

"Ultimately, however, this line of research may result in advances for treatment," she concluded. "There may be ways that we can enhance extinction learning—perhaps through medications or with other modifications to existing behavioral treatments."

Chapter 2

Self-Examinations Recommended for Men

Chapter Contents

Section 2.1—Breast Self-Examination 26

Section 2.2—Oral Cancer Self-Examination 28

Section 2.3—Skin Cancer Self-Examination 30

Section 2.4—Testicular Self-Examination................................. 33

Section 2.1

Breast Self-Examination

"Breast Self-Examination," © 2017 Omnigraphics.
Reviewed August 2016.

Many people are not aware that men can develop breast cancer. Males do have breast tissue, however, and malignant (cancerous) cells can develop there—just as they can in any other part of the body. Although less than 1% of all cases of breast cancer occur in males, several factors may increase the risk of male breast cancer, including:

- inherited gene mutations, such as BRCA1 or BRCA2;

- a family history of breast cancer;

- exposure to radiation;

- high levels of estrogen;

- advanced age (most cases are detected in men between the ages of 60 and 70).

Since early detection of male breast cancer can lead to improved treatment options and prognosis, many healthcare practitioners and cancer-prevention organizations recommend that men with an increased risk of breast cancer perform monthly breast self-examinations.

Breast self-examination is a technique people can use to visually and manually check their own breast tissue for lumps or other changes. People who conduct regular self-exams become familiar with the normal appearance and feel of their breast tissue, which enables them to recognize changes and discover lumps that may require medical attention. Some of the changes that should be checked by a doctor include:

- hard lumps or new areas of thickness, which may or may not be painful;

- discharge of fluid from the nipples;

- dimpling, puckering, rashes, or other changes to the skin;

- changes to the size or shape of the breast.

How to Perform a Breast Self-Examination

Doctors recommend that men at risk of breast cancer perform a regular breast self-examination once per month. It should cover the entire surface area of each breast, from the collarbone down to the abdomen, and from the armpit across to the center of the chest. Perhaps the easiest way for men to examine their breast area is in the shower. Using soap and water to create a slippery surface allows the fingers to slide easily over the breast tissue.

The main steps in performing a male breast self-examination are as follows:

1. Raise your right arm and place it behind or on top of your head.

2. Use the pads of the three middle fingers on your left hand to examine your right breast.

3. Move your fingers in small circles, about the size of a quarter.

4. Begin under the armpit and work from top to bottom along the outer part of your breast.

5. After completing one vertical strip, move over one finger width and begin a new strip, working from bottom to top. Do not lift the fingers between rows.

6. Check the entire breast area in an up-and-down pattern, as if mowing a lawn.

7. Repeat the process by using the left hand to examine the right breast.

8. Gently squeeze each nipple between your fingers to check for any fluid discharge, puckering, or retraction.

9. After stepping out of the shower and drying off, visually examine your breasts in front of a mirror. They should appear symmetrical in size and shape, and the skin should not show signs of dimpling, puckering, or rashes.

Men who find a lump or notice other changes in their breast tissue during a self-examination should not become alarmed. Around 80% of all breast lumps are not cancerous. In addition, most lumps or inflammation detected in male breasts are due to a benign condition called gynecomastia. This condition is commonly associated with the hormonal changes of puberty, but it may also occur as a side effect of certain medications. Still, any hard lumps or other areas of concern should be checked by a medical practitioner.

References

1. "Check Yourself for Male Breast Cancer," MaleCare, 2016.

2. Stephan, Pam. "Male Breast Self-Examination," VeryWell, December 16, 2014.

Section 2.2

Oral Cancer Self-Examination

This section contains text excerpted from the following sources: Text beginning with the heading "What Is Oral Cancer?" is excerpted from "Oral Cancer: Causes and Symptoms and the Oral Cancer Exam," National Institute of Dental and Craniofacial Research (NIDCR), July 1, 2016; Text under the heading "The Oral Cancer Exam" is excerpted from "The Oral Cancer Exam," National Institute of Dental and Craniofacial Research (NIDCR), July 1, 2016.

What Is Oral Cancer?

The term oral cancer includes cancers of the mouth and the pharynx (the back of the throat).

What Puts Someone at Risk for Developing Oral Cancer?

Tobacco and alcohol use. Most cases of oral cancer are linked to cigarette smoking, heavy alcohol use, or the use of both tobacco and alcohol together. *Using tobacco plus alcohol poses a much greater risk than using either substance alone.*

HPV. Infection with the sexually transmitted human papillomavirus (specifically the HPV 16 type) has been linked to a subset of oral cancers.

Age. Risk increases with age. Oral cancer most often occurs in people over the age of 40.

Sun exposure. Cancer of the lip can be caused by sun exposure.

Diet. A diet low in fruits and vegetables may play a role in oral cancer development.

What Are the Possible Signs and Symptoms of Oral Cancer?

- A sore, irritation, lump or thick patch in the mouth, lip, or throat
- A white or red patch in the mouth
- A feeling that something is caught in the throat
- Difficulty chewing or swallowing
- Difficulty moving the jaw or tongue
- Numbness in the tongue or other areas of the mouth
- Swelling of the jaw that causes dentures to fit poorly or become uncomfortable
- Pain in one ear without hearing loss

A person who has any of these symptoms for more than 2 weeks should see a dentist or doctor for an oral cancer exam. Most often, symptoms like those listed above do not mean cancer. An infection or another problem can cause the same symptoms. *But it's important to have the symptoms checked out—because if it is cancer, it can be treated more successfully if it's caught early.*

What Is the Oral Cancer Exam?

An oral cancer examination can detect early signs of cancer. The exam is painless and takes only a few minutes.

During the exam, a dentist or doctor checks the face, neck, lips, tongue, mouth, and the back of the throat for possible signs of cancer.

The Oral Cancer Exam

An oral cancer exam is painless and quick—it takes only a few minutes. Here's what to expect:

- Preparing for the exam: If you have dentures (plates) or partials, you will be asked to remove them.
- Your doctor or dentist will inspect your face, neck, lips and mouth.

- With both hands, he or she will feel the area under your jaw and the side of your neck, checking for unusual lumps.

- Next, your doctor or dentist will have you stick out your tongue to check for swelling or abnormal color or texture.

- Using gauze, he or she will then gently pull your tongue to one side, then the other, to check the base of your tongue. The underside of your tongue will also be checked.

- In addition, he or she will look at the roof and floor of your mouth, as well as the back of your throat.

- He or she will then look at and feel the insides of your lips and cheeks to check for possible signs of cancer, such as red and/or white patches.

- Finally, your doctor or dentist will put one finger on the floor of your mouth and, with the other hand under your chin, gently press down to check for unusual lumps or sensitivity.

Section 2.3

Skin Cancer Self-Examination

"Skin Cancer Self-Examination," © 2017 Omnigraphics.
Reviewed August 2016.

When potential skin cancers are found and treated early, they can usually be cured. Early detection is thus a major priority. Doctors and cancer-fighting organizations recommend conducting a thorough, head-to-toe skin cancer self-examination every month as a way to help people notice changes in their skin and identify suspicious moles, growths, or lesions that should be checked by a physician.

Medical professionals have developed two main strategies to help people recognize malignant melanoma—the deadliest form of skin cancer—as well as non-melanoma skin cancers, such as basal cell carcinoma and squamous cell carcinoma. These early recognition strategies, the ABCDEs and the Ugly Duckling sign, can be applied by individuals examining their own skin as well as by healthcare professionals.

How to Conduct a Self-Examination

Medical practitioners and skin cancer awareness organizations recommend that people conduct a head-to-toe self-examination once per month to check for unusual moles or lesions on their skin. A complete examination should include the following areas:

1. Face—use a mirror to examine the nose, mouth, and ears.

2. Scalp—use a blow dryer to expose various sections of the scalp for inspection or ask a friend or family member to help.

3. Hands—check the palms as well as the backs of the hands, and look between the fingers and under the fingernails.

4. Arms—begin by inspecting the wrists and forearms, then use a mirror to check the elbows, upper arms, and underarms.

5. Chest—examine the neck, collarbone, chest, and torso.

6. Back—using a full-length mirror and a hand mirror, check the back of the neck, shoulders, upper back, and lower back.

7. Genitals—use a hand mirror to examine the buttocks and genital area.

8. Legs—inspect the front and back of each leg, including thigh, shin, calf, and ankle.

9. Feet—check the top and bottom of each foot, as well as between the toes and under toenails.

What to Look for in a Self-Examination

Most people have ordinary, harmless moles or spots on their skin. Also known as nevi, moles are common skin growths in which pigment cells form a cluster. A typical nevus may appear black, brown, tan, pink, or red. It may be flat or slightly raised, and it may be round or oval in shape. The goal of a skin cancer self-examination is to identify atypical moles (dysplastic nevi) that may be pre-cancerous or cancerous. The two main strategies to help people distinguish between harmless and suspicious moles are the ABCDEs and the Ugly Duckling sign.

The ABCDEs

The acronym ABCDE is a valuable tool for helping people evaluate moles, spots, and other skin growths. Each letter represents a specific

31

warning sign that a mole may potentially be cancerous and should be checked by a doctor:

- Asymmetry—benign (non-cancerous) moles tend to be symmetrical, meaning that the two halves match; asymmetry is a warning sign for melanoma.

- Border irregularity—typical moles tend to have smooth, regular borders, while melanomas usually have rough, uneven, notched, or scalloped edges.

- Color variation—benign moles tend to be all one color, while melanomas often have a number of different shades of brown, tan, black, red, or white.

- Diameter—benign moles are typically smaller than 6 mm in diameter (about the size of the eraser on a pencil), while melanomas tend to be larger in diameter.

- Evolution—the appearance of common moles tends to remain the same over time, so any changes or evolution in a mole's size, shape, color, or other characteristics (such as itching, crusting, bleeding, or failing to heal) should be considered a warning sign.

The Ugly Duckling Sign

Although the ABCDEs are helpful in identifying potential skin cancers, even experts may find it challenging to distinguish melanomas from harmless moles that display some of the warning signs. Given the importance of early detection, skin cancer specialists developed a second tool—the Ugly Duckling sign—to aid in screening and diagnosis.

The Ugly Duckling sign is based on the fact that all of the moles on the skin of a specific person tend to resemble one another. Whether a person has a dozen moles or a hundred moles, most will be of a similar shape, color, and size. As a result, part of the skin cancer self-examination should involve comparing each mole to surrounding moles and looking for outliers—or "ugly ducklings"—that do not fit into the usual pattern. For instance, a mole that stands out from the background because it is larger or a different color than most others should be considered suspicious and checked by a doctor.

Section 2.4

Testicular Self-Examination

Although testicular cancer has a relatively low rate of occurrence, accounting for just one percent of malignancies in all men, it is the most common neoplasm, or abnormal growth, in adolescent males and young men under 35 years of age. Testicular cancer is easily diagnosable and can be successfully treated, with a high survival rate of more than ten years in nearly 90 percent of patients. As with most types of cancer, the prognosis is particularly good with early detection. While significant advances have been made in developing treatments for testicular cancer in the last few decades, the benefits of early detection through self-examination have not received much attention, often resulting in delays before medical attention is sought.

Importance of Testicular Self-Examination (TSE)

In the absence of a standard or routine screening for testicular cancer, the condition is most often detected either by a doctor during a routine physical examination, or by an individual during the course of a self-exam. The outlook for testicular cancer depends on whether or not the disease has metastasized to lymph nodes, tissues, and organs, and this underscores the importance of early detection by TSE. Early detection involves the diagnosis of testicular cancer through Stages 1 and 2. Stage 1 refers to a "localized" tumor restricted to the primary site, the testes. Stage 2 is the term for a "regional" tumor, one that has spread to other areas. An early diagnosis resulting from a self-exam can greatly enhance treatment outcomes and also reduce the side effects commonly associated with chemotherapy, radiation, and surgery.

How to Perform a Self-Exam

It is important to perform a self-examination every month. This allows you to familiarize yourself with the size, shape, and consistency of your testes and sensitize you to any abnormality in the future. This also helps you to distinguish the epididymis—a highly coiled duct behind the testis for the temporary storage of sperm—from an abnormal lump or growth. Further, it is quite normal for most men to have testicular asymmetry. Differently sized testes with one hanging lower than the other is a normal anatomical feature and should not be construed as a sign of abnormality.

The ideal time to perform a self-exam is right after a warm shower when the scrotum is relaxed and can be easily drawn back to examine the testicles.

TSE is a simple procedure that takes no more than a couple of minutes:

- Hold the penis away from the scrotum to enable close examination of the testes.

- Hold the testicles between your thumb and fingers and roll gently.

- Feel each testicle for any painless lump, usually grain or pea-sized, in the front or sides, taking care not to confuse a lump with supporting tissues and blood vessels.

- If you detect any thickening, discomfort, or pain in the testicles or groin, contact your healthcare professional immediately.

Studies show that men often delay seeking medical attention because early symptoms are typically mild, and many men tend to believe that a lump is benign or harmless and may go away on its own. Concerns about loss of sexuality, or sterility, may also get in the way of seeking professional help when an abnormality is detected.

While the majority of scrotal and testicular irregularities may not be associated with malignancy, it is important for all men—especially those who carry a high risk for testicular tumors—to perform regular self-exams. A family history of testicular cancer and previous history of malignant tumors in one or both of the testes are regarded as high-risk factors, as are conditions such as *cryptorchidism*, a common birth defect associated with undescended testes.

References

1. "How to Perform a Testicular Self-Examination," The Nemours Foundation, 2012.

2. "Testicular Examination and Testicular Self-Examination (TSE)," Healthwise, Incorporated, June 4, 2014.

3. "SEER Stat Fact Sheets: Testis Cancer," National Institutes of Health (NIH), April 2016.

Chapter 3

Recommended Screening Tests for Men

Chapter Contents

Section 3.1—Screening Tests for Men: What You
Need and When 36

Section 3.2—Abdominal Aortic Aneurysm Screening 39

Section 3.3—Blood Pressure Screening 41

Section 3.4—Cholesterol Screening 44

Section 3.5—Colorectal Cancer Screening.................................... 47

Section 3.6—Osteoporosis Screening 52

Section 3.7—Prostate Cancer Screening 53

Section 3.1

Screening Tests for Men:
What You Need and When

This section includes text excerpted from "Men: Stay Healthy at Any Age," Agency for Healthcare Research and Quality (AHRQ), U.S. Department of Health and Human Services (HHS), March 2014.

Get the Screenings You Need

Screenings are tests that look for diseases before you have symptoms. Blood pressure checks and tests for high blood cholesterol are examples of screenings.

You can get some screenings, such as blood pressure readings, in your doctor's office. Others, such as colonoscopy, a test for colon cancer, need special equipment, so you may need to go to a different office.

After a screening test, ask when you will see the results and who you should talk to about them.

Abdominal Aortic Aneurysm. If you are between the ages of 65 and 75 and have ever been a smoker, (smoked 100 or more cigarettes in your lifetime) get screened once for abdominal aortic aneurysm (AAA). AAA is a bulging in your abdominal aorta, your largest artery. An AAA may burst, which can cause dangerous bleeding and death.

An ultrasound, a painless procedure in which you lie on a table while a technician slides a medical device over your abdomen, will show whether an aneurysm is present.

Colon Cancer. Have a screening test for colorectal cancer starting at age 50. If you have a family history of colorectal cancer, you may need to be screened earlier. Several different tests can detect this cancer. Your doctor can help you decide which is best for you.

Depression. Your emotional health is as important as your physical health. Talk to your doctor or nurse about being screened for depression, especially if during the last 2 weeks:

- You have felt down, sad, or hopeless.

- You have felt little interest or pleasure in doing things.

Diabetes. Get screened for diabetes (high blood sugar) if you have high blood pressure or if you take medication for high blood pressure.

Diabetes can cause problems with your heart, brain, eyes, feet, kidneys, nerves, and other body parts.

Hepatitis C virus (HCV). Get screened one time for HCV infection if:

- You were born between 1945 and 1965.

- You have ever injected drugs.

- You received a blood transfusion before 1992.

If you currently are an injection drug user, you should be screened regularly.

High Blood Cholesterol. If you are 35 or older, have your blood cholesterol checked regularly with a blood test. High cholesterol increases your chance of heart disease, stroke, and poor circulation. Talk to your doctor or nurse about having your cholesterol checked starting at age 20 if:

- You use tobacco.

- You are overweight or obese.

- You have diabetes or high blood pressure.

- You have a history of heart disease or blocked arteries.

- A man in your family had a heart attack before age 50 or a woman, before age 60.

High Blood Pressure. Have your blood pressure checked at least every 2 years. High blood pressure can cause strokes, heart attacks, kidney and eye problems, and heart failure.

HIV. If you are 65 or younger, get screened for HIV. If you are older than 65, ask your doctor or nurse whether you should be screened.

Lung Cancer: Talk to your doctor or nurse about getting screened for lung cancer if you are between the ages of 55 and 80, have a 30 pack-year smoking history, and smoke now or have quit within the past 15 years. (Your pack-year history is the number of packs of cigarettes smoked per day times the number of years you have smoked.) Know that quitting smoking is the best thing you can do for your health.

Overweight and Obesity. The best way to learn if you are overweight or obese is to find your body mass index (BMI).

A BMI between 18.5 and 25 indicates a normal weight. Persons with a BMI of 30 or higher may be obese. If you are obese, talk to your doctor or nurse about getting intensive counseling and help with changing your behaviors to lose weight. Overweight and obesity can lead to diabetes and cardiovascular disease.

Get Preventive Medicines If You Need Them

Aspirin. If you are 45 or older, your doctor or nurse can help you decide whether taking aspirin to prevent a heart attack is right for you.

Vitamin D to Avoid Falls. If you are 65 or older and have a history of falls, mobility problems, or other risks for falling, ask your doctor about taking a vitamin D supplement to help reduce your chances of falling. Exercise and physical therapy may also help.

Immunizations:

- Get a flu shot every year.

- If you are 60 or older, get a shot to prevent shingles.

- If you are 65 or older, get a pneumonia shot.

- Get a shot for tetanus, diphtheria, and whooping cough. Get a tetanus booster if it has been more than 10 years since your last shot.

- Talk with your healthcare team about whether you need other vaccinations.

Section 3.2

Abdominal Aortic Aneurysm Screening

This section includes text excerpted from "Talk to Your Doctor
about Abdominal Aortic Aneurysm," Office of Disease Prevention
and Health Promotion (ODPHP), U.S. Department of Health and
Human Services (HHS), March 29, 2016.

The Basics

If you are a man age 65 to 75 and have ever smoked, ask your doctor
about getting screened (tested) for abdominal aortic aneurysm (AAA).
If AAA isn't found and treated early, it can be deadly.

Am I at risk for AAA?

Men over age 65 who have smoked at any point in their lives have
the highest risk of AAA.

Risk factors for AAA include:

- Close family history

- Smoking

- Older age

- High blood pressure

- Heart disease or vascular disease (problems with blood vessels)

If you think you may be at risk for AAA, talk to your doctor.

What is AAA?

The aorta is your body's main artery. An artery is a blood vessel (or
tube) that carries blood from your heart. The aorta carries blood from
your heart to your abdomen (belly), pelvis, and legs.

If the wall of your aorta is weak, it can swell like a balloon. This
balloon-like swelling is called an aneurysm. AAA is an aneurysm that
occurs in the part of the aorta running through the abdomen.

Why do I need to talk to the doctor?

Aneurysms usually grow slowly without any symptoms. When aneurysms grow large enough to burst (break open), they can cause dangerous bleeding inside the body that can lead to death.

If AAA is found early, it can be treated before it bursts. That's why it's so important to ask the doctor about your risk.

How do I know if I have AAA?

To check for AAA, your doctor may order an ultrasound test. An ultrasound uses sound waves to look inside the body. It can help your doctor see if there is any swelling of the aorta. Most types of ultrasounds are painless.

What are the symptoms of AAA?

There are usually no symptoms of AAA. Blood vessels like the aorta can swell up slowly over time. That's why it's important to talk with your doctor about AAA to see if you are at risk.

A torn or bleeding aneurysm is a medical emergency. If this happens, you may suddenly have:

- Pain in your lower back, abdomen, or legs
- Nausea (feeling like you are going to throw up) and vomiting (throwing up)
- Clammy (sweaty) skin

You will need surgery right away.

Take Action!

Talk with your doctor about your risk for AAA.

Here are some questions you might want to ask your doctor or nurse:

- Do I need to get screened (tested) for AAA?
- How can I get help to quit smoking?
- What are my blood pressure numbers and cholesterol levels?
- What other steps can I take to keep my heart and blood vessels healthy?

What about the cost of screening?

Thanks to the Affordable Care Act, the healthcare reform law passed in 2010, insurance plans must cover AAA screening for men ages 65 to 75 who have ever smoked. This means you may be able to get screened at no cost to you.

- If you have Medicare, find out about Medicare coverage for AAA screening.

- If you have private insurance, talk to your insurance provider about what's included in your plan. Ask about the Affordable Care Act.

Make changes to lower your risk for AAA

It's never too late to take steps to lower your risk for AAA.

- quit smoking
- check your blood pressure
- get your cholesterol checked

Section 3.3

Blood Pressure Screening

This section includes text excerpted from "Get Your Blood Pressure Checked," Office of Disease Prevention and Health Promotion (ODPHP), February 25, 2016.

The Basics

One in 3 Americans have high blood pressure. Get your blood pressure checked regularly starting at age 18.

How Often Do I Need to Get My Blood Pressure Checked?

If you are age 40 or older, or if you are at higher risk for high blood pressure, get your blood pressure checked once a year.

If you are age 18 to 40 and you aren't at higher risk for high blood pressure, get your blood pressure checked every 3 to 5 years.

What Puts Me at Higher Risk for High Blood Pressure?

You are at higher risk for high blood pressure if you:

- Are African American
- Are overweight or obese
- Have blood pressure that's a little higher than usual (called high normal blood pressure)

What Is Blood Pressure?

Blood pressure is how hard your blood pushes against the walls of your arteries when your heart pumps blood. Arteries are the tubes that carry blood away from your heart. Every time your heart beats, it pumps blood through your arteries to the rest of your body.

What Is Hypertension?

Hypertension is the medical term for high blood pressure. High blood pressure has no signs or symptoms. The only way to know if you have high blood pressure is to get tested.

By taking steps to lower your blood pressure, you can reduce your risk of heart disease, stroke, and kidney failure. Lowering your blood pressure can help you live a longer, healthier life.

What Do Blood Pressure Numbers Mean?

A blood pressure test measures how hard your heart is working to pump blood through your body.

Blood pressure is measured with 2 numbers. The first number is the pressure in your arteries when your heart beats. The second number is the pressure in your arteries between each beat, when your heart relaxes.

Compare your blood pressure to these numbers:

- Normal blood pressure is lower than 120/80 (said "120 over 80").
- High blood pressure is 140/90 or higher.
- Blood pressure that's between normal and high (for example, 130/85) is called prehypertension, or high normal blood pressure.

How Can I Get My Blood Pressure Checked?

To test your blood pressure, a nurse or doctor will put a cuff around your upper arm. The cuff will be pumped with air until it feels tight, then the air will be slowly let out.

This won't take more than a few minutes. The nurse or doctor can tell you what your blood pressure numbers are right after the test is over.

If the test shows that your blood pressure is high, ask the doctor what to do next. Blood pressure can go up and down, so you may need to get it checked it more than once.

Can I Check My Blood Pressure by Myself?

Yes—you can check your own blood pressure with a blood pressure machine. You can find blood pressure machines in shopping malls, pharmacies, and grocery stores. If the test shows that your blood pressure is high, talk to a doctor.

What If I Have High Blood Pressure?

If you have high blood pressure, you may need medicine to control your blood pressure.

Take these steps to lower your blood pressure:

- Eat healthy foods that are low in saturated fat and sodium (salt).

- Get active. Aim for 2 hours and 30 minutes a week of moderate aerobic activity.

- Watch your weight by eating healthy and getting active.

- Remember to take medicines as prescribed (ordered) by your doctor.

Small changes can add up. For example, losing just 10 pounds can help lower your blood pressure.

Take Action!

Take steps to prevent or lower high blood pressure. To start, get your blood pressure checked as soon as possible.

- check your blood pressure regularly
- eat less sodium
- watch your weight

- get active

- drink alcohol only in moderation

- manage your stress

- quit smoking

Section 3.4

Cholesterol Screening

This section includes text excerpted from "Get Your Cholesterol Checked," Office of Disease Prevention and Health Promotion (ODPHP), June 27, 2016.

The Basics

Too much cholesterol in your blood can cause a heart attack or a stroke. You could have high cholesterol and not know it.

The good news is that it's easy to get your cholesterol checked—and if your cholesterol is high, you can take steps to control it.

Who Needs to Get Their Cholesterol Checked?

- All men age 35 and older

- Men ages 20 to 35 who have heart disease or risk factors for heart disease

Talk to your doctor or nurse about your risk factors for heart disease. Ask if you need to get your cholesterol checked.

What Are the Risk Factors for Heart Disease?

Risk factors for heart disease include:

- high blood pressure

- a family history of heart disease

- hardening of the arteries (called atherosclerosis)

- smoking
- diabetes
- being overweight or obese
- not getting enough physical activity

What Is Cholesterol?

Cholesterol is a waxy substance (material) that's found naturally in your blood. Your body makes cholesterol and uses it to do important things, like making hormones and digesting fatty foods.

You also get cholesterol by eating foods like egg yolks, fatty meats, and regular cheese.

If you have too much cholesterol in your body, it can build up inside your blood vessels and make it hard for blood to flow through them. Over time, this can lead to a heart attack or a stroke.

What Are the Symptoms of High Cholesterol?

There are no signs or symptoms of high cholesterol. That's why it's so important to get your cholesterol checked.

How Often Do I Need to Get My Cholesterol Checked?

The general recommendation is to get your cholesterol checked every 5 years. Some people may need to get their cholesterol checked more or less often. Talk to your doctor about what's best for you.

How Can I Get My Cholesterol Checked?

Cholesterol is checked with a blood test called a lipid profile. During the test, a nurse will take a small sample of blood from your finger or arm.

Be sure to find out how to get ready for the test. For example, you may need to fast (not eat or drink anything except water) for 9 to 12 hours before the test.

There are other blood tests that can check cholesterol, but a lipid profile gives the most information.

What Do the Test Results Mean?

If you get a lipid profile test, the results will show 4 numbers. A lipid profile measures:

- Total cholesterol

- HDL (good) cholesterol
- LDL (bad) cholesterol
- Triglycerides

Total cholesterol is a measure of all the cholesterol in your blood. It's based on the HDL, LDL, and triglycerides numbers.

HDL cholesterol is the good type of cholesterol—so a higher level is better for you. Having a low HDL cholesterol level can increase your risk for heart disease.

LDL cholesterol is the bad type of cholesterol that can block your arteries—so a lower level is better for you.

Triglycerides are a type of fat in your blood that can increase your risk for heart attack and stroke.

What Can Cause Unhealthy Cholesterol Levels?

Causes of unhealthy HDL cholesterol levels include:

- genetic (inherited) factors
- type 2 diabetes
- smoking
- being overweight
- not getting enough physical activity
- taking certain medicines

Causes of unhealthy LDL cholesterol levels include:

- Having a family history of high LDL cholesterol
- Eating too much saturated fat, *trans* fat, and cholesterol

What If My Cholesterol Levels Aren't Healthy?

As your LDL cholesterol gets higher, so does your risk of heart disease. Take these steps to lower your cholesterol and reduce your risk of heart disease:

- eat heart-healthy foods
- get active
- if you smoke, quit

Ask your doctor if you also need to take medicine to help lower your cholesterol.

Section 3.5

Colorectal Cancer Screening

This section includes text excerpted from "Colorectal Cancer Screening (PDQ®)–Patient Version," National Cancer Institute (NCI), July 23, 2015.

Colorectal Cancer Is a Disease in Which Malignant (Cancer) Cells Form in the Tissues of the Colon or the Rectum

The colon and rectum are parts of the body's digestive system. The digestive system removes and processes nutrients (vitamins, minerals, carbohydrates, fats, proteins, and water) from foods and helps pass waste material out of the body. The digestive system is made up of the mouth, throat, esophagus, stomach, and the small and large intestines. The colon (large bowel) is the first part of the large intestine and is about 5 feet long. Together, the rectum and anal canal make up the last part of the large intestine and are 6–8 inches long. The anal canal ends at the anus (the opening of the large intestine to the outside of the body).

Cancer that begins in the colon is called colon cancer, and cancer that begins in the rectum is called rectal cancer. Cancer that begins in either of these organs may also be called colorectal cancer.

Colorectal Cancer Is the Second Leading Cause of Death from Cancer in the United States

The number of new colorectal cancer cases and the number of deaths from colorectal cancer are decreasing a little bit each year. But in adults younger than 50 years, there has been a small increase in the number of new cases each year since 1998. Colorectal cancer is found more often in men than in women.

47

Age and Health History Can Affect the Risk of Developing Colon Cancer

Anything that increases a person's chance of getting a disease is called a risk factor. Risk factors for colorectal cancer include the following:

- Being older than 50 years of age.
- Having a personal history of any of the following:
  - Colorectal cancer
  - Polyps in the colon or rectum
  - Cancer of the breast
  - Ulcerative colitis or Crohn disease
- Having a parent, brother, sister, or child with colorectal cancer
- Having certain hereditary conditions, such as familial adenomatous polyposis (FAP) and hereditary nonpolyposis colon cancer (HNPCC; Lynch Syndrome)

Tests Are Used to Screen for Different Types of Cancer

Some screening tests are used because they have been shown to be helpful both in finding cancers early and decreasing the chance of dying from these cancers. Other tests are used because they have been shown to find cancer in some people; however, it has not been proven in clinical trials that use of these tests will decrease the risk of dying from cancer.

Scientists study screening tests to find those with the fewest risks and most benefits. Cancer screening trials also are meant to show whether early detection (finding cancer before it causes symptoms) decreases a person's chance of dying from the disease. For some types of cancer, finding and treating the disease at an early stage may result in a better chance of recovery.

Studies Show That Screening for Colorectal Cancer Helps Decrease the Number of Deaths from the Disease

Four Tests Are Used to Screen for Colorectal Cancer

Fecal Occult Blood Test

A fecal occult blood test (FOBT) is a test to check stool (solid waste) for blood that can only be seen with a microscope. Small samples of stool are placed on special cards and returned to the doctor or laboratory for testing. Blood in the stool may be a sign of polyps or cancer.

A new colorectal cancer screening test called immunochemical FOBT (iFOBT) is being studied to see if it is better at finding advanced polyps or cancer than the FOBT.

Sigmoidoscopy

Sigmoidoscopy is a procedure to look inside the rectum and sigmoid (lower) colon for polyps, abnormal areas, or cancer. A sigmoidoscope is inserted through the rectum into the sigmoid colon. A sigmoidoscope is a thin, tube-like instrument with a light and a lens for viewing. It may also have a tool to remove polyps or tissue samples, which are checked under a microscope for signs of cancer.

Barium Enema

A barium enema is a series of X-rays of the lower gastrointestinal tract. A liquid that contains barium (a silver-white metallic compound) is put into the rectum. The barium coats the lower gastrointestinal tract and X-rays are taken. This procedure is also called a lower GI series.

Colonoscopy

Colonoscopy is a procedure to look inside the rectum and colon for polyps, abnormal areas, or cancer. A colonoscope is inserted through the rectum into the colon. A colonoscope is a thin, tube-like instrument with a light and a lens for viewing. It may also have a tool to remove polyps or tissue samples, which are checked under a microscope for signs of cancer.

Studies Have Not Shown That Screening for Colorectal Cancer Using Digital Rectal Exam Helps Decrease the Number of Deaths from the Disease

A digital rectal exam (DRE) may be done as part of a routine physical exam. A digital rectal exam is an exam of the rectum. A doctor or nurse inserts a lubricated, gloved finger into the lower part of the rectum to feel for lumps or anything else that seems unusual. Study results have shown that there is no evidence to support DRE as a screening method for colorectal cancer.

New Screening Tests Are Being Studied in Clinical Trials

Virtual Colonoscopy

Virtual colonoscopy is a procedure that uses a series of X-rays called computed tomography to make a series of pictures of the colon. A computer puts the pictures together to create detailed images that may show polyps and anything else that seems unusual on the inside surface of the colon. This test is also called colonography or CT colonography. Clinical trials are comparing virtual colonoscopy with commonly used colorectal cancer screening tests. Other clinical trials are testing whether drinking a contrast material that coats the stool, instead of using laxatives to clear the colon, shows polyps clearly.

DNA Stool Test

This test checks DNA in stool cells for genetic changes that may be a sign of colorectal cancer.

Screening Tests Have Risks

Decisions about screening tests can be difficult. Not all screening tests are helpful and most have risks. Before having any screening test, you may want to discuss the test with your doctor. It is important to know the risks of the test and whether it has been proven to reduce the risk of dying from cancer.

False-Negative Test Results Can Occur

Screening test results may appear to be normal even though colorectal cancer is present. A person who receives a false-negative test result (one that shows there is no cancer when there really is) may delay seeking medical care even if there are symptoms.

False-Positive Test Results Can Occur

Screening test results may appear to be abnormal even though no cancer is present. A false-positive test result (one that shows there is cancer when there really isn't) can cause anxiety and is usually followed by more tests (such as biopsy), which also have risks.

The following colorectal cancer screening tests have risks:

Fecal Occult Blood Testing

The results of fecal occult blood testing may appear to be abnormal even though no cancer is present. A false-positive test result can cause anxiety and lead to more testing, including colonoscopy or barium enema with sigmoidoscopy.

Sigmoidoscopy

There can be discomfort or pain during sigmoidoscopy. Tears in the lining of the colon and bleeding also may occur.

Colonoscopy

Serious complications from colonoscopy are rare, but can include tears in the lining of the colon, bleeding, and problems with the heart or blood vessels. These complications may occur more often in older patients.

Virtual Colonoscopy

Virtual colonoscopy often finds problems with organs other than the colon, including the kidneys, chest, liver, ovaries, spleen, and pancreas. Some of these findings lead to more testing. The risks and benefits of this follow-up testing are being studied.

Your doctor can advise you about your risk for colorectal cancer and your need for screening tests.

Section 3.6

Osteoporosis Screening

This section includes text excerpted from "Get a Bone Density Test," Office of Disease Prevention and Health Promotion (ODPHP), July 1, 2016.

The Basics

A bone density test measures how strong your bones are. The test will tell you if you have osteoporosis, or weak bones.

- If you are a woman age 65 or older, schedule a bone density test.
- If you are a woman age 50 to 64, ask your doctor if you need a bone density test.

If you are at risk for osteoporosis, your doctor or nurse may recommend getting a bone density test every 2 years.

Men can get osteoporosis, too. If you are a man over age 65 and you are concerned about your bone strength, talk with your doctor or nurse.

What Is Osteoporosis?

Osteoporosis is a bone disease. It means your bones are weak and more likely to break. People with osteoporosis most often break bones in the hip, spine, and wrist.

There are no signs or symptoms of osteoporosis. You might not know you have the disease until you break a bone. That's why it's so important to get a bone density test to measure your bone strength.

What Happens during a Bone Density Test?

A bone density test is like an X-ray or scan of your body. A bone density test doesn't hurt. It only takes about 15 minutes.

Am I at Risk for Osteoporosis?

Anyone can get osteoporosis, but it's most common in older women. The older you are, the greater your risk for osteoporosis.These things can also increase your risk for osteoporosis:

- hormone changes

- not getting enough calcium and Vitamin D

- taking certain medicines

- smoking cigarettes or drinking too much alcohol

- not getting enough physical activity

What If I Have Osteoporosis?

If you have osteoporosis, you can still slow down bone loss. Finding and treating it early can keep you healthier and more active—and lower your chances of breaking a bone.

Depending on the results of your bone density test, you may need to:

- add more calcium and vitamin D to your diet

- exercise more to strengthen your bones

- take medicine to stop bone loss

Section 3.7

Prostate Cancer Screening

This section includes text excerpted from "Prostate Cancer Screening (PDQ®)–Patient Version," National Cancer Institute (NCI), July 31, 2015.

Prostate Cancer Is a Disease in Which Malignant (Cancer) Cells Form in the Tissues of the Prostate

The prostate is a gland in the male reproductive system located just below the bladder (the organ that collects and empties urine) and in front of the rectum (the lower part of the intestine). It is about the size of a walnut and surrounds part of the urethra (the tube that empties urine from the bladder). The prostate gland produces fluid that makes up part of semen.

53

As men age, the prostate may get bigger. A bigger prostate may block the flow of urine from the bladder and cause problems with sexual function. This condition is called benign prostatic hyperplasia (BPH), and although it is not cancer, surgery may be needed to correct it. The symptoms of benign prostatic hyperplasia or of other problems in the prostate may be similar to symptoms of prostate cancer.

Prostate Cancer Is the Most Common Nonskin Cancer among Men in the United States

Prostate cancer is found mainly in older men. Although the number of men with prostate cancer is large, most men diagnosed with this disease do not die from it. Prostate cancer occurs more often in African-American men than in white men. African-American men with prostate cancer are more likely to die from the disease than white men with prostate cancer.

Age, Race, and Family History of Prostate Cancer Can Affect the Risk of Developing Prostate Cancer

Anything that increases a person's chance of developing a disease is called a risk factor. Risk factors for prostate cancer include the following:

- being 50 years of age or older
- being black
- having a brother, son, or father who had prostate cancer
- eating a diet high in fat or drinking alcoholic beverages

Tests Are Used to Screen for Different Types of Cancer

Some screening tests are used because they have been shown to be helpful both in finding cancers early and decreasing the chance of dying from these cancers. Other tests are used because they have been shown to find cancer in some people; however, it has not been proven in clinical trials that use of these tests will decrease the risk of dying from cancer.

Scientists study screening tests to find those with the fewest risks and most benefits. Cancer screening trials also are meant to show whether early detection (finding cancer before it causes symptoms) decreases a person's chance of dying from the disease. For some types of cancer, finding and treating the disease at an early stage may result in a better chance of recovery.

There Is No Standard or Routine Screening Test for Prostate Cancer

Screening tests for prostate cancer are under study, and there are screening clinical trials taking place in many parts of the country.

Tests to detect (find) prostate cancer that are being studied include the following:

Digital Rectal Exam

Digital rectal exam (DRE) is an exam of the rectum. The doctor or nurse inserts a lubricated, gloved finger into the lower part of the rectum to feel the prostate for lumps or anything else that seems unusual.

Prostate-Specific Antigen Test

A prostate-specific antigen (PSA) test is a test that measures the level of PSA in the blood. PSA is a substance made mostly by the prostate that may be found in an increased amount in the blood of men who have prostate cancer. The level of PSA may also be high in men who have an infection or inflammation of the prostate or benign prostatic hyperplasia (BPH; an enlarged, but noncancerous, prostate).

If a man has a high PSA level and a biopsy of the prostate does not show cancer, a prostate cancer gene 3 (PCA3) test may be done. This test measures the amount of PCA3 in the urine. If the PCA3 level is high, another biopsy may help diagnose prostate cancer.

Scientists are studying the combination of PSA testing and digital rectal exam as a way to get more accurate results from the screening tests.

Screening Tests Have Risks

Decisions about screening tests can be difficult. Not all screening tests are helpful and most have risks. Before having any screening test, you may want to discuss the test with your doctor. It is important to know the risks of the test and whether it has been proven to reduce the risk of dying from cancer.

The risks of prostate screening include the following:

Finding Prostate Cancer May Not Improve Health or Help a Man Live Longer

Screening may not improve your health or help you live longer if you have cancer that has already spread to the area outside of the prostate or to other places in your body.

Some cancers never cause symptoms or become life-threatening, but if found by a screening test, the cancer may be treated. Finding these cancers is called overdiagnosis. It is not known if treatment of these cancers would help you live longer than if no treatment were given, and treatments for cancer, such as surgery and radiation therapy, may have serious side effects.

Some studies of patients with prostate cancer showed these patients had a higher risk of death from cardiovascular (heart and blood vessel) disease or suicide. The risk was greatest the first year after diagnosis.

Follow-Up Tests, Such as a Biopsy, May Be Done to Diagnose Cancer

If a PSA test is higher than normal, a biopsy of the prostate may be done. Complications from a biopsy of the prostate may include fever, pain, blood in the urine or semen, and urinary tract infection. Even if a biopsy shows that a patient does not have prostate cancer, he may worry more about developing prostate cancer in the future.

False-Negative Test Results Can Occur

Screening test results may appear to be normal even though prostate cancer is present. A man who receives a false-negative test result (one that shows there is no cancer when there really is) may delay seeking medical care even if he has symptoms.

False-Positive Test Results Can Occur

Screening test results may appear to be abnormal even though no cancer is present. A false-positive test result (one that shows there is cancer when there really isn't) can cause anxiety and is usually followed by more tests, (such as biopsy) which also have risks.

Your doctor can advise you about your risk for prostate cancer and your need for screening tests.

Chapter 4

Vaccinations for Men

Chapter Contents

Section 4.1—Recommended Vaccinations for Adults.................. 58

Section 4.2—Human Papillomavirus Vaccination 61

Section 4.3—Seasonal Influenza Vaccination 63

Section 4.1

Recommended Vaccinations for Adults

This section includes text excerpted from "Vaccine
Information for Adults," Centers for Disease Control
and Prevention (CDC), May 2, 2016.

What Vaccines Are Recommended for You

Immunizations are not just for children. Protection from some
childhood vaccines can wear off over time. You may also be at risk for
vaccine-preventable disease due to your age, job, lifestyle, travel, or
health conditions.

**All adults need immunizations to help them prevent getting
and spreading serious diseases that could result in poor health,
missed work, medical bills, and not being able to care for family.**

- All adults need a seasonal flu (influenza) vaccine every year. Flu
  vaccine is especially important for people with chronic health
  conditions and older adults.

- Every adult should get the Tdap vaccine once if they did not receive
  it as an adolescent to protect against pertussis (whooping cough),
  and then a Td (tetanus, diphtheria) booster shot every 10 years.

Adults 19–26 Years Old

In addition to seasonal flu (influenza) vaccine and Td or Tdap vaccine (Tetanus, diphtheria, and pertussis), you should also get:

- HPV vaccinewhich protects against the human papillomaviruses
  that causes most anal cancer, and genital warts. It is recommended for:

  - men up to age 21 years

  - men ages 22–26 who have sex with men

Some vaccines may be recommended for adults because of particular job or school-related requirements, health conditions, lifestyle
or other factors. For example, some states require students entering

colleges and universities to be vaccinated against certain diseases like meningitis due to increased risk among college students living in residential housing.

Talk with your doctor or other healthcare professional to find out which vaccines are recommended for you at your next medical appointment.

Under the Affordable Care Act, insurance plans that cover children now allow parents to add or keep children on the health insurance policy until they turn 26 years old.

Adults 60 Years or Older

An estimated 1 million Americans get shingles every year, and about half of them are 60 years old or older. Additionally, over 60 percent of seasonal flu-related hospitalizations occur in people 65 years and older.

As we get older, our immune systems tend to weaken over time, putting us at higher risk for certain diseases. This is why, in addition to seasonal flu (influenza) vaccine and Td or Tdap vaccine (tetanus, diphtheria, and pertussis), you should also get:

- Pneumococcal vaccines, which protect against pneumococcal disease, including infections in the lungs and bloodstream (recommended for all adults over 65 years old, and for adults younger than 65 years who have certain chronic health conditions)

- Zoster vaccine, which protects against shingles (recommended for adults 60 years or older)

Talk with your doctor or other healthcare professional to find out which vaccines are recommended for you at your next medical appointment.

Adults with Health Conditions

All adults need a seasonal flu (influenza) vaccine and Td or Tdap vaccine (Tetanus, diphtheria, and pertussis) but there may be additional vaccines recommended for you.

Talk with your doctor or other healthcare professional to find out which vaccines are recommended for you based on your specific health status, age, and lifestyle.

Healthcare Workers

Healthcare workers (HCWs) are at risk for exposure to serious, and sometimes deadly, diseases. If you work directly with patients or handle material that could spread infection, you should get appropriate vaccines to reduce the chance that you will get or spread vaccine-preventable diseases.

In addition to seasonal flu (influenza) vaccine and Td or Tdap vaccine (Tetanus, diphtheria, and pertussis), you should also get:

- **Hepatitis B:** If you don't have documented evidence of a complete hepB vaccine series, or if you don't have an up-to-date blood test that shows you are immune to hepatitis B (i.e., no serologic evidence of immunity or prior vaccination) then you should get the 3-dose series (dose #1 now, #2 in 1 month, #3 approximately 5 months after #2). Get anti-HBs serologic tested 1–2 months after dose #3.

- **MMR (Measles, Mumps, and Rubella):** If you were born in 1957 or later and have not had the MMR vaccine, or if you don't have an up-to-date blood test that shows you are immune to measles, mumps, and rubella (i.e., no serologic evidence of immunity or prior vaccination), get 2 doses of MMR, 4 weeks apart.

- **Varicella (Chickenpox):** If you have not had chickenpox (varicella), if you haven't had varicella vaccine, or if you don't have an up-to-date blood test that shows you are immune to varicella (i.e., no serologic evidence of immunity or prior vaccination) get 2 doses of varicella vaccine, 4 weeks apart.

- **Meningococcal:** Those who are routinely exposed to isolates of *N. meningitidis* should get one dose.

International Travelers

If you are planning on visiting or living abroad you may need certain vaccinations.

Get the vaccines you need:

STEP 1: Make sure you are up-to-date with all recommended vaccinations. Take this the adult vaccination quiz to determine which vaccines you need and create a customized printout to take with you to your next medical appointment. Talk with your doctor or healthcare professional and get any vaccines that you may have missed.

STEP 2: Visit the CDC Travel Health site for more information about recommendations and requirements for the locations you will be visiting during your travel.

STEP 3: Make an appointment to get recommended vaccines at least 4 to 6 weeks before your trip. Planning ahead will give you enough time to build up immunity and get best protection from vaccines that may require multiple doses.

Many state and local health departments throughout the United States provide travel vaccinations.

Section 4.2

Human Papillomavirus Vaccination

This section includes text excerpted from "HPV Vaccine Is Recommended for Boys," Centers for Disease Control and Prevention (CDC), December 2, 2015.

HPV Vaccine is Recommended for Boys

Boys need HPV vaccine, too. Here's why.

Many people think the HPV vaccine only protects girls, but this vaccine protects boys against certain HPV-related cancers, too!

Girls aren't the only ones affected by HPV, also known as human papillomavirus. HPV is common in both males and females. Every year, over 9,000 males are affected by cancers caused by HPV infections that don't go away. HPV can cause cancers of the anus, mouth/throat (oropharynx), and penis in males.

Cases of anal cancer and cancers of the mouth/throat are on the rise. In fact, if current trends continue, the annual number of cancers of the mouth/throat attributed to HPV is expected to surpass the annual number of cervical cancers by 2020.

Many of the cancers caused by HPV infection could be prevented by HPV vaccination.

HPV vaccination is recommended by doctors and other health experts for boys at ages 11–12. HPV vaccination of boys is also likely to benefit girls by reducing the spread of HPV infection.

HPV Vaccine Is Recommended for Boys at 11 or 12 Years

HPV vaccine is recommended at ages 11–12 for two reasons:

1. HPV vaccine must be given before exposure to virus for it to be effective in preventing cancers and other diseases caused by HPV.

2. HPV vaccine produces a high immune response at this age.

If you haven't already vaccinated your preteens and teens, it's not too late. Ask your child's doctor at their next appointment about getting HPV vaccine. The series is three shots over six months' time. Take advantage of any visit to the doctor—such as an annual health checkup or physicals for sports, camp, or college—to ask the doctor about what shots your preteens and teens need.

HPV Vaccine Is Safe

HPV vaccine has been studied very carefully and shown to be safe. Nearly 80 million doses of HPV vaccine have been distributed in the U.S. since 2006, and no serious safety concerns have been linked to HPV vaccination. Common, mild side effects reported include pain in the arm where the shot was given, fever, dizziness, and nausea.

Some preteens and teens might faint after getting a shot, including HPV vaccine. Preteens and teens should sit or lie down when they get a shot and stay like that for about 15 minutes after the shot. This can help prevent fainting and any injury that could happen while fainting.

How Can I Get Help Paying for HPV Vaccine?

Families who need help paying for vaccines should ask their doctor or other healthcare professional about Vaccines for Children (VFC). The VFC program provides vaccines at no cost to children younger than 19 years who are uninsured, Medicaid-eligible, American Indian, or Alaska Native.

Section 4.3

Seasonal Influenza Vaccination

This section includes text excerpted from "Influenza (Flu)," Centers for Disease Control and Prevention (CDC), September 16, 2015.

Get Vaccinated

Everyone 6 months of age and older should get a flu vaccine every season. Vaccination to prevent influenza is particularly important for people who are at high risk of serious complications from influenza.

Flu vaccination has important benefits. It can reduce flu illnesses, doctors' visits, and missed work and school due to flu, as well as prevent flu-related hospitalizations.

Different flu vaccines are approved for use in different groups of people. Factors that can determine a person's suitability for vaccination, or vaccination with a particular vaccine, include a person's age, health (current and past) and any relevant allergies.

Flu shots are approved for use in people with chronic health conditions. There are flu shots that also are approved for use in people as young as 6 months of age and up.

The nasal spray vaccine is approved for use in people 2 years through 49 years of age.

Who Should Not Receive a Flu Shot

- People who cannot get a flu shot

  - Children younger than 6 months old

  - People with severe, life-threatening allergies to flu vaccine or any of its ingredients

Note: There are certain flu shots that have different age indications. For example people younger than 65 years of age should not get the high-dose flu shot and people who are younger than 18 years old or older than 64 years old should not get the intradermal flu shot.

- People who should talk to their doctor before getting the flu shot
  - People who have an allergy to eggs or other vaccine ingredients
  - People who have ever had Guillain-Barre Syndrome (GBS)
  - People who are feeling ill

Who Should Not Receive Nasal Spray Vaccine

- People who cannot get a nasal spray vaccine
  - Children younger than 2 years old
  - Adults 50 years and older
  - People who have a history of severe allergic reactions to any component of the vaccine or to a previous dose of any influenza vaccine
  - People who are allergic to eggs
  - Children age 2–17 receiving aspirin therapy
  - People with weakened immune systems
  - Children age 2–4 who have asthma or history of wheezing in past 12 months
  - People who have taken flu antivirals drugs in the previous 48 hours
  - People who care for severely immunocompromised persons who require a protective environment (or otherwise avoid contact with those persons for 7 days after getting the nasal spray vaccine).
- People who should talk to their doctor before getting the nasal spray vaccine
  - People with Asthma
  - People with a chronic condition
  - People who have ever had Guillain-Barre Syndrome (GBS)
  - People who are feeling ill
  - People who have gotten other vaccines in the past 4 weeks

When Should I Get Vaccinated?

CDC recommends that people get vaccinated against flu soon after vaccine becomes available, if possible by October. It takes about two weeks after vaccination for antibodies to develop in the body and provide protection against the flu.

People who have ever had a severe allergic reaction to eggs can get recombinant flu vaccine if they are 18 years and older or they should get the regular flu shot (IIV) given by a medical doctor with experience in management of severe allergic conditions. People who have had a mild reaction to egg—that is, one which only involved hives—may get a flu shot with additional safety measures. Recombinant flu vaccines also are an option for people if they are 18 years and older and they do not have any contraindications to that vaccine. Make sure your doctor or healthcare professional knows about any allergic reactions. Most, but not all, types of flu vaccine contain a small amount of egg.

Preventive Steps

Take Time to Get a Flu Vaccine

- CDC recommends a yearly flu vaccine as the first and most important step in protecting against flu viruses.

- While there are many different flu viruses, a flu vaccine protects against the viruses that research suggests will be most common.

- Flu vaccination can reduce flu illnesses, doctors' visits, and missed work and school due to flu, as well as prevent flu-related hospitalizations.

- Everyone 6 months of age and older should get a flu vaccine as soon as the current season's vaccines are available.

- Vaccination of high risk persons is especially important to decrease their risk of severe flu illness.

- People at high risk of serious flu complications include young children, people with chronic health conditions like asthma, diabetes or heart and lung disease and people 65 years and older.

- Vaccination also is important for healthcare workers, and other people who live with or care for high risk people to keep from spreading flu to them.

- Children younger than 6 months are at high risk of serious flu illness, but are too young to be vaccinated. People who care for infants should be vaccinated instead.

Take Everyday Preventive Actions to Stop the Spread of Germs

- Try to avoid close contact with sick people.

- While sick, limit contact with others as much as possible to keep from infecting them.

- If you are sick with flu-like illness, CDC recommends that you stay home for at least 24 hours after your fever is gone except to get medical care or for other necessities. (Your fever should be gone for 24 hours without the use of a fever-reducing medicine.)

- Cover your nose and mouth with a tissue when you cough or sneeze. Throw the tissue in the trash after you use it.

- Wash your hands often with soap and water. If soap and water are not available, use an alcohol-based hand rub.

- Avoid touching your eyes, nose and mouth. Germs spread this way.

- Clean and disinfect surfaces and objects that may be contaminated with germs like the flu.

Take Flu Antiviral Drugs If Your Doctor Prescribes Them

- If you get the flu, antiviral drugs can be used to treat your illness.

- Antiviral drugs are different from antibiotics. They are prescription medicines (pills, liquid or an inhaled powder) and are not available over-the-counter.

- Antiviral drugs can make illness milder and shorten the time you are sick. They may also prevent serious flu complications. For people with high-risk factors, treatment with an antiviral drug can mean the difference between having a milder illness versus a very serious illness that could result in a hospital stay.

- Studies show that flu antiviral drugs work best for treatment when they are started within 2 days of getting sick, but starting them later can still be helpful, especially if the sick person has a high-risk health condition or is very sick from the flu. Follow your doctor's instructions for taking this drug.

- Flu-like symptoms include fever, cough, sore throat, runny or stuffy nose, body aches, headache, chills and fatigue. Some people also may have vomiting and diarrhea. People may be infected with the flu, and have respiratory symptoms without a fever.

Chapter 5

Managing Common Disease Risk Factors

Chapter Contents

Section 5.1—Preventing High Blood Pressure 68

Section 5.2—Preventing High Cholesterol 70

Section 5.3—Ensuring Adequate Sleep 72

Section 5.4—Managing Stress 75

Section 5.1

Preventing High Blood Pressure

This section includes text excerpted from "High Blood Pressure,"
National Institute on Aging (NIA), National Institutes of
Health (NIH), March 2015.

What Is Blood Pressure?

Blood pressure is the force of blood pushing against the walls of arteries. When the doctor measures your blood pressure, the results are given in two numbers. The first number, called systolic blood pressure, is the pressure caused by your heart pushing out blood. The second number, called diastolic blood pressure, is the pressure when your heart fills with blood. The safest range, often called normal blood pressure, is a systolic blood pressure of less than 120 and a diastolic blood pressure of less than 80. This is stated as 120/80.

Do You Have High Blood Pressure?

One reason to have regular visits to the doctor is to have your blood pressure checked. The doctor will say your blood pressure is high when it measures 140/90 or higher at two or more checkups. He or she may ask you to check your blood pressure at home at different times of the day. If the pressure stays high, even when you are relaxed, the doctor may suggest exercise, changes in your diet, and medications.

The term "prehypertension" describes people whose blood pressure is slightly higher than normal—for example, the first number (systolic) is between 120 and 139, or the second number (diastolic) is between 80 and 89. Prehypertension can put you at risk for developing high blood pressure. Your doctor will probably want you to make changes in your day-to-day habits to try to lower your blood pressure.

How Can I Control My Blood Pressure?

High blood pressure is very common in older people—over time most people find that aging causes changes to their heart. This is true even for people who have heart healthy habits. The good news is that blood pressure can be controlled in most people.

There are many lifestyle changes you can make to lower your risk of high blood pressure, including:

- **Keep a healthy weight.** Being overweight adds to your risk of high blood pressure. Ask your doctor if you need to lose weight.

- **Exercise every day.** Moderate exercise can lower your risk of high blood pressure. Set some goals for yourself so that you can exercise safely and work your way up to exercising at least 30 minutes a day most days of the week. You should check with your doctor before starting an exercise plan if you have any health problems that are not being treated.

- **Eat a healthy diet.** A diet rich in fruits, vegetables, whole grains, and low-fat dairy products may help to lower blood pressure. Ask your doctor about following a healthy diet.

- **Cut down on salt.** Many Americans eat more salt (sodium) than they need. Most of the salt comes from processed food (for example, soup and baked goods). A low-salt diet might help lower your blood pressure. Talk with your doctor about eating less salt.

- **Drink less alcohol.** Drinking alcohol can affect your blood pressure. Most men should not have more than two drinks a day.

- **Don't smoke.** Smoking increases your risk for high blood pressure, heart disease, stroke, and other health problems. If you smoke, quit.

- **Get a good night's sleep.** Tell your doctor if you've been told you snore or sound like you stop breathing for moments when you sleep. This may be a sign of a problem called sleep apnea. Treating sleep apnea and getting a good night's sleep can help to lower blood pressure.

If these lifestyle changes don't lower your blood pressure enough to a safe level, your doctor will also prescribe medicine. You may try several kinds or combinations of medicines before finding a plan that works best for you. Medicine can control your blood pressure, but it can't cure it. You will likely need to take medicine for the rest of your life. Plan with your doctor how to manage your blood pressure.

Section 5.2

Preventing High Cholesterol

This section contains text excerpted from the following sources:
Text under the heading "About High Cholesterol" is excerpted
from "Cholesterol," Centers for Disease Control and Prevention
(CDC), March 16, 2015; Text beginning with the heading
"Preventing or Managing High Cholesterol: Healthy Living Habits"
is excerpted from "Cholesterol," Centers for Disease Control and
Prevention (CDC), December 11, 2015.

About High Cholesterol

Cholesterol is a waxy, fat-like substance that travels through the
blood on proteins called lipoproteins. It comes from two sources:

1. It's made by your body and used to do important things, like
   make hormones and digest fatty foods.

2. It's found in many foods, like egg yolks, fatty meats, and regular cheese.

When your body has too much cholesterol, it can build up on the
walls of your blood vessels. These deposits are called plaque.

As your blood vessels build up plaque deposits over time, the inside
of the vessels narrow and allows less blood to flow through to your
heart and other organs.

When plaque buildup totally blocks a coronary artery carrying blood
to the heart, it causes a heart attack. Another cause of heart attack is
when a plaque deposit bursts and releases a clot in a coronary artery.

Angina is caused by plaque partially blocking a coronary artery,
reducing blood flow to the heart and causing chest pain.

Preventing or Managing High Cholesterol: Healthy Living Habits

By living a healthy lifestyle, you can help keep your cholesterol in
a healthy range and lower your risk for heart disease and stroke. A
healthy lifestyle includes:

1. Eating a healthy diet.

2. Maintaining a healthy weight.

3. Getting enough physical activity.

4. Not smoking.

5. Limiting alcohol use.

Healthy Diet

Choosing healthy meal and snack options can help you avoid high low-density lipoprotein (LDL) cholesterol and its complications. Be sure to eat plenty of fresh fruits and vegetables.

Eating foods low in saturated fats, trans fat, and cholesterol as well as foods high in fiber, monounsaturated fats, and polyunsaturated fats can help prevent and manage high levels of "bad" LDL cholesterol and triglycerides while increasing "good" high-density lipoprotein cholesterol levels. Try to:

- Eat less saturated fats, which comes from animal products (like cheese, fatty meats, and dairy desserts) and tropical oils (like palm oil).

- Stay away from trans fats, which may be in baked goods (like cookies and cake), snack foods (like microwave popcorn), fried foods, and margarines.

- Limit foods that are high in cholesterol, including fatty meats and organ meat (like liver and kidney).

- Choose low-fat or fat-free milk, cheese, and yogurt.

- Eat more foods that are high in fiber, like oatmeal, oat bran, beans, and lentils.

- Eat a heart-healthy diet that includes plenty of vegetables and fruits and is low in salt and sugar.

Maintain a Healthy Weight

Being overweight or obese increases your risk for high cholesterol. To determine if your weight is in a healthy range, doctors often calculate your body mass index (BMI). If you know your weight and height, you can calculate your BMI. Doctors sometimes also use waist and hip measurements to measure excess body fat.

Physical Activity

Physical activity can help you maintain a healthy weight and lower your cholesterol and blood pressure levels. For adults, the Surgeon General recommends 2 hours and 30 minutes of moderate-intensity exercise, like brisk walking or bicycling, every week. Children and adolescents should get 1 hour of physical activity every day.

No Smoking

Cigarette smoking damages your blood vessels, speeds up the hardening of the arteries, and greatly increases your risk for heart disease. If you don't smoke, don't start. If you do smoke, quitting will lower your risk for heart disease. Your doctor can suggest ways to help you quit.

Limited Alcohol

Avoid drinking too much alcohol, which can raise your cholesterol. Men should have no more than 2 drinks per day.

Section 5.3

Ensuring Adequate Sleep

This section includes text excerpted from "Get Enough Sleep," Office of Disease Prevention and Health Promotion (ODPHP), U.S. Department of Health and Human Services (HHS), February 24, 2016.

The Basics

Everyone needs to get enough sleep. Sleep helps keep your mind and body healthy.

How Much Sleep Do I Need?

Most adults need 7 to 8 hours of good quality sleep on a regular schedule each night. Make changes to your routine if you can't find enough time to sleep.

Getting enough sleep isn't only about total hours of sleep. It's also important to get good quality sleep so you feel rested when you wake up.

If you often have trouble sleeping—or if you don't feel well rested after sleeping—talk with your doctor.

How Much Sleep Do Children Need?

Kids need even more sleep than adults.

- Teens need at least 9 hours of sleep each night.
- School-aged children need at least 10 hours of sleep each night.
- Preschoolers need to sleep between 11 and 12 hours a day.
- Newborns need to sleep between 16 and 18 hours a day.

Why Is Getting Enough Sleep Important?

Getting enough sleep has many benefits. It can help you:

- Get sick less often.
- Stay at a healthy weight.
- Lower your risk of high blood pressure and diabetes.
- Reduce stress and improve your mood.
- Think more clearly and do better in school and at work.
- Get along better with people.
- Make good decisions and avoid injuries (For example, sleepy drivers cause thousands of car crashes every year).

Does It Matter When I Sleep?

Yes. Your body sets your "biological clock" according to the pattern of daylight where you live. This helps you naturally get sleepy at night and stay alert during the day.

When people have to work at night and sleep during the day, they can have trouble getting enough sleep. When people travel to a different time zone, they can also have trouble sleeping.

Why Can't I Fall Asleep?

Many things can make it harder for you to sleep, including:

- stress

- pain
- certain health conditions
- some medicines
- caffeine (usually from coffee, tea, and soda)
- alcohol and other drugs
- untreated sleep disorders, like sleep apnea or insomnia

If you are having trouble sleeping, make changes to your routine to get the sleep you need. For example, try to:

- Follow a regular sleep schedule.
- Stay away from caffeine in the afternoon.
- Take a hot bath before bed to relax.

How Can I Tell If I Have a Sleep Disorder?

Signs of a sleep disorder can include:

- Difficulty falling asleep.
- Trouble staying asleep.
- Sleepiness during the day that makes it difficult to do tasks like driving a car.
- Frequent loud snoring.
- Pauses in breathing or gasping while sleeping.
- Pain or itchy feelings in your legs or arms at night that feel better when you move or massage the area.

If you have any of these signs, talk to a doctor or nurse. You may need to be tested or treated for a sleep disorder.

Section 5.4

Managing Stress

This section includes text excerpted from "Coping with Stress,"
Centers for Disease Control and Prevention (CDC), October 2, 2015.

Everyone—adults, teens, and even children—experiences stress at times. Stress can be beneficial by helping people develop the skills they need to cope with and adapt to new and potentially threatening situations throughout life. However, the beneficial aspects of stress diminish when it is severe enough to overwhelm a person's ability to take care of themselves and family. Using healthy ways to cope and getting the right care and support can put problems in perspective and help stressful feelings and symptoms subside.

Stress is a condition that is often characterized by symptoms of physical or emotional tension. It is a reaction to a situation where a person feels threatened or anxious. Stress can be positive (e.g., preparing for a wedding) or negative (e.g., dealing with a natural disaster).

Sometimes after experiencing a traumatic event that is especially frightening—including personal or environmental disasters, or being threatened with an assault—people have a strong and lingering stress reaction to the event. Strong emotions, jitters, sadness, or depression may all be part of this normal and temporary reaction to the stress of an overwhelming event.

Common reactions to a stressful event can include:

- Disbelief, shock, and numbness

- Feeling sad, frustrated, and helpless

- Fear and anxiety about the future

- Feeling guilty

- Anger, tension, and irritability

- Difficulty concentrating and making decisions

- Crying

- Reduced interest in usual activities

- Wanting to be alone
- Loss of appetite
- Sleeping too much or too little
- Nightmares or bad memories
- Reoccurring thoughts of the event
- Headaches, back pains, and stomach problems
- Increased heart rate, difficulty breathing
- Smoking or use of alcohol or drugs

Healthy Ways to Cope with Stress

Feeling emotional and nervous or having trouble sleeping and eating can all be normal reactions to stress. Engaging in healthy activities and getting the right care and support can put problems in perspective and help stressful feelings subside in a few days or weeks. Some tips for beginning to feel better are:

- Take care of yourself.
  - Eat healthy, well-balanced meals.
  - Exercise on a regular basis.
  - Get plenty of sleep.
  - Give yourself a break if you feel stressed out.
- Talk to others. Share your problems and how you are feeling and coping with a parent, friend, counselor, doctor, or pastor.
- Avoid drugs and alcohol. Drugs and alcohol may seem to help with the stress. In the long run, they create additional problems and increase the stress you are already feeling.
- Take a break. If your stress is caused by a national or local event, take breaks from listening to the news stories, which can increase your stress.

Recognize when you need more help. If problems continue or you are thinking about suicide, talk to a psychologist, social worker, or professional counselor.

If you or someone you know needs immediate help, please contact the one of the following crisis hotlines:

Disaster Distress Helpline: 1-800-985-5990
National Suicide Prevention Lifeline: 1-800-273-TALK (1-888-628-9454 for Spanish-speaking callers)
Youth Mental Health Line: 1-888-568-1112
Child-Help USA: 1-800-422-4453 (24-hour toll free) Coping With Stress

Helping Youth Cope with Stress

Because of their level of development, children and adolescents often struggle with how to cope well with stress. Youth can be particularly overwhelmed when their stress is connected to a traumatic event—like a natural disaster (earthquakes, tornados, wildfires), family loss, school shootings, or community violence. Parents and educators can take steps to provide stability and support that help young people feel better.

Tips

Tips for Parents

It is natural for children to worry, especially when scary or stressful events happen in their lives. Talking with children about these stressful events and monitoring what children watch or hear about the events can help put frightening information into a more balanced context. Some suggestions to help children cope are:

- **Maintain a normal routine.** Helping children wake up, go to sleep, and eat meals at regular times provide them a sense of stability. Going to school and participating in typical after-school activities also provide stability and extra support.

- **Talk, listen, and encourage expression.** Create opportunities to have your children talk, but do not force them. Listen to your child's thoughts and feelings and share some of yours. After a traumatic event, it is important for children to feel like they can share their feelings and to know that their fears and worries are understandable. Keep these conversations going by asking them how they feel in a week, then in a month, and so on.

- **Watch and listen.** Be alert for any change in behavior. Are children sleeping more or less? Are they withdrawing from friends or family? Are they behaving in any way out of the ordinary? Any changes in behavior, even small changes, may be signs that the child is having trouble coming to terms with the event and may support.

- **Reassure.** Stressful events can challenge a child's sense of physical and emotional safety and security. Take opportunities to reassure your child about his or her safety and well-being and discuss ways that you, the school, and the community are taking steps to keep them safe.

- **Connect with others.** Make an on-going effort to talk to other parents and your child's teachers about concerns and ways to help your child cope. You do not have to deal with problems alone-it is often helpful for parents, schools, and health professionals to work together to support and ensuring the well-being of all children in stressful times.

Tips for Kids and Teens

After a traumatic or violent event, it is normal to feel anxious about your safety and security. Even if you were not directly involved, you may worry about whether this type of event may someday affect you. How can you deal with these fears? Start by looking at the tips below for some ideas.

- **Talk to and stay connected to others.** This connection might be your parent, another relative, a friend, neighbor, teacher, coach, school nurse, counselor, family doctor, or member of your church or temple. Talking with someone can help you make sense out of your experience and figure out ways to feel better. If you are not sure where to turn, call your local crisis intervention center or a national hotline.

- **Get active.** Go for a walk, play sports, write a play or poem, play a musical instrument, or join an after-school program. Volunteer with a community group that promotes nonviolence or another school or community activity that you care about. Trying any of these can be a positive way to handle your feelings and to see that things are going to get better.

- **Take care of yourself.** As much as possible, try to get enough sleep, eat right, exercise, and keep a normal routine. It may be hard to do, but by keeping yourself healthy you will be better able to handle a tough time.

- **Take information breaks.** Pictures and stories about a disaster can increase worry and other stressful feelings. Taking breaks from the news, Internet, and conversations about the disaster can help calm you down.

Tips for School Personnel

Kids and teens who experience a stressful event, or see it on television, may react with shock, sadness, anger, fear, and confusion. They may be reluctant to be alone or fearful of leaving secure areas such as the house or classroom. School personnel can help their students restore their sense of safety by talking with the children about their fears. Other tips for school personnel include:

- **Reach out and talk.** Create opportunities to have students talk, but do not force them. Try asking questions like, what do you think about these events, or how do you think these things happen? You can be a model by sharing some of your own thoughts as well as correct misinformation. Children talking about their feelings can help them cope and to know that different feelings are normal.

- **Watch and listen.** Be alert for any change in behavior. Are students talking more or less? Withdrawing from friends? Acting out? Are they behaving in any way out of the ordinary? These changes may be early warning signs that a student is struggling and needs extra support from the school and family.

- **Maintain normal routines.** A regular classroom and school schedule can provide reassurance and promote a sense of stability and safety. Encourage students to keep up with their schoolwork and extracurricular activities but do not push them if they seem overwhelmed.

- **Take care of yourself.** You are better able to support your students if you are healthy, coping well, and taking care of yourself first.

  - Eat healthy, well-balanced meals

  - Exercise on a regular basis

  - Get plenty of sleep

  - Give yourself a break if you feel stressed out

Chapter 6

Aim for a Healthy Weight

Chapter Contents

Section 6.1—Assessing Your Weight and Health Risk............... 82

Section 6.2—About Body Mass Index (BMI) 84

Section 6.3—Health Risks of Overweight and Obesity............... 88

Section 6.4—Tips for Healthy Weight Loss 92

Section 6.5—Choosing a Safe and Successful
Weight-Loss Program 97

Section 6.1

Assessing Your Weight and Health Risk

This section includes text excerpted from "Aim for a Healthy Weight,"
National Heart, Lung, and Blood Institute (NHLBI), August 2014.

Assessment of weight and health risk involves using three key
measures:

1. Body mass index (BMI)

2. Waist circumference

3. Risk factors for diseases and conditions associated with obesity

Body Mass Index (BMI)

BMI is a useful measure of overweight and obesity. It is calculated
from your height and weight. BMI is an estimate of body fat and a
good gauge of your risk for diseases that can occur with more body
fat. The higher your BMI, the higher your risk for certain diseases
such as heart disease, high blood pressure, type 2 diabetes, gallstones,
breathing problems, and certain cancers.

Although BMI can be used for most men and women, it does have
some limits:

- It may overestimate body fat in athletes and others who have a
  muscular build.

- It may underestimate body fat in older persons and others who
  have lost muscle.

Use the BMI Calculator or BMI Tables to estimate your body fat.
The BMI score means the following:

Table 6.1. BMI Score

	BMI
Underweight	Below 18.5
Normal	18.5–24.9

Table 6.1. Continued

	BMI
Overweight	25.0–29.9
Obesity	30.0 and Above

Waist Circumference

Measuring waist circumference helps screen for possible health risks that come with overweight and obesity. If most of your fat is around your waist rather than at your hips, you're at a higher risk for heart disease and type 2 diabetes. This risk goes up with a waist size that is greater than 40 inches for men. To correctly measure your waist, stand and place a tape measure around your middle, just above your hipbones. Measure your waist just after you breathe out.

Risk Factors for Health Topics Associated with Obesity

Along with being overweight or obese, the following conditions will put you at greater risk for heart disease and other conditions:

- high blood pressure (hypertension)
- high LDL cholesterol ("bad" cholesterol)
- low HDL cholesterol ("good" cholesterol)
- high triglycerides
- high blood glucose (sugar)
- family history of premature heart disease
- physical inactivity
- cigarette smoking

For people who are considered obese (BMI greater than or equal to 30) or those who are overweight (BMI of 25 to 29.9) and have two or more risk factors, it is recommended that you lose weight. Even a small weight loss (between 5 and 10 percent of your current weight) will help lower your risk of developing diseases associated with obesity. People who are overweight, do not have a high waist measurement, and have fewer than two risk factors may need to prevent further weight gain rather than lose weight.

Talk to your doctor to see whether you are at an increased risk and whether you should lose weight. Your doctor will evaluate your BMI, waist measurement, and other risk factors for heart disease.

The good news is even a small weight loss (between 5 and 10 percent of your current weight) will help lower your risk of developing those diseases.

Section 6.2

About Body Mass Index (BMI)

This section includes text excerpted from "Healthy Weight," Centers for Disease Control and Prevention (CDC), May 15, 2015.

What Is Body Mass Index (BMI)?

BMI is a person's weight in kilograms divided by the square of height in meters. BMI does not measure body fat directly, but research has shown that BMI is moderately correlated with more direct measures of body fat obtained from skinfold thickness measurements, bioelectrical impedance, densitometry (underwater weighing), dual energy X-ray absorptiometry (DXA) and other methods. Furthermore, BMI appears to be as strongly correlated with various metabolic and disease outcome as are these more direct measures of body fatness. In general, BMI is an inexpensive and easy-to-perform method of screening for weight category, for example underweight, normal or healthy weight, overweight, and obesity.

How Is BMI Used?

A high BMI can be an indicator of high body fatness. BMI can be used as a screening tool but is not diagnostic of the body fatness or health of an individual.

To determine if a high BMI is a health risk, a healthcare provider would need to perform further assessments. These assessments might include skinfold thickness measurements, evaluations of diet, physical activity, family history, and other appropriate health screenings.

What Are the BMI Trends for Adults in the United States?

The prevalence of adult BMI greater than or equal to 30 kg/m^2 (obese status) has greatly increased since the 1970s. Recently, however, this trend has leveled off, except for older women. Obesity has continued to increase in adult women who are age 60 years and older.

Why Is BMI Used to Measure Overweight and Obesity?

BMI can be used for population assessment of overweight and obesity. Because calculation requires only height and weight, it is inexpensive and easy to use for clinicians and for the general public. BMI can be used as a screening tool for body fatness but is not diagnostic.

What Are Some of the Other Ways to Assess Excess Body Fatness besides BMI?

Other methods to measure body fatness include skinfold thickness measurements (with calipers), underwater weighing, bioelectrical impedance, dual-energy X-ray absorptiometry (DXA), and isotope dilution. However, these methods are not always readily available, and they are either expensive or need to be conducted by highly trained personnel. Furthermore, many of these methods can be difficult to standardize across observers or machines, complicating comparisons across studies and time periods.

How Is BMI calculated?

BMI is calculated the same way for both adults and children. The calculation is based on the following formulas:

Table 6.2. Calculating BMI

Measurement Units	Formula and Calculation
Kilograms and meters (or centimeters)	Formula: weight (kg) / [height (m)]^2 With the metric system, the formula for BMI is weight in kilograms divided by height in meters squared. Because height is commonly measured in centimeters, divide height in centimeters by 100 to obtain height in meters. Example: Weight = 68 kg, Height = 165 cm (1.65 m) Calculation: $68 \div (1.65)^2 = 24.98$

Table 6.2. Continued

Measurement Units	Formula and Calculation
Pounds and inches	Formula: weight (lb) / [height (in)]^2 x 703 Calculate BMI by dividing weight in pounds (lbs) by height in inches (in) squared and multiplying by a conversion factor of 703. Example: Weight = 150 lbs, Height = 5'5" (65") Calculation: [150 ÷ (65)^2] x 703 = 24.96

How Is BMI Interpreted for Adults?

For adults 20 years old and older, BMI is interpreted using standard weight status categories. These categories are the same for men and women of all body types and ages.

The standard weight status categories associated with BMI ranges for adults are shown in the following table.

Table 6.3. The standard weight status categories and thier BMI ranges

BMI	Weight Status
Below 18.5	Underweight
18.5–24.9	Normal or Healthy Weight
25.0–29.9	Overweight
30.0 and Above	Obese

For example, here are the weight ranges, the corresponding BMI ranges, and the weight status categories for a person who is 5' 9".

Table 6.4. Weight ranges, corresponding BMI ranges, and weight status categories for a person who is 5' 9"

Height	Weight Range	BMI	Weight Status
5' 9"	124 lbs or less	Below 18.5	Underweight
	125 lbs to 168 lbs	18.5 to 24.9	Normal or Healthy Weight
	169 lbs to 202 lbs	25.0 to 29.9	Overweight
	203 lbs or more	30 or higher	Obese

For children and teens, the interpretation of BMI depends upon age and sex.

Is BMI Interpreted the Same Way for Children and Teens as It Is for Adults?

BMI is interpreted differently for children and teens, even though it is calculated using the same formula as adult BMI. Children and teen's BMI need to be age and sex-specific because the amount of body fat changes with age and the amount of body fat differs between girls and boys. The CDC BMI-for-age growth charts take into account these differences and visually show BMI as a percentile ranking. These percentiles were determined using representative data of the U.S. population of 2- to 19-year-olds that was collected in various surveys from 1963–65 to 1988–9411.

Obesity among 2- to 19-year-olds is defined as a BMI at or above the 95th percentile of children of the same age and sex in this 1963 to 1994 reference population. For example, a 10-year-old boy of average height (56 inches) who weighs 102 pounds would have a BMI of 22.9 kg/m². This would place the boy in the 95th percentile for BMI—meaning that his BMI is greater than that of 95% of similarly aged boys in this reference population—and he would be considered to have obesity.

How Good Is BMI as an Indicator of Body Fatness?

The correlation between the BMI and body fatness is fairly strong, but even if 2 people have the same BMI, their level of body fatness may differ.

In general,

- At the same BMI, women tend to have more body fat than men.

- At the same BMI, Blacks have less body fat than do Whites, and Asians have more body fat than do Whites

- At the same BMI, older people, on average, tend to have more body fat than younger adults.

- At the same BMI, athletes have less body fat than do non-athletes.

The accuracy of BMI as an indicator of body fatness also appears to be higher in persons with higher levels of BMI and body fatness. While, a person with a very high BMI (e.g., 35 kg/m²) is very likely to have high body fat, a relatively high BMI can be the results of either high body fat or high lean body mass (muscle and bone). A trained healthcare provider should perform appropriate health assessments in order to evaluate an individual's health status and risks.

If an Athlete or Other Person with a Lot of Muscle Has a BMI over 25, Is That Person Still Considered to Be Overweight?

According to the BMI weight status categories, anyone with a BMI between 25 and 29.9 would be classified as overweight and anyone with a BMI over 30 would be classified as obese.

However, athletes may have a high BMI because of increased muscularity rather than increased body fatness. In general, a person who has a high BMI is likely to have body fatness and would be considered to be overweight or obese, but this may not apply to athletes. A trained healthcare provider should perform appropriate health assessments in order to evaluate an individual's health status and risks.

Section 6.3

Health Risks of Overweight and Obesity

This section includes text excerpted from "Overweight and Obesity,"
Centers for Disease Control and Prevention (CDC), June 16, 2015.

Obesity is a complex health issue to address. Obesity results from a combination of causes and contributing factors, including individual factors such as behavior and genetics. Behaviors can include dietary patterns, physical activity, inactivity, medication use, and other exposures. Additional contributing factors in our society include the food and physical activity environment, education and skills, and food marketing and promotion.

Obesity is a serious concern because it is associated with poorer mental health outcomes, reduced quality of life, and the leading causes of death in the United States and worldwide, including diabetes, heart disease, stroke, and some types of cancer.

Behavior

Healthy behaviors include a healthy diet pattern and regular physical activity. Energy balance of the number of calories consumed from foods and beverages with the number of calories the body uses for activity plays a role in preventing excess weight gain. A healthy diet pattern follows the Dietary Guidelines for Americans which emphasizes eating whole grains, fruits, vegetables, lean protein, low-fat and fat-free dairy products and drinking water. The Physical Activity Guidelines for Americans recommends adults do at least 150 minutes of moderate intensity activity or 75 minutes of vigorous intensity activity, or a combination of both, along with 2 days of strength training per week.

Having a healthy diet pattern and regular physical activity is also important for long term health benefits and prevention of chronic diseases such as Type 2 diabetes and heart disease.

Community Environment

People and families may make decisions based on their environment or community. For example, a person may choose not to walk or bike to the store or to work because of a lack of sidewalks or safe bike trails. Community, home, child care, school, healthcare, and workplace settings can all influence people's daily behaviors. Therefore, it is important to create environments in these locations that make it easier to engage in physical activity and eat a healthy diet.

Genetics

Do Genes Have a Role in Obesity?

Genetic changes in human populations occur too slowly to be responsible for the obesity epidemic. Nevertheless, the variation in how people respond to the environment that promotes physical inactivity and intake of high-calorie foods suggests that genes do play a role in the development of obesity.

How Could Genes Influence Obesity?

Genes give the body instructions for responding to changes in its environment. Studies have identified variants in several genes that may contribute to obesity by increasing hunger and food intake.

Rarely, a clear pattern of inherited obesity within a family is caused by a specific variant of a single gene (monogenic obesity). Most obesity, however, probably results from complex interactions among multiple genes and environmental factors that remain poorly understood (multifactorial obesity).

What about Family History?

Healthcare practitioners routinely collect family health history to help identify people at high risk of obesity-related diseases such as diabetes, cardiovascular diseases, and some forms of cancer. Family health history reflects the effects of shared genetics and environment among close relatives. Families can't change their genes but they can change the family environment to encourage healthy eating habits and physical activity. Those changes can improve the health of family members—and improve the family health history of the next generation.

Other Factors: Diseases and Drugs

Some illnesses may lead to obesity or weight gain. These may include Cushing disease, and polycystic ovary syndrome. Drugs such as steroids and some antidepressants may also cause weight gain. The science continues to emerge on the role of other factors in energy balance and weight gain such as chemical exposures and the role of the microbiome.

A healthcare provider can help you learn more about your health habits and history in order to tell you whether behaviors, illnesses, medications, and/or psychological factors are contributing to weight gain or making weight loss hard.

Consequences of Obesity

Health Consequences

People who are obese, compared to those with a normal or healthy weight, are at increased risk for many serious diseases and health conditions, including the following:

- all-causes of death (mortality)
- high blood pressure (Hypertension)
- high LDL cholesterol, low HDL cholesterol, or high levels of triglycerides (Dyslipidemia)
- type 2 diabetes
- coronary heart disease
- stroke
- gallbladder disease
- osteoarthritis (a breakdown of cartilage and bone within a joint)

- sleep apnea and breathing problems

- some cancers (breast, colon, kidney, gallbladder, and liver)

- low quality of life

- mental illness such as clinical depression, anxiety, and other mental disorders

- body pain and difficulty with physical functioning

Economic and Societal Consequences

Obesity and its associated health problems have a significant economic impact on the U.S. healthcare system. Medical costs associated with overweight and obesity may involve direct and indirect costs. Direct medical costs may include preventive, diagnostic, and treatment services related to obesity. Indirect costs relate to morbidity and mortality costs including productivity. Productivity measures include 'absenteeism' (costs due to employees being absent from work for obesity-related health reasons) and 'presenteeism' (decreased productivity of employees while at work) as well as premature mortality and disability.

Section 6.4

Tips for Healthy Weight Loss

This section contains text excerpted from the following sources:
Text beginning with the heading "Interested in Losing Weight?" is
excerpted from "Interested in Losing Weight?" Nutrition.gov, U.S.
Department of Agriculture (USDA), July 27, 2016; Text beginning
with the heading "If You Need to Lose Weight" is excerpted
from "If You Need to Lose Weight," Office on Women's Health
(OWH), U.S. Department of Health and Human Services (HHS),
November 5, 2013. Reviewed August 2016.

Interested in Losing Weight?

What You Need to Know Before Getting Started

Weight loss can be achieved either by eating fewer calories or by
burning more calories with physical activity, preferably both.

A healthy weight loss program consists of:

- A reasonable, realistic weight loss goal.

- A reduced calorie, nutritionally-balanced eating plan.

- Regular physical activity.

- A behavior change plan to help you stay on track with your
  goals.

Keep in Mind

- Calories count.

- Portions count.

- Nutrition counts.

- Even a small amount of weight loss can lead to big health
  benefits.

- Strive to develop good habits to last a lifetime.

- Discuss weight loss with your doctor before getting started.

Getting Started

- Check your body mass index (BMI)—an indicator of body fat— and see where it fits within the BMI categories.

- Discuss weight loss with your doctor and decide on a goal. If you have a lot of weight to lose, set a realistic intermediate goal, maybe to lose 10 pounds. Remember that even a small amount of weight loss can lead to big health benefits.

- Estimate your calorie needs. Using U.S. Department of Agriculture's (USDA) online Adult Energy Needs and BMI Calculator, you can determine the number of calories needed each day to maintain your current weight. To lose about 1 pound per week, subtract 500 calories each day from the daily amount. To lose about 2 pounds per week, subtract 1000 calories daily.

- Score your current food intake and physical activity level using MyPlate SuperTracker (www.supertracker.usda.gov). Taking a good look at your current habits will help you determine what changes you might make as well as what you are doing right.

How Do I Know Which Weight Loss Plan is Right For Me?

- Keep in mind that you want to develop lifestyle habits that will help you maintain your weight in a healthy range. A short-term "diet" that you "go on" and then "go off" is not the answer to long-term weight management.

- In choosing how to go about losing weight, keep in mind key habits of people who have lost weight and kept in off. These people are called "Successful Losers" by the weight control experts who have studied them.

Key Behaviors of Successful Losers*

- Getting regular physical activity.

- Reducing calorie and fat intake.

- Eating regular meals, including breakfast.

- Weighing themselves regularly.

- Not letting small "slips" turn into large weight regain.

*From The National Weight Control Registry.

Ask your doctor if you should have a referral to a Registered Dietitian (RD). An RD can provide personalized dietary advice taking into consideration other health issues, lifestyle, and food likes and dislikes.

Staying on Track with Your Goals

Setting realistic goals and tracking your progress are key to your success. In fact, research has shown that those who keep track of their behaviors are more likely to take off weight and keep it off. A reasonable rate of weight loss is 1 to 2 pounds per week.

If You Need to Lose Weight

Lots of people need to lose some weight. If your doctor tells you that you are overweight or obese, it's important that you try to lose weight. You can ask your doctor and perhaps a dietitian about ways to lose weight. It can be a bit harder for some people to lose weight because of their genes or because of things around them, such as the food choices in their house. But with the right support and a good plan, you can get to a healthy weight. Learn more about losing weight:

Great Ways to Lose Weight

You don't need a special diet like a low-carb or high-protein diet to lose weight. The best way to lose weight is to get the right mix of nutrients and energy your body needs. Here are some tips for losing weight in a healthy way:

- **Follow a food guide.** It can be hard to know which foods to choose. The MyPlate guide can be a big help. It will encourage you to eat whole grains, vegetables, and fruits. These foods are full of fiber, which can help you feel full. And keeping a record can help, so try the ChooseMyPlate tracking tool.

- **Cut back on fats.** You need some fat, but even small amounts of fats have lots of calories. Read labels to see how much fat a food has. And try to cut back on fried foods and on meats that are high in fat, such as burgers.

- **Eat fewer sweets and unhealthy snacks.** Candy, cookies, and cakes often have a lot of sugar and fat and not many nutrients.

- **Avoid sugary drinks.** Try not to drink a lot of sugary sodas, energy drinks, and sports drinks. They can add a lot of calories.

(There are about 10 packets of sugar in 12 ounces of soda.) Also try not to drink a lot of fruit juice. Water is a great choice instead. Add a piece of lemon or a splash of juice for more flavor.

- **Get enough sleep at night.** Staying up late often increases night-time snacking and low energy the next morning (which you might be tempted to beat with some extra food).

- **Limit fast food meals.** Studies show that the more fast food you eat each week, the greater the risk of gaining extra weight. So try to limit fast food meals to once a week or less.

- **Tackle hunger with fiber and protein.** Don't wait until you are so hungry that it gets hard to make smart food choices. Instead, when you start to feel hungry, eat a small snack that combines a protein with a food that's high in fiber, such as a whole-grain cracker with low-fat cheese. These are filling but not packed with calories.

- **Be aware of how much you are eating.** If you're not sure how much is considered one serving, you can learn how to read labels. You also may eat less if you use a smaller plate. Try not to eat straight from a big package of food—it's easy to lose track that way. And if you're at a restaurant, see if you can take home some leftovers.

- **Think about why you are eating.** Sometimes we eat to fill needs other than hunger, such as being bored, stressed, or lonely. If you do that, see if you can think of some other ways to meet those needs. Consider calling a friend or listening to some great music. And if think you may be having emotional problems, talk to an adult you trust.

- **Get moving.** One great way to lose weight is by being physically active. You should aim for a total of 60 minutes of moderate or vigorous physical activity each day. If you haven't been active in a while, start slowly.

- **Cut down on sitting around.** This means less TV, Internet, and other forms of screen time.

Remember that losing weight is about making healthy changes in your life that you can stick with—and not just a one-time diet.

How Not to Lose Weight

It can be tempting to look for a quick fix if you need to lose weight. Remember, though, that if something sounds too good to be true, it probably is. Keep these tips in mind:

- **Avoid fad diets.** Fad diets often allow only a few types of food. That means you are not getting all the nutrients you need. And these diets may cause you to lose weight for a short time, but then you likely will gain it back quickly.

- **Avoid weight-loss pills and other quick-loss products.** Most weight-loss pills, drinks, supplements, and other products you can buy without a prescription have not been shown to work. And they can actually be very dangerous. If you are thinking about taking weight-loss pills or similar products, talk to your doctor first.

- **Don't eat too little.** Your body needs fuel to grow and be healthy. If you eat fewer than 1,600 calories each day, you may not get the nutrients you need. And don't skip breakfast.

- **Don't try to get rid of food you eat.** Some people think they can lose weight by making themselves vomit or taking laxatives (pills that make you go to the bathroom). These are very dangerous steps and signs of eating disorders. Your body is too precious to treat this way, so get help if you think you may have an eating disorder.

- **Don't expect to lose weight quickly.** Losing about one to two pounds a week is a healthy rate of weight loss. If you are taking extreme steps to lose weight faster, you will probably gain most or all of it back.

Section 6.5

Choosing a Safe and Successful Weight-Loss Program

This section includes text excerpted from "Weight Management," National Institute of Diabetes and Digestive and Kidney Diseases (NIDDK), December 2012. Reviewed August 2016.

Do you need to lose weight? Have you been thinking about trying a weight-loss program? Diets and programs that promise to help you lose weight are advertised everywhere—through magazines and newspapers, radio, TV, and websites. Are these programs safe? Will they work for you?

This section provides tips on how to identify a weight-loss program that may help you lose weight safely and keep the weight off over time. It also suggests ways to talk to your healthcare provider about your weight. He or she may be able to help you control your weight by making changes to your eating and physical activity habits. If these changes are not enough, you may want to consider a weight-loss program or other types of treatment.

Where Do I Start?

Talking to your healthcare provider about your weight is an important first step. Doctors do not always address issues such as healthy eating, physical activity, and weight control during general office visits. It is important for you to bring up these issues to get the help you need. Even if you feel uneasy talking about your weight with your doctor, remember that he or she is there to help you improve your health.

Prepare for the visit:

- Write down your questions in advance.

- Bring pen and paper to take notes.

- Invite a family member or friend along for support if this will make you feel better.

Talk to your doctor about safe and effective ways to control your weight.

He or she can review any medical problems that you have and any drugs that you take to help you set goals for controlling your weight. Make sure you understand what your doctor is saying. Ask questions if you do not understand something.

You may want to ask your doctor to recommend a weight-loss program or specialist. If you do start a weight-loss program, discuss your choice of program with your doctor, especially if you have any health problems.

Questions to Ask Your Healthcare Provider

About Your Weight

- What is a healthy weight for me?

- Do I need to lose weight?

- How much weight should I lose?

- Could my extra weight be caused by a health problem or by a medicine I am taking?

About Ways to Lose Weight

- What kind of eating habits may help me control my weight?

- How much physical activity do I need?

- How can I exercise safely?

- Could a weight-loss program help me?

- Should I take weight-loss drugs?

- Is weight-loss surgery right for me?

What Should I Look for in a Weight-Loss Program?

Successful, long-term weight control must focus on your overall health, not just on what you eat. Changing your lifestyle is not easy, but adopting healthy habits may help you manage your weight in the long run.

Effective weight-loss programs include ways to keep the weight off for good. These programs promote healthy behaviors that help you lose weight and that you can stick with every day.

Safe and effective weight-loss programs should include

- a plan to keep the weight off over the long run

- guidance on how to develop healthier eating and physical activity habits

- ongoing feedback, monitoring, and support

- slow and steady weight-loss goals—usually ½ to 2 pounds per week (though weight loss may be faster at the start of a program)

Some weight-loss programs may use very low-calorie diets (up to 800 calories per day) to promote rapid weight loss among people who have a lot of excess weight. This type of diet requires close medical supervision through frequent office visits and medical tests.

What If the Program Is Offered Online?

Many weight-loss programs are now being offered online—either fully or partly. Not much is known about how well these programs work. However, experts suggest that online weight-loss programs should provide the following:

- structured, weekly lessons offered online or by podcasts support tailored to your personal goals

- support tailored to your personal goals

- self-monitoring of eating and physical activity using handheld devices, such as cell phones or online journals

- regular feedback from a counselor on goals, progress, and results, given by email, phone, or text messages

- social support from a group through bulletin boards, chat rooms, and/or online meetings

Whether the program is online or in person, you should get as much background as you can before deciding to join.

If It Seems Too Good to Be True...It Probably Is!

In choosing a weight-loss program, watch out for these false claims:

- Lose weight without diet or exercise!

- Lose weight while eating all of your favorite foods!

- Lose 30 pounds in 30 days!

- Lose weight in specific problem areas of your body!

Other warning signs include:

- very small print
- asterisks and footnotes
- before-and-after photos that seem too good to be true

What Questions Should I Ask about the Program?

Professionals working for weight-loss programs should be able to answer questions about the program's features, safety, costs, and results. The following are sample questions you may want to ask.

What Does the Weight-Loss Program Include?

- Does the program offer group classes or one-on-one counseling that will help me develop healthier habits?
- Do I have to follow a specific meal plan or keep food records?
- Do I have to buy special meals or supplements?
- If the program requires special foods, can I make changes based on my likes, dislikes, and food allergies (if any)?
- Will the program help me be more physically active, follow a specific physical activity plan, or provide exercise guidelines?
- Will the program work with my lifestyle and cultural needs? Does the program provide ways to deal with such issues as social or holiday eating, changes to work schedules, lack of motivation, and injury or illness?
- Does the program include a plan to help me keep the weight off once I've lost weight?

What Are the Staff Credentials?

- Who supervises the program?
- What type of weight-control certifications, education, experience, and training do the staff have?

Does the Product or Program Carry Any Risks?

- Could the program hurt me?
- Could the suggested drugs or supplements harm my health?

- Do the people involved in the program get to talk with a doctor?

- Does a doctor or other certified health professional run the program?

- Will the program's doctor or staff work with my healthcare provider if needed (for example, to address how the program may affect an existing medical issue)?

- Is there ongoing input and follow-up from a healthcare provider to ensure my safety while I take part in the program?

How Much Does the Program Cost?

- What is the total cost of the program?

- Are there other costs, such as membership fees, fees for weekly visits, and payments for food, meal replacements, supplements, or other products?

- Are there other fees for medical tests?

- Are there fees for a follow-up program after I lose weight?

What Results Do People in the Program Typically Have?

- How much weight does the average person lose?

- How long does the average person keep the weight off?

- Do you have written information on these results?

What If I Need More Help?

If a weight-loss program is not a good option for you, ask your healthcare provider about other types of treatment. Prescription drugs, combined with lifestyle changes, may help some people lose weight. For some people who have obesity, bariatric surgery on the stomach and/or intestines may be an option.

Chapter 7

Nutrition Tips for Men

Chapter Contents

Section 7.1—Healthy Eating for Men 104

Section 7.2—Nutrition Tips for Building Strength
and Increasing Muscle Mass 106

Section 7.1

Healthy Eating for Men

This section contains text excerpted from the following sources:
Text in this section begins with excerpts from "Men and Women,"
U.S. Department of Agriculture (USDA), June 26, 2015; Text under
the heading "Get the Facts to Feel and Look Better" is excerpted
from "Get the Facts to Feel and Look Better," U.S. Department of
Agriculture (USDA), January 2014.

Adults of all ages have different nutrition and physical activity
needs as their lives and bodies change. A strong and healthy body can
provide many benefits. As you age, maintaining healthy habits is an
important way to lower your risk for cancer, diabetes, heart disease
and hypertension. Make your food and beverage choices a priority and
be physically active to feel and look better.

Eat a Healthy Diet

Fruits, vegetables, whole grains, and fat-free or low-fat dairy products are healthy choices. Include protein foods such as poultry, fish,
beans, eggs, nuts and lean meats. Choose foods that are low in saturated fats, sodium, and added sugars.

Be Physically Active

Jogging, playing team sports, and biking are just a few examples
of how you can get moving. Start small and work up to 150 minutes
of moderate-intensity physical activity per week if you are not already
physically active.

Know Your BMI

Knowing your body mass index (BMI) can be an important first step
in adopting a realistic diet and physical activity plan to help you get
to and maintain a healthy weight.

Stay at a Healthy Weight

As you age, manage your calories to stay at a healthy weight. This will prevent gradual weight gain over time. Balance the calories you take in with the calories you burn through physical activities. Periodically track what you eat and drink as well as your physical activity to keep you focused. Use online tools available on your phone, tablet or computer to accurately monitor your food and physical activity. Use the daily food plans below to find out how many calories you need to maintain or achieve your goals.

Get the Facts to Feel and Look Better

- There's no magic food or way to eat. There are some foods men need to eat such as vegetables; fruits; whole grains; protein foods like beans, eggs, or lean meats; and dairy like 1% milk. You'll get nutrients you need for good health? including magnesium, potassium, calcium, vitamin D, fiber, and protein.

- Keep healthy foods in your kitchen that need little preparation. Keep your fridge filled with carrots, apples, oranges, low-fat yogurt, and eggs. Stock up on fresh, canned, or frozen vegetables and fruits, lean meats, canned beans, and tuna or salmon. Find healthier heat-and-eat options to replace heating up a frozen pizza.

- Make sure half your grains are whole grains. Whole grains can help give a feeling of fullness and key nutrients. Choose whole-wheat breads, pasta, and crackers; brown rice; and oatmeal instead of white bread, rice, or other refined-grain products.

- Cut calories by skipping foods high in solid fats and added sugar. Limit fatty meats like ribs, bacon, and hot dogs. Cakes, cookies, candies, and ice cream should be just occasional treats. Use smaller plates to adjust the amount of food you eat.

- Water is a better choice than many routine drink choices. Beverages can add about 400 calories a day to men's diets. So limit high-calorie beverages, including those with alcohol. Skip soda, fruit drinks, energy drinks, sports drinks, and other sugary drinks.

- Men's energy needs differ from women's needs. Find exactly how much and what foods you need, based on your height, weight, age, and physical activity level at www.SuperTracker.usda.gov.

- Start cooking more often. Try steaming vegetables, roasting a chicken, and making a tasty veggie sauce for spaghetti from scratch. Eating your own home-cooked meals allows you to control what and how much you eat.

- Use both Nutrition Facts and ingredient labels to discover what nutrients foods and beverages contain. Cut back on foods that have sugar or fat as the first ingredient. Use SuperTracker's Food-A-Pedia to compare more than 8,000 foods.

- Be active whenever you can. Have friends or family join you when you go for a long walk, bike, or jog. Vary activities to stay motivated. Set a goal of 2½ hours or more of moderate physical activity a week. Include strengthening your arms, legs, and core muscles at least 2 days a week. Being active just 10 minutes at a time makes a difference.

Section 7.2

Nutrition Tips for Building Strength and Increasing Muscle Mass

This section includes text excerpted from "Healthy Muscles Matter,"
National Institute of Arthritis and Musculoskeletal and Skin
Diseases (NIAMS), October 2015.

Basic Facts about Muscles

Did you know you have more than 600 muscles in your body? These muscles help you move, lift things, pump blood through your body, and even help you breathe.

When you think about your muscles, you probably think most about the ones you can control. These are your voluntary muscles, which means you can control their movements. They are also called skeletal muscles, because they attach to your bones and work together with your bones to help you walk, run, pick up things, play an instrument, throw a baseball, kick a soccer ball, push a lawnmower, or ride a bicycle. The muscles of your mouth and throat even help you talk!

Keeping your muscles healthy will help you to be able to walk, run, jump, lift things, play sports, and do all the other things you love to do. Exercising, getting enough rest, and eating a balanced diet will help to keep your muscles healthy for life.

Different Kinds of Muscles Have Different Jobs

Skeletal muscles are connected to your bones by tough cords of tissue called tendons. As the muscle contracts, it pulls on the tendon, which moves the bone. Bones are connected to other bones by ligaments, which are like tendons and help hold your skeleton together.

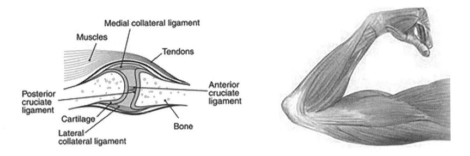

Figure 7.1. *Muscles of the Arm*

A joint showing muscles, ligaments, and tendons

Smooth muscles are also called involuntary muscles since you have no control over them. Smooth muscles work in your digestive system to move food along and push waste out of your body. They also help keep your eyes focused without your having to think about it.

Cardiac muscle. Did you know your heart is also a muscle? It is a specialized type of involuntary muscle. It pumps blood through your body, changing its speed to keep up with the demands you put on it. It pumps more slowly when you're sitting or lying down, and faster when you're running or playing sports and your skeletal muscles need more blood to help them do their work.

Why Healthy Muscles Matter to You

Healthy muscles let you move freely and keep your body strong. They help you to enjoy playing sports, dancing, walking the dog, swimming, and other fun activities. And they help you do those other (not so fun) things that you have to do, like making the bed, vacuuming the carpet, or mowing the lawn.

Strong muscles also help to keep your joints in good shape. If the muscles around your knee, for example, get weak, you may be more likely to injure that knee. Strong muscles also help you keep your balance, so you are less likely to slip or fall.

And remember—the activities that make your skeletal muscles strong will also help to keep your heart muscle strong!

What Can Go Wrong?

Injuries

Almost everyone has had sore muscles after exercising or working too much. Some soreness can be a normal part of healthy exercise. But, in other cases, muscles can become strained. Muscle strains can be mild (the muscle has just been stretched too much) to severe (the muscle actually tears). Maybe you lifted something that was too heavy and the muscles in your arms were stretched too far. Lifting heavy things in the wrong way can also strain the muscles in your back. This can be very painful and can even cause an injury that will last a long time and make it hard to do everyday things.

The tendons that connect the muscles to the bones can also be strained if they are pulled or stretched too much. If ligaments (remember, they connect bones to bones) are stretched or pulled too much, the injury is called a sprain. Most people are familiar with the pain of a sprained ankle.

Contact sports like soccer, football, hockey, and wrestling can often cause strains. Sports in which you grip something (like gymnastics or tennis) can lead to strains in your hand or forearm.

How Do I Keep My Muscles Healthy?

Physical Activity

When you make your muscles work by being physically active, they respond by growing stronger. They may even get bigger by adding more muscle tissue. This is how bodybuilders get such big muscles, but your muscles can be healthy without getting that big.

There are lots of activities you can do to for your muscles. Walking, jogging, lifting weights, playing tennis, climbing stairs, jumping, and dancing are all good ways to exercise your muscles. Swimming and biking will also give your muscles a good workout. It's important to do different kinds of activities to work all your muscles. And any activity that makes you breathe harder and faster will help exercise that important heart muscle as well!

Get 60 minutes of physical activity every day. It doesn't have to be all at once, but it does need to be in at least 10-minute increments to count toward your 60 minutes of physical activity per day.

Eat a Healthy Diet

You really don't need a special diet to keep your muscles in good health. Eating a balanced diet will help manage your weight and provide a variety of nutrients for your muscles and overall health. A balanced diet:

- Emphasizes fruits, vegetables, whole grains, and fat-free or low-fat dairy products like milk, cheese, and yogurt.

- Includes protein from lean meats, poultry, seafood, beans, eggs, and nuts.

- Is low in solid fats, saturated fats, cholesterol, salt (sodium), added sugars, and refined grains.

- Is as low as possible in trans fats.

- Balances calories taken in through food with calories burned in physical activity to help maintain a healthy weight.

As you grow and become an adult, iron is an important nutrient, especially for girls. Not getting enough iron can cause anemia, which can make you feel weak and tired, because your muscles don't get enough oxygen. This can also keep you from getting enough activity to keep your muscles healthy. You can get iron from foods like lean beef, chicken, and turkey; beans and peas; spinach; and iron-enriched breads and cereals. You can also get iron from dietary supplements, but it's always good to check with a doctor first.

Some people think that supplements will make their muscles bigger and stronger. However, supplements like creatine can cause serious side effects, and protein and amino acid supplements are no better than getting protein from your food. Using steroids to increase your muscles is illegal (unless a doctor has prescribed them for a medical problem), and can have dangerous side effects. No muscles-building supplement can take the place of good nutrition and proper training.

Prevent Injuries

To help prevent sprains, strains, and other muscle injuries:

- **Warm up and cool down.** Before exercising or playing sports, warm-up exercises, such as stretching and light jogging, may make it less likely that you'll strain a muscle. They are called warm-up exercises because they make the muscles warmer—and more flexible. Cool-down exercises loosen muscles that have tightened during exercise.

- **Wear the proper protective gear** for your sport, for example pads or helmets. This will help reduce your risk for injuring your muscles or joints.

- Remember to **drink lots of water** while you're playing or exercising, especially in warm weather. If your body's water level gets too low (dehydration), you could get dizzy or even pass out. Dehydration can cause many medical problems.

- **Don't try to "play through the pain."** If something starts to hurt, STOP exercising or playing. You might need to see a doctor, or you might just need to rest the injured part for a while.

- If you have been inactive, **"start low and go slow"** by gradually increasing how often and how long activities are done. Increase physical activity gradually over time.

- **Be careful when you lift heavy objects.** Keep your back straight and bend your knees to lift the object. This will protect the muscles in your back and put most of the weight on the strong muscles in your legs. Get someone to help you lift something heavy.

Start Now

Keeping your muscles healthy will help you have more fun and enjoy the things you do. Healthy muscles will help you look your best and feel full of energy. Start good habits now, while you are young, and you'll have a better chance of keeping your muscles healthy for the rest of your life.

Chapter 8

Physical Activity: Key to a Healthy Life

Chapter Contents

Section 8.1—How Much Physical Activity
      Do Adults Need?.. 112

Section 8.2—The Benefits of Physical Activity 115

Section 8.1

How Much Physical Activity Do Adults Need?

This section includes text excerpted from "How Much Physical Activity Do Adults Need?" Centers for Disease Control and Prevention (CDC), June 4, 2015.

Physical activity is anything that gets your body moving. According to the 2008 *Physical Activity Guidelines for Americans*, you need to do two types of physical activity each week to improve your health—aerobic and muscle-strengthening.

For Important Health Benefits

Adults Need at Least

- 2 hours and 30 minutes (150 minutes) of moderate-intensity aerobic activity (i.e., brisk walking) every week and muscle-strengthening activities on 2 or more days a week that work all major muscle groups (legs, hips, back, abdomen, chest, shoulders, and arms). **OR**

- 1 hour and 15 minutes (75 minutes) of vigorous-intensity aerobic activity (i.e., jogging or running) every week and muscle-strengthening activities on 2 or more days a week that work all major muscle groups (legs, hips, back, abdomen, chest, shoulders, and arms). **OR**

- An equivalent mix of moderate- and vigorous-intensity aerobic activity and muscle-strengthening activities on 2 or more days a week that work all major muscle groups (legs, hips, back, abdomen, chest, shoulders, and arms).

For Even Greater Health Benefits

Older Adults Should Increase Their Activity To

- 5 hours (300 minutes) each week of moderate-intensity aerobic activity and muscle-strengthening activities on 2 or more days a week that work all major muscle groups (legs, hips, back, abdomen, chest, shoulders, and arms). **OR**

- 2 hours and 30 minutes (150 minutes) each week of vigrous-intensity aerobic activity and muscle-strengthening activities on 2 or more days a week that work all major muscle groups (legs, hips, back, abdomen, chest, shoulders, and arms). **OR**

- An equivalent mix of moderate-and vigorous-intensity aerobic activity and muscle-strengthening activities on 2 or more days a week that work all major muscle groups (legs, hips, back, abdomen, chest, shoulders, and arms).

Aerobic Activity—What Counts?

Aerobic activity or "cardio" gets you breathing harder and your heart beating faster. From pushing a lawn mower, to taking a dance class, to biking to the store—all types of activities count. As long as you're doing them at a moderate or vigorous intensity for **at least 10 minutes at a time.**

Intensity is how hard your body is working during aerobic activity.

How Do You Know If You're Doing Light, Moderate, or Vigorous Intensity Aerobic Activities?

For most people, light daily activities such as shopping, cooking, or doing the laundry doesn't count toward the guidelines. Why? Your body isn't working hard enough to get your heart rate up.

Moderate-intensity aerobic activity means you're working hard enough to raise your heart rate and break a sweat. One way to tell is that you'll be able to talk, but not sing the words to your favorite song. Here are some examples of activities that require moderate effort:

- walking fast

- doing water aerobics

- riding a bike on level ground or with few hills

- playing doubles tennis

- pushing a lawn mower

Vigorous-intensity aerobic activity means you're breathing hard and fast, and your heart rate has gone up quite a bit. If you're working at this level, you won't be able to say more than a few words without pausing for a breath. Here are some examples of activities that require vigorous effort:

- jogging or running
- swimming laps
- riding a bike fast or on hills
- playing singles tennis
- playing basketball

You can do moderate- or vigorous-intensity aerobic activity, or a mix of the two each week. A rule of thumb is that **1 minute of vigorous-intensity activity is about the same as 2 minutes of moderate-intensity activity**.

Some people like to do vigorous types of activity because it gives them about the same health benefits in half the time. If you haven't been very active lately, increase your activity level slowly. You need to feel comfortable doing moderate-intensity activities before you move on to more vigorous ones. The guidelines are about doing physical activity that is right for you.

Muscle-Strengthening Activities—What Counts?

Besides aerobic activity, you need to do things to strengthen your muscles at least 2 days a week. These activities should work all the major muscle groups of your body (legs, hips, back, chest, abdomen, shoulders, and arms).

To gain health benefits, muscle-strengthening activities need to be done to the point where it's hard for you to do another repetition without help. A **repetition** is one complete movement of an activity, like lifting a weight or doing a sit-up. Try to do 8–12 repetitions per activity that count as 1 **set**. Try to do at least 1 set of muscle-strengthening activities, but to gain even more benefits, do 2 or 3 sets.

You can do activities that strengthen your muscles on the same or different days that you do aerobic activity, whatever works best. Just keep in mind that muscle-strengthening activities don't count toward your aerobic activity total.

There are many ways you can strengthen your muscles, whether it's at home or the gym. You may want to try the following:

- lifting weights
- working with resistance bands

- doing exercises that use your body weight for resistance (i.e., push ups, sit ups)

- heavy gardening (i.e., digging, shoveling)

- yoga

Section 8.2

The Benefits of Physical Activity

This section includes text excerpted from "Benefits of Physical Activity," National Heart, Lung, and Blood Institute (NHLBI), June 22, 2016.

Physical activity has many health benefits. These benefits apply to people of all ages and races and both sexes.

For example, physical activity helps you maintain a healthy weight and makes it easier to do daily tasks, such as climbing stairs and shopping.

Physically active adults are at lower risk for depression and declines in cognitive function as they get older. (Cognitive function includes thinking, learning, and judgment skills.) Physically active children and teens may have fewer symptoms of depression than their peers.

Physical activity also lowers your risk for many diseases, such as coronary heart disease (CHD), diabetes, and cancer.

Many studies have shown the clear benefits of physical activity for your heart and lungs.

Physical Activity Strengthens Your Heart and Improves Lung Function

When done regularly, moderate- and vigorous-intensity physical activity strengthens your heart muscle. This improves your heart's ability to pump blood to your lungs and throughout your body. As a result, more blood flows to your muscles, and oxygen levels in your blood rise.

Capillaries, your body's tiny blood vessels, also widen. This allows them to deliver more oxygen to your body and carry away waste products.

Physical Activity Reduces Coronary Heart Disease Risk Factors

When done regularly, moderate- and vigorous-intensity aerobic activity can lower your risk for CHD. CHD is a condition in which a waxy substance called plaque builds up inside your coronary arteries. These arteries supply your heart muscle with oxygen-rich blood.

Plaque narrows the arteries and reduces blood flow to your heart muscle. Eventually, an area of plaque can rupture (break open). This causes a blood clot to form on the surface of the plaque.

If the clot becomes large enough, it can mostly or completely block blood flow through a coronary artery. Blocked blood flow to the heart muscle causes a heart attack.

Certain traits, conditions, or habits may raise your risk for CHD. Physical activity can help control some of these risk factors because it:

- Can lower blood pressure and triglyceride. Triglycerides are a type of fat in the blood.

- Can raise HDL cholesterol levels. HDL sometimes is called "good" cholesterol.

- Helps your body manage blood sugar and insulin levels, which lowers your risk for type 2 diabetes.

- Reduces levels of C-reactive protein (CRP) in your body. This protein is a sign of inflammation. High levels of CRP may suggest an increased risk for CHD.

- Helps reduce overweight and obesity when combined with a reduced-calorie diet. Physical activity also helps you maintain a healthy weight over time once you have lost weight.

- May help you quit smoking. Smoking is a major risk factor for CHD.

Inactive people are more likely to develop CHD than people who are physically active. Studies suggest that inactivity is a major risk factor for CHD, just like high blood pressure, high blood cholesterol, and smoking.

Physical Activity Reduces Heart Attack Risk

For people who have CHD, aerobic activity done regularly helps the heart work better. It also may reduce the risk of a second heart attack in people who already have had heart attacks.

Vigorous aerobic activity may not be safe for people who have CHD. Ask your doctor what types of activity are safe for you.

Part Two

Leading Causes
of Death in Men

Chapter 9

Mortality in the United States

Chapter Contents

Section 9.1—Causes of Death: A Statistical Overview 122

Section 9.2—Cancer among Men: Some Statistics.................... 124

Section 9.1

Causes of Death: A Statistical Overview

This section includes text excerpted from "Mortality in the
United States, 2014," Centers for Disease Control and
Prevention (CDC), November 6, 2015.

Key findings

Data from the National Vital Statistics System, Mortality

- Life expectancy for the U.S. population in 2014 was unchanged
  from 2013 at 78.8 years.

- The age-adjusted death rate decreased 1.0% to 724.6 deaths per
  100,000 standard population in 2014 from 731.9 in 2013.

- The 10 leading causes of death in 2014 remained the same as
  in 2013. Age-adjusted death rates significantly decreased for 5
  leading causes and significantly increased for 4 leading causes.

- The infant mortality rate decreased 2.3% to a historic low of
  582.1 infant deaths per 100,000 live births. The 10 leading
  causes of infant death in 2014 remained the same as in 2013.

This report presents 2014 U.S. final mortality data on deaths and
death rates by demographic and medical characteristics. These data
provide information on mortality patterns among U.S. residents by
such variables as sex, race and ethnicity, and cause of death. Information on mortality patterns is key to understanding changes in the
health and well-being of the U.S. population. Life expectancy estimates, age-adjusted death rates by race and ethnicity and sex, the 10
leading causes of death, and the 10 leading causes of infant death were
analyzed by comparing 2014 final data with 2013 final data.

How Long Can We Expect to Live?

Life expectancy at birth represents the average number of years
that a group of infants would live if the group was to experience,
throughout life, the age-specific death rates present in the year of

birth. In 2014, life expectancy at birth was 78.8 years for the total U.S. population—81.2 years for females and 76.4 years for males, the same as in 2013. Life expectancy for females was consistently higher than life expectancy for males. In 2014, the difference in life expectancy between females and males was 4.8 years, the same as in 2013.

Life expectancy at age 65 for the total population was 19.3 years, the same as in 2013. Life expectancy at age 65 was 20.5 years for females, unchanged from 2013, and 18.0 years for males, a 0.1-year increase from 2013. The difference in life expectancy at age 65 between females and males decreased 0.1 year, to 2.5 years in 2014 from 2.6 years in 2013.

Which Population Groups Experienced Reductions in Mortality?

The age-adjusted death rate for the total population decreased 1.0% to a record low of 724.6 deaths per 100,000 standard population in 2014 from 731.9 in 2013. Age-adjusted death rates decreased significantly in 2014 from 2013 for non-Hispanic black males (2.1%), non-Hispanic black females (1.3%), non-Hispanic white males (0.5%), non-Hispanic white females (0.7%), Hispanic males (2.0%), and Hispanic females (2.5%).

What Are the Leading Causes of Death?

In 2014, the 10 leading causes of death—heart disease, cancer, chronic lower respiratory diseases, unintentional injuries, stroke, Alzheimer disease, diabetes, influenza and pneumonia, kidney disease, and suicide—remained the same as in 2013. The 10 leading causes accounted for 73.8% of all deaths in the United States in 2014.

From 2013 to 2014, age-adjusted death rates significantly decreased for 5 of the 10 leading causes of death and significantly increased for 4 leading causes. The rate decreased by 1.6% for heart disease, 1.2% for cancer, 3.8% for chronic lower respiratory diseases, 1.4% for diabetes, and 5.0% for influenza and pneumonia. The rate increased by 2.8% for unintentional injuries, 0.8% for stroke, 8.1% for Alzheimer disease, and 3.2% for suicide. The rate for kidney disease in 2014 remained the same as in 2013.

Section 9.2

Cancer among Men: Some Statistics

This section includes text excerpted from "Cancer among Men,"
Centers for Disease Control and Prevention (CDC), August 20, 2015.

Cancer among Men

Three Most Common Cancers among Men

Prostate cancer (101.6)

- First among men of all races and Hispanic* origin populations.

Lung cancer (69.8)

- Second among white, black, American Indian/Alaska Native, and Asian/Pacific Islander men.

- Third among Hispanic* men.

Colorectal cancer (44.2)

- Second among Hispanic* men.

- Third among white, black, American Indian/Alaska Native, and Asian/Pacific Islander men.

Leading Causes of Cancer Death among Men

Lung cancer (53.9)

- First among men of all races and Hispanic* origin populations.

Prostate cancer (19.2)

- Second among white, black, and Hispanic* men.

- Third among American Indian/Alaska Native men.

- Fourth among Asian/Pacific Islander men.

*Hispanic origin is not mutually exclusive from race categories (white, black, Asian/Pacific Islander, American Indian/Alaska Native).

Colorectal cancer (17.3)

- Second among American Indian/Alaska Native men.
- Third among white, black, Asian/Pacific Islander, and Hispanic* men.

Liver cancer (9.5)

- Second among Asian/Pacific Islander men.

Chapter 10

Alzheimer Disease

Alzheimer disease (AD) is an irreversible, progressive brain disorder that slowly destroys memory and thinking skills, and eventually the ability to carry out the simplest tasks. In most people with AD, symptoms first appear in their mid-60s. Estimates vary, but experts suggest that more than 5 million Americans may have AD.

AD is currently ranked as the sixth leading cause of death in the United States, but recent estimates indicate that the disorder may rank third, just behind heart disease and cancer, as a cause of death for older people.

AD is the most common cause of dementia among older adults. Dementia is the loss of cognitive functioning—thinking, remembering, and reasoning—and behavioral abilities to such an extent that it interferes with a person's daily life and activities. Dementia ranges in severity from the mildest stage, when it is just beginning to affect a person's functioning, to the most severe stage, when the person must depend completely on others for basic activities of daily living.

The causes of dementia can vary, depending on the types of brain changes that may be taking place. Other dementias include Lewy body dementia, frontotemporal disorders, and vascular dementia. It is common for people to have mixed dementia—a combination of two or more disorders, at least one of which is dementia. For example, some people have both AD and vascular dementia.

Alzheimer disease is named after Dr. Alois Alzheimer. In 1906, Dr. Alzheimer noticed changes in the brain tissue of a woman who had

---

This chapter includes text excerpted from "Alzheimer's Disease Fact Sheet," National Institute on Aging (NIA), May 2015.

died of an unusual mental illness. Her symptoms included memory loss, language problems, and unpredictable behavior. After she died, he examined her brain and found many abnormal clumps (now called amyloid plaques) and tangled bundles of fibers (now called neurofibrillary, or tau, tangles).

These plaques and tangles in the brain are still considered some of the main features of AD. Another feature is the loss of connections between nerve cells (neurons) in the brain. Neurons transmit messages between different parts of the brain, and from the brain to muscles and organs in the body.

Changes in the Brain

Scientists continue to unravel the complex brain changes involved in the onset and progression of AD. It seems likely that damage to the brain starts a decade or more before memory and other cognitive problems appear. During this preclinical stage of Alzheimer disease, people seem to be symptom-free, but toxic changes are taking place in the brain. Abnormal deposits of proteins form amyloid plaques and tau tangles throughout the brain, and once-healthy neurons stop functioning, lose connections with other neurons, and die.

The damage initially appears to take place in the hippocampus, the part of the brain essential in forming memories. As more neurons die, additional parts of the brain are affected, and they begin to shrink. By the final stage of AD, damage is widespread, and brain tissue has shrunk significantly.

Signs and Symptoms

Memory problems are typically one of the first signs of cognitive impairment related to AD. Some people with memory problems have a condition called mild cognitive impairment (MCI). In MCI, people have more memory problems than normal for their age, but their symptoms do not interfere with their everyday lives. Movement difficulties and problems with the sense of smell have also been linked to MCI. Older people with MCI are at greater risk for developing AD, but not all of them do. Some may even go back to normal cognition.

The first symptoms of AD vary from person to person. For many, decline in non-memory aspects of cognition, such as word-finding, vision/spatial issues, and impaired reasoning or judgment, may signal the very early stages of AD. Researchers are studying biomarkers (biological signs of disease found in brain images, cerebrospinal fluid, and blood) to see if they can detect early changes in the brains of people with MCI and in cognitively normal people who may be at greater risk for AD. Studies indicate that such early detection may be possible, but more research is needed before these techniques can be relied upon to diagnose AD in everyday medical practice.

Mild Alzheimer Disease

As AD progresses, people experience greater memory loss and other cognitive difficulties. Problems can include wandering and getting lost, trouble handling money and paying bills, repeating questions, taking longer to complete normal daily tasks, and personality and behavior changes. People are often diagnosed in this stage.

Moderate Alzheimer Disease

In this stage, damage occurs in areas of the brain that control language, reasoning, sensory processing, and conscious thought. Memory loss and confusion grow worse, and people begin to have problems recognizing family and friends. They may be unable to learn new things, carry out multistep tasks such as getting dressed, or cope with new situations. In addition, people at this stage may have hallucinations, delusions, and paranoia and may behave impulsively.

Severe Alzheimer Disease

Ultimately, plaques and tangles spread throughout the brain, and brain tissue shrinks significantly. People with severe AD cannot communicate and are completely dependent on others for their care. Near the end, the person may be in bed most or all of the time as the body shuts down.

What Causes Alzheimer Disease

Scientists don't yet fully understand what causes AD in most people. In people with early-onset AD, a genetic mutation is usually the cause. Late-onset AD arises from a complex series of brain changes that occur over decades. The causes probably include a combination of genetic, environmental, and lifestyle factors. The importance of any one of these factors in increasing or decreasing the risk of developing AD may differ from person to person.

The Basics of Alzheimer Disease

One of the great mysteries of AD is why it largely strikes older adults. Research on normal brain aging is shedding light on this question. For example, scientists are learning how age-related changes in the brain may harm neurons and contribute to AD damage. These age-related changes include atrophy (shrinking) of certain parts of the brain, inflammation, production of unstable molecules called free radicals, and mitochondrial dysfunction (a breakdown of energy production within a cell).

Genetics

Most people with AD have the late-onset form of the disease, in which symptoms become apparent in their mid-60s. The apolipoprotein E (*APOE*) gene is involved in late-onset AD. This gene has several forms. One of them, *APOE ε4*, increases a person's risk of developing the disease and is also associated with an earlier age of disease onset. However, carrying the *APOE ε4* form of the gene does not mean that a person will definitely develop AD, and some people with no *APOE ε4* may also develop the disease.

Also, scientists have identified a number of regions of interest in the genome (an organism's complete set of DNA) that may increase a person's risk for late-onset AD to varying degrees.

Early-onset AD occurs in people age 30 to 60 and represents less than 5 percent of all people with AD. Most cases are caused by an inherited change in one of three genes, resulting in a type known as early-onset familial AD, or FAD. For others, the disease appears to develop without any specific, known cause, much as it does for people with late-onset disease.

Most people with Down syndrome develop AD. This may be because people with Down syndrome have an extra copy of chromosome 21, which contains the gene that generates harmful amyloid.

Health, Environmental, and Lifestyle Factors

Research suggests that a host of factors beyond genetics may play a role in the development and course of AD. There is a great deal of interest, for example, in the relationship between cognitive decline and vascular conditions such as heart disease, stroke, and high blood pressure, as well as metabolic conditions such as diabetes and obesity. Ongoing research will help us understand whether and how reducing risk factors for these conditions may also reduce the risk of AD.

A nutritious diet, physical activity, social engagement, and mentally stimulating pursuits have all been associated with helping people stay healthy as they age. These factors might also help reduce the risk of cognitive decline and AD. Clinical trials are testing some of these possibilities.

Diagnosis of Alzheimer Disease

Doctors use several methods and tools to help determine whether a person who is having memory problems has "possible AD dementia" (dementia may be due to another cause) or "probable AD dementia" (no other cause for dementia can be found).

To diagnose AD, doctors may:

- Ask the person and a family member or friend questions about overall health, past medical problems, ability to carry out daily activities, and changes in behavior and personality.

- Conduct tests of memory, problem solving, attention, counting, and language.

- Carry out standard medical tests, such as blood and urine tests, to identify other possible causes of the problem.

- Perform brain scans, such as computed tomography (CT), magnetic resonance imaging (MRI), or positron emission tomography (PET), to rule out other possible causes for symptoms.

These tests may be repeated to give doctors information about how the person's memory and other cognitive functions are changing over time.

AD disease can be *definitely* diagnosed only after death, by linking clinical measures with an examination of brain tissue in an autopsy.

People with memory and thinking concerns should talk to their doctor to find out whether their symptoms are due to AD or another cause, such as stroke, tumor, Parkinson's disease, sleep disturbances, side effects of medication, an infection, or a non-AD dementia. Some of these conditions may be treatable and possibly reversible.

If the diagnosis is AD, beginning treatment early in the disease process may help preserve daily functioning for some time, even though the underlying disease process cannot be stopped or reversed. An early diagnosis also helps families plan for the future. They can take care of financial and legal matters, address potential safety issues, learn about living arrangements, and develop support networks.

In addition, an early diagnosis gives people greater opportunities to participate in clinical trials that are testing possible new treatments for AD or other research studies.

Treatment of Alzheimer Disease

AD is complex, and it is unlikely that any one drug or other intervention can successfully treat it. Current approaches focus on helping people maintain mental function, manage behavioral symptoms, and slow or delay the symptoms of disease. Researchers hope to develop therapies targeting specific genetic, molecular, and cellular mechanisms so that the actual underlying cause of the disease can be stopped or prevented.

Maintaining Mental Function

Several medications are approved by the U.S. Food and Drug Administration (FDA) to treat symptoms of AD. Donepezil (Aricept®), rivastigmine (Exelon®), and galantamine (Razadyne®) are used to treat mild to moderate AD (donepezil can be used for severe AD as well). Memantine (Namenda®) is used to treat moderate to severe AD. These drugs work by regulating neurotransmitters, the chemicals that transmit messages between neurons. They may help maintain thinking, memory, and communication skills, and help with certain behavioral problems. However, these drugs don't change the underlying disease process. They are effective for some but not all people, and may help only for a limited time.

Managing Behavior

Common behavioral symptoms of AD include sleeplessness, wandering, agitation, anxiety, and aggression. Scientists are learning why these symptoms occur and are studying new treatments—drug and non-drug—to manage them. Research has shown that treating behavioral symptoms can make people with AD more comfortable and makes things easier for caregivers.

Looking for New Treatments

AD research has developed to a point where scientists can look beyond treating symptoms to think about addressing underlying disease processes. In ongoing clinical trials, scientists are developing and testing several possible interventions, including immunization therapy, drug therapies, cognitive training, physical activity, and treatments used for cardiovascular and diabetes.

Chapter 11

Chronic Liver Disease

Chapter Contents

Section 11.1—Viral Hepatitis.. 134
Section 11.2—Cirrhosis 140

Section 11.1

Viral Hepatitis

This section includes text excerpted from "Viral Hepatitis," Centers for Disease Control and Prevention (CDC), May 26, 2016.

What Is Viral Hepatitis?

"Hepatitis" means inflammation of the liver. The liver is a vital organ that processes nutrients, filters the blood, and fights infections. When the liver is inflamed or damaged, its function can be affected. Heavy alcohol use, toxins, some medications, and certain medical conditions can cause hepatitis. However, hepatitis is most often caused by a virus. In the United States, the most common types of viral hepatitis are Hepatitis A, Hepatitis B, and Hepatitis C.

Hepatitis A

What Causes It?

Hepatitis A virus

Number of U.S. Cases

About 2,500 new infections each year.

Key Facts

- Effective vaccine available.

- Outbreaks still occur in the United States.

- Common in many countries, especially those without modern sanitation.

How Long Does It Last?

Hepatitis A can last from a few weeks to several months.

How Is It Spread?

Hepatitis A is spread when a person ingests fecal matter—even in microscopic amounts—from contact with objects, food, or drinks contaminated by feces or stool from an infected person.

Who Should Be Vaccinated?

- All children at age 1.
- Travelers to regions where Hepatitis A is common.
- Family and caregivers of recent adoptees from countries where Hepatitis A is common.
- Men who have sex with men.
- Users of certain recreation drugs, whether injected or not.
- People with certain medical conditions including chronic liver disease, clotting-factor disorders.

How Serious Is It?

- People can be sick for a few weeks to a few months.
- Most recover with no lasting liver damage.
- Although very rare, death can occur.

Treatment

Supportive treatment for symptoms.

Who Should Be Tested?

Testing for Hepatitis A is not routinely recommended.

Hepatitis B

What Causes It?

Hepatitis B virus

Number of U.S. Cases

- Estimated 850,000–2.2 million people living with chronic Hepatitis B.

- About 19,200 new infections each year.

Key Facts

- About 2 in 3 people with Hepatitis B do not know they are infected.
- 1 in 12 Asian Americans has chronic Hepatitis B.
- Hepatitis B is a leading cause of liver cancer.

How Long Does It Last?

Hepatitis B can range from a mild illness, lasting a few weeks, to a serious life-long or chronic condition.

More than 90% of unimmunized infants who get infected develop a chronic infection occurs, whereas 6%–10% of older children and adults who get infected develop chronic Hepatitis B.

How Is It Spread?

Hepatitis B is primarily spread when blood, semen, or certain other body fluids from a person infected with the Hepatitis B virus — even in microscopic amounts — enters the body of someone who is not infected.

The Hepatitis B virus can also be transmitted from:

- Birth to an infected mother.
- Sex with an infected person.
- Sharing equipment that has been contaminated with blood from an infected person, such as needles, syringes, and even medical equipment, such as glucose monitors.
- Sharing personal items such as toothbrushes or razors.
- Poor infection control has resulted in outbreaks in healthcare facilities.

Who Should Be Vaccinated?

- All infants at birth.
- Unvaccinated adults with diabetes.
- Uninfected household members and sexual partners with Hepatitis B.
- Persons with multiple sex partners.

- Persons seeking evaluation or treatment for an STD.
- Men who have sex with men.
- People who inject drugs.
- People with certain medical conditions, including HIV, chronic liver disease.
- Travelers to regions where Hepatitis B is common.

How Serious Is It?

- The risk for chronic infection depends on age when infected. When infected as an infant, 90% will develop a chronic infection.
- 15%–25% of chronically infected people develop chronic liver disease, including cirrhosis, liver failure, or liver cancer.

Treatment

Acute: No medication available; best addressed through supportive care

Chronic: Regular monitoring for signs of liver disease progression; some patients are treated with antiviral drugs.

Who Should Be Tested?

- People born in regions with moderate or high rates of Hepatitis B.
- U.S.–born people not vaccinated as infants whose parents were born in regions with high rates of Hepatitis B
- Household, needle-sharing, or sex contacts of anyone with Hepatitis B.
- Men who have sex with men.
- People who inject drugs.
- Patients with abnormal liver tests.
- Hemodialysis patients.
- People needing immunosuppressive or cytotoxic therapy.
- HIV-infected people.

Hepatitis C

What Causes It?

Hepatitis C virus

Number of U.S. Cases

- Estimated 2.7–3.9 million people living with chronic Hepatitis C.
- About 30,500 new infections each year.

Key Facts

- About 50% of people with Hepatitis C do not know they are infected.
- 3 in 4 people with Hepatitis C were born from 1945–1965.
- Hepatitis C is a leading cause of liver transplants and liver cancer.

How Long Does It Last?

Hepatitis C can range from a mild illness, lasting a few weeks, to a serious life-long infection. Most people who get infected develop chronic Hepatitis C.

How Is It Spread?

Hepatitis C is spread when blood from a person infected with the Hepatitis C virus—even in microscopic amounts—enters the body of someone who is not infected.

This can happen through multiple ways including:

- Sharing equipment that has been contaminated with blood from an infected person, such as needles and syringes.
- Receiving a blood transfusion or organ transplant before 1992 (when widespread screening virtually eliminated Hepatitis C from the blood supply).
- Poor infection control has resulted in outbreaks in healthcare facilities.

Who Should Be Vaccinated?

There is no vaccine available for Hepatitis C.

How Serious Is It?

- 75%–85% of people who get infected with the Hepatitis C virus develop a chronic infection.

- 5%–20% of people with chronic Hepatitis C develop cirrhosis.

- 1%–5% will die from cirrhosis or liver cancer.

Treatment

Acute: Antivirals and supportive care.

Chronic: Regular monitoring for signs of liver disease progression; Some patients are treated with antiviral drugs including new medications that can cure.

Hepatitis C and offer shorter length of treatment and increased effectiveness.

Who Should Be Tested?

- People born during 1945–1965.

- Recipients of clotting factor concentrates before 1987.

- Recipients of blood transfusions or donated organs before July 1992.

- People who have injected drugs.

- Long-term hemodialysis patients.

- People with known exposures to Hepatitis C (e.g., healthcare workers after needlesticks, recipients of blood or organs from a donor who later tested positive for Hepatitis C).

- HIV-infected persons.

- People with signs or symptoms of liver disease.

Symptoms

Many people with hepatitis do not have symptoms and do not know they are infected. If symptoms occur with an acute infection, they can appear anytime from 2 weeks to 6 months after exposure. Symptoms of chronic viral hepatitis can take decades to develop.

Symptoms of hepatitis can include: fever, fatigue, loss of appetite, nausea, vomiting, abdominal pain, dark urine, grey-colored stools, joint pain, and jaundice.

Section 11.2

Cirrhosis

This section includes text excerpted from "Cirrhosis,"
National Institute of Diabetes and Digestive and
Kidney Diseases (NIDDK), April 2014.

What Is Cirrhosis?

Cirrhosis is a condition in which the liver slowly deteriorates and is unable to function normally due to chronic, or long lasting, injury. Scar tissue replaces healthy liver tissue and partially blocks the flow of blood through the liver.

The liver is the body's largest internal organ. The liver is called the body's metabolic factory because of the important role it plays in metabolism—the way cells change food into energy after food is digested and absorbed into the blood. The liver has many functions, including

- Taking up, storing, and processing nutrients from food—including fat, sugar, and protein—and delivering them to the rest of the body when needed.

- Making new proteins, such as clotting factors and immune factors.

- Producing bile, which helps the body absorb fats, cholesterol, and fat-soluble vitamins.

- Removing waste products the kidneys cannot remove, such as fats, cholesterol, toxins, and medications.

A healthy liver is necessary for survival. The liver can regenerate most of its own cells when they become damaged. However, if injury to the liver is too severe or long lasting, regeneration is incomplete, and the liver creates scar tissue. Scarring of the liver, also called fibrosis, may lead to cirrhosis.

The buildup of scar tissue that causes cirrhosis is usually a slow and gradual process. In the early stages of cirrhosis, the liver continues to function. However, as cirrhosis gets worse and scar tissue replaces more healthy tissue, the liver will begin to fail. Chronic liver failure, which is also called end-stage liver disease, progresses over months, years, or even decades. With end-stage liver disease, the liver can no longer perform important functions or effectively replace damaged cells.

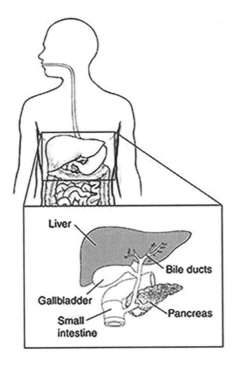

Figure 11.1. *Cirrhosis*

Cirrhosis is a condition in which the liver slowly deteriorates and is unable to function normally due to chronic injury.

Cirrhosis is the 12th leading cause of death in the United States, accounting for nearly 32,000 deaths each year. More men die of cirrhosis than women.

What Causes Cirrhosis?

Cirrhosis has various causes. Many people with cirrhosis have more than one cause of liver damage.

The list below shows common causes of cirrhosis in the United States. While chronic hepatitis C and alcohol-related liver disease are the most common causes of cirrhosis, the incidence of cirrhosis caused by nonalcoholic fatty liver disease is rising due to increasing rates of obesity.

Most Common Causes of Cirrhosis

- Chronic hepatitis C
- Alcohol-related liver disease
- Nonalcoholic fatty liver disease (NAFLD) and nonalcoholic steatohepatitis (NASH)
- Chronic hepatitis B

Less Common Causes of Cirrhosis

Less common causes of cirrhosis include the following:

- Autoimmune hepatitis
- Diseases that damage, destroy, or block the bile ducts
  - Alagille syndrome
  - Biliary atresia
  - Cystic fibrosis
- Inherited diseases that affect the liver
- Rare viral infections of the liver

Other causes. Other causes of cirrhosis may include

- Reactions to medications taken over a period of time.
- Prolonged exposure to toxic chemicals.
- Parasitic infections.
- Chronic heart failure with liver congestion, a condition in which blood flow out of the liver is slowed. Liver congestion can also occur after surgery to correct a congenital heart problem—a heart problem that is present at birth.

Trauma to the liver or other acute, or short term, causes of damage do not cause cirrhosis. Usually, years of chronic injury are required to cause cirrhosis.

What Are the Signs and Symptoms of Cirrhosis?

Many people with cirrhosis have no symptoms in the early stages of the disease. However, as the disease progresses, a person may experience the following symptoms:

- fatigue, or feeling tired

- weakness

- itching

- loss of appetite

- weight loss

- nausea

- bloating of the abdomen from ascites—a buildup of fluid in the abdomen

- edema—swelling due to a buildup of fluid—in the feet, ankles, or legs

- spiderlike blood vessels, called spider angiomas, on the skin

- jaundice, a condition that causes the skin and whites of the eyes to turn yellow

What Are the Complications of Cirrhosis?

As the liver fails, complications may develop. In some people, complications may be the first signs of the disease. Complications of cirrhosis may include the following:

Portal hypertension. The portal vein carries blood from the stomach, intestines, spleen, gallbladder, and pancreas to the liver. In cirrhosis, scar tissue partially blocks the normal flow of blood, which increases the pressure in the portal vein. This condition is called portal hypertension. Portal hypertension is a common complication of cirrhosis. This condition may lead to other complications, such as

- fluid buildup leading to edema and ascites

- enlarged blood vessels, called varices, in the esophagus, stomach, or both

- an enlarged spleen, called splenomegaly

- mental confusion due to a buildup of toxins that are ordinarily removed by the liver, a condition called hepatic encephalopathy

Edema and ascites. Liver failure causes fluid buildup that results in edema and ascites. Ascites can lead to spontaneous bacterial peritonitis, a serious infection that requires immediate medical attention.

Varices. Portal hypertension may cause enlarged blood vessels in the esophagus, stomach, or both. These enlarged blood vessels, called esophageal or gastric varices, cause the vessel walls to become thin and blood pressure to increase, making the blood vessels more likely to burst. If they burst, serious bleeding can occur in the esophagus or upper stomach, requiring immediate medical attention.

Splenomegaly. Portal hypertension may cause the spleen to enlarge and retain white blood cells and platelets, reducing the numbers of these cells and platelets in the blood. A low platelet count may be the first evidence that a person has developed cirrhosis.

Hepatic encephalopathy. A failing liver cannot remove toxins from the blood, so they eventually accumulate in the brain. The buildup of toxins in the brain is called hepatic encephalopathy. This condition can decrease mental function and cause stupor and even coma. Stupor is an unconscious, sleeplike state from which a person can only be aroused briefly by a strong stimulus, such as a sharp pain. Coma is an unconscious, sleeplike state from which a person cannot be aroused. Signs of decreased mental function include

- confusion
- personality changes
- memory loss
- trouble concentrating
- a change in sleep habits

Metabolic bone diseases. Some people with cirrhosis develop a metabolic bone disease, which is a disorder of bone strength usually caused by abnormalities of vitamin D, bone mass, bone structure, or minerals, such as calcium and phosphorous. Osteopenia is a condition in which the bones become less dense, making them weaker. When bone loss becomes more severe, the condition is referred to as osteoporosis. People with these conditions are more likely to develop bone fractures.

Gallstones and bile duct stones. If cirrhosis prevents bile from flowing freely to and from the gallbladder, the bile hardens into gallstones. Symptoms of gallstones include abdominal pain and recurrent bacterial cholangitis—irritated or infected bile ducts. Stones may also form in and block the bile ducts, causing pain, jaundice, and bacterial cholangitis.

Bruising and bleeding. When the liver slows the production of or stops producing the proteins needed for blood clotting, a person will bruise or bleed easily.

Sensitivity to medications. Cirrhosis slows the liver's ability to filter medications from the blood. When this slowdown occurs, medications act longer than expected and build up in the body. For example, some pain medications may have a stronger effect or produce more side effects in people with cirrhosis than in people with a healthy liver.

Insulin resistance and type 2 diabetes. Cirrhosis causes resistance to insulin. The pancreas tries to keep up with the demand for insulin by producing more; however, extra glucose builds up in the bloodstream, causing type 2 diabetes.

Liver cancer. Liver cancer is common in people with cirrhosis. Liver cancer has a high mortality rate. Current treatments are limited and only fully successful if a healthcare provider detects the cancer early, before the tumor is too large. For this reason, healthcare providers should check people with cirrhosis for signs of liver cancer every 6 to 12 months. Healthcare providers use blood tests, ultrasound, or both to check for signs of liver cancer.

Other complications. Cirrhosis can cause immune system dysfunction, leading to an increased chance of infection. Cirrhosis can also cause kidney and lung failure, known as hepatorenal and hepatopulmonary syndromes.

How Is Cirrhosis Diagnosed?

A healthcare provider usually diagnoses cirrhosis based on the presence of conditions that increase its likelihood, such as heavy alcohol use or obesity, and symptoms. A healthcare provider may test for cirrhosis based on the presence of these conditions alone because many people do not have symptoms in the early stages of the disease. A healthcare provider may confirm the diagnosis with

- a medical and family history
- a physical exam
- a blood test
- imaging tests
- a liver biopsy

Medical and family history. Taking a medical and family history is one of the first things a healthcare provider may do to help diagnose cirrhosis. He or she will ask the patient to provide a medical and family history.

Physical exam. A physical exam may help diagnose cirrhosis. During a physical exam, a healthcare provider usually

- examines a patient's body

- uses a stethoscope to listen to sounds in the abdomen

- taps on specific areas of the patient's body

Blood test. A blood test involves drawing blood at a healthcare provider's office or a commercial facility and sending the sample to a lab for analysis. Blood tests can show abnormal liver enzyme levels or abnormal numbers of blood cells or platelets.

Imaging tests. Imaging tests can show signs of advanced cirrhosis, such as irregularities in the liver surface, gastric varices, and splenomegaly. These tests can also detect signs of complications, such as ascites and liver cancer.

- Ultrasound

- Computerized tomography (CT) scans

- Magnetic resonance imaging (MRI)

- Elastography

Liver biopsy. A liver biopsy is a procedure that involves taking a piece of liver tissue for examination with a microscope for signs of damage or disease.

How Is Cirrhosis Treated?

Treatment for cirrhosis depends on the cause of the disease and whether complications are present. In the early stages of cirrhosis, the goals of treatment are to slow the progression of tissue scarring in the liver and prevent complications. As cirrhosis progresses, a person may need additional treatments and hospitalization to manage complications. Treatment may include the following:

- avoiding alcohol and illegal substances

- preventing problems with medications

- viral hepatitis vaccination and screening

- treating causes of cirrhosis

Treating Symptoms and Complications of Cirrhosis

Itching and abdominal pain. A healthcare provider may give medications to treat various symptoms of cirrhosis, such as itching and abdominal pain.

Portal hypertension. A healthcare provider may prescribe a beta-blocker or nitrate to treat portal hypertension. Beta blockers lower blood pressure by helping the heart beat slower and with less force, and nitrates relax and widen blood vessels to let more blood flow to the heart and reduce the heart's workload.

Varices. Beta blockers can lower the pressure in varices and reduce the likelihood of bleeding. Bleeding in the stomach or esophagus requires an immediate upper endoscopy. This procedure involves using an endoscope—a small, flexible tube with a light—to look for varices. The healthcare provider may use the endoscope to perform a band ligation, a procedure that involves placing a special rubber band around the varices that causes the tissue to die and fall off. A gastroenterologist—a doctor who specializes in digestive diseases—performs the procedure at a hospital or an outpatient center. People who have had varices in the past may need to take medication to prevent future episodes.

Edema and ascites. Healthcare providers prescribe diuretics—medications that remove fluid from the body—to treat edema and ascites. A healthcare provider may remove large amounts of ascitic fluid from the abdomen and check for spontaneous bacterial peritonitis. A healthcare provider may prescribe bacteria-fighting medications called antibiotics to prevent infection. He or she may prescribe oral antibiotics; however, severe infection with ascites requires intravenous (IV) antibiotics.

Hepatic encephalopathy. A healthcare provider treats hepatic encephalopathy by cleansing the bowel with lactulose, a laxative given orally or as an enema—a liquid put into the rectum. A healthcare provider may also add antibiotics to the treatment. Hepatic encephalopathy may improve as other complications of cirrhosis are controlled.

Hepatorenal syndrome. Some people with cirrhosis who develop hepatorenal syndrome must undergo regular dialysis treatment, which filters wastes and extra fluid from the body by means other than the

147

kidneys. People may also need medications to improve blood flow through the kidneys.

Osteoporosis. A healthcare provider may prescribe bisphosphonate medications to improve bone density.

Gallstones and bile duct stones. A healthcare provider may use surgery to remove gallstones. He or she may use endoscopic retrograde cholangiopancreatography, which uses balloons and basketlike devices, to retrieve the bile duct stones.

Liver cancer. A healthcare provider may recommend screening tests every 6 to 12 months to check for signs of liver cancer. Screening tests can find cancer before the person has symptoms of the disease. Cancer treatment is usually more effective when the healthcare provider finds the disease early. Healthcare providers use blood tests, ultrasound, or both to screen for liver cancer in people with cirrhosis. He or she may treat cancer with a combination of surgery, radiation, and chemotherapy.

When Is a Liver Transplant Considered for Cirrhosis?

A healthcare provider may consider a liver transplant when cirrhosis leads to liver failure or treatment for complications is ineffective. Liver transplantation is surgery to remove a diseased or an injured liver and replace it with a healthy whole liver or part of a liver from another person, called a donor.

Chapter 12

Chronic Obstructive Pulmonary Disease (COPD)

What Is COPD?

COPD, or chronic obstructive pulmonary disease, is a progressive disease that makes it hard to breathe. "Progressive" means the disease gets worse over time.

COPD can cause coughing that produces large amounts of mucus (a slimy substance), wheezing, shortness of breath, chest tightness, and other symptoms.

Cigarette smoking is the leading cause of COPD. Most people who have COPD smoke or used to smoke. Long-term exposure to other lung irritants—such as air pollution, chemical fumes, or dust—also may contribute to COPD.

Other Names for COPD

- Chronic bronchitis

- Chronic obstructive airway disease

- Chronic obstructive lung disease

- Emphysema

This chapter includes text excerpted from "COPD," National Heart, Lung, and Blood Institute (NHLBI), July 31, 2013. Reviewed August 2016.

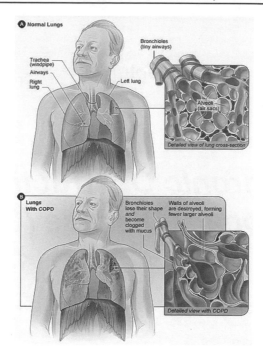

Figure 12.1. *Normal Lungs and Lungs with COPD*

Figure A shows the location of the lungs and airways in the body. The inset image shows a detailed cross-section of the bronchioles and alveoli. Figure B shows lungs damaged by COPD. The inset image shows a detailed cross-section of the damaged bronchioles and alveolar walls.

What Causes COPD?

Long-term exposure to lung irritants that damage the lungs and the airways usually is the cause of COPD.

In the United States, the most common irritant that causes COPD is cigarette smoke. Pipe, cigar, and other types of tobacco smoke also can cause COPD, especially if the smoke is inhaled.

Breathing in secondhand smoke, air pollution, or chemical fumes or dust from the environment or workplace also can contribute to COPD. (Secondhand smoke is smoke in the air from other people smoking.)

Rarely, a genetic condition called alpha-1 antitrypsin deficiency may play a role in causing COPD. People who have this condition have low levels of alpha-1 antitrypsin (AAT)—a protein made in the liver.

Having a low level of the AAT protein can lead to lung damage and COPD if you're exposed to smoke or other lung irritants. If you have this condition and smoke, COPD can worsen very quickly.

Although uncommon, some people who have asthma can develop COPD. Asthma is a chronic (long-term) lung disease that inflames and narrows the airways. Treatment usually can reverse the inflammation and narrowing. However, if not, COPD can develop.

Who Is at Risk for COPD?

The main risk factor for COPD is smoking. Most people who have COPD smoke or used to smoke. People who have a family history of COPD are more likely to develop the disease if they smoke.

Long-term exposure to other lung irritants also is a risk factor for COPD. Examples of other lung irritants include secondhand smoke, air pollution, and chemical fumes and dust from the environment or workplace. (Secondhand smoke is smoke in the air from other people smoking.)

Most people who have COPD are at least 40 years old when symptoms begin. Although uncommon, people younger than 40 can have COPD. For example, this may happen if a person has alpha-1 antitrypsin deficiency, a genetic condition.

What Are the Signs and Symptoms of COPD?

At first, COPD may cause no symptoms or only mild symptoms. As the disease gets worse, symptoms usually become more severe. Common signs and symptoms of COPD include:

- an ongoing cough or a cough that produces a lot of mucus (often called "smoker's cough")
- shortness of breath, especially with physical activity
- wheezing (a whistling or squeaky sound when you breathe)
- chest tightness

If you have COPD, you also may have colds or the flu (influenza) often.

Not everyone who has the symptoms above has COPD. Likewise, not everyone who has COPD has these symptoms. Some of the symptoms of COPD are similar to the symptoms of other diseases and conditions. Your doctor can find out whether you have COPD.

If your symptoms are mild, you may not notice them, or you may adjust your lifestyle to make breathing easier. For example, you may take the elevator instead of the stairs.

Over time, symptoms may become severe enough to see a doctor. For example, you may get short of breath during physical exertion.

The severity of your symptoms will depend on how much lung damage you have. If you keep smoking, the damage will occur faster than if you stop smoking.

Severe COPD can cause other symptoms, such as swelling in your ankles, feet, or legs; weight loss; and lower muscle endurance.

Some severe symptoms may require treatment in a hospital. You—with the help of family members or friends, if you're unable—should seek emergency care if:

- You're having a hard time catching your breath or talking.

- Your lips or fingernails turn blue or gray. (This is a sign of a low oxygen level in your blood.)

- You're not mentally alert.

- Your heartbeat is very fast.

- The recommended treatment for symptoms that are getting worse isn't working.

How Is COPD Diagnosed?

Your doctor will diagnose COPD based on your signs and symptoms, your medical and family histories, and test results.

Your doctor may ask whether you smoke or have had contact with lung irritants, such as secondhand smoke, air pollution, chemical fumes, or dust.

If you have an ongoing cough, let your doctor know how long you've had it, how much you cough, and how much mucus comes up when you cough. Also, let your doctor know whether you have a family history of COPD.

Your doctor will examine you and use a stethoscope to listen for wheezing or other abnormal chest sounds. He or she also may recommend one or more tests to diagnose COPD.

Lung Function Tests

Lung function tests measure how much air you can breathe in and out, how fast you can breathe air out, and how well your lungs deliver oxygen to your blood.

The main test for COPD is spirometry. Other lung function tests, such as a lung diffusion capacity test, also might be used.

Spirometry

During this painless test, a technician will ask you to take a deep breath in. Then, you'll blow as hard as you can into a tube connected to a small machine. The machine is called a spirometer.

The machine measures how much air you breathe out. It also measures how fast you can blow air out.

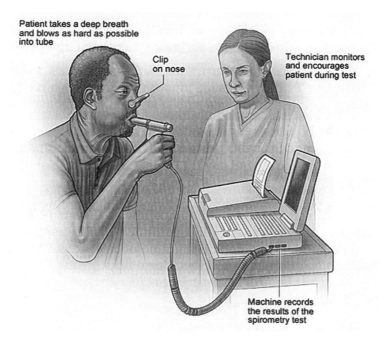

Patient takes a deep breath and blows as hard as possible into tube

Clip on nose

Technician monitors and encourages patient during test

Machine records the results of the spirometry test

Figure 12.2. *Spirometry*

The image shows how spirometry is done. The patient takes a deep breath and blows as hard as possible into a tube connected to a spirometer. The spirometer measures the amount of air breathed out. It also measures how fast the air was blown out.

Your doctor may have you inhale medicine that helps open your airways and then blow into the tube again. He or she can then compare your test results before and after taking the medicine.

Spirometry can detect COPD before symptoms develop. Your doctor also might use the test results to find out how severe your COPD is and to help set your treatment goals.

The test results also may help find out whether another condition, such as asthma or heart failure, is causing your symptoms.

Other Tests

Your doctor may recommend other tests, such as:

- A chest X-ray or chest CT scan

- An arterial blood gas test

How Is COPD Treated?

COPD has no cure yet. However, lifestyle changes and treatments can help you feel better, stay more active, and slow the progress of the disease.

The goals of COPD treatment include:

- relieving your symptoms

- slowing the progress of the disease

- improving your exercise tolerance (your ability to stay active)

- preventing and treating complications

- improving your overall health

To assist with your treatment, your family doctor may advise you to see a pulmonologist. This is a doctor who specializes in treating lung disorders.

Lifestyle Changes

Quit Smoking and Avoid Lung Irritants

Quitting smoking is the most important step you can take to treat COPD. Talk with your doctor about programs and products that can help you quit.

If you have trouble quitting smoking on your own, consider joining a support group. Many hospitals, workplaces, and community groups offer classes to help people quit smoking. Ask your family members and friends to support you in your efforts to quit.

Also, try to avoid secondhand smoke and places with dust, fumes, or other toxic substances that you may inhale.

Other Lifestyle Changes

If you have COPD, you may have trouble eating enough because of your symptoms, such as shortness of breath and fatigue. (This issue is more common with severe disease.)

As a result, you may not get all of the calories and nutrients you need, which can worsen your symptoms and raise your risk for infections.

Talk with your doctor about following an eating plan that will meet your nutritional needs. Your doctor may suggest eating smaller, more frequent meals; resting before eating; and taking vitamins or nutritional supplements.

Also, talk with your doctor about what types of activity are safe for you. You may find it hard to be active with your symptoms. However, physical activity can strengthen the muscles that help you breathe and improve your overall wellness.

Medicines

Bronchodilators

Bronchodilators relax the muscles around your airways. This helps open your airways and makes breathing easier.

Depending on the severity of your COPD, your doctor may prescribe short-acting or long-acting bronchodilators. Short-acting bronchodilators last about 4–6 hours and should be used only when needed. Long-acting bronchodilators last about 12 hours or more and are used every day.

Most bronchodilators are taken using a device called an inhaler. This device allows the medicine to go straight to your lungs. Not all inhalers are used the same way. Ask your healthcare team to show you the correct way to use your inhaler.

If your COPD is mild, your doctor may only prescribe a short-acting inhaled bronchodilator. In this case, you may use the medicine only when symptoms occur.

If your COPD is moderate or severe, your doctor may prescribe regular treatment with short- and long-acting bronchodilators.

Combination Bronchodilators Plus Inhaled Glucocorticosteroids (Steroids)

If your COPD is more severe, or if your symptoms flare up often, your doctor may prescribe a combination of medicines that includes a bronchodilator and an inhaled steroid. Steroids help reduce airway inflammation.

In general, using inhaled steroids alone is not a preferred treatment.

Your doctor may ask you to try inhaled steroids with the bronchodilator for a trial period of 6 weeks to 3 months to see whether the addition of the steroid helps relieve your breathing problems.

Vaccines

Flu Shots

The flu (influenza) can cause serious problems for people who have COPD. Flu shots can reduce your risk of getting the flu. Talk with your doctor about getting a yearly flu shot.

Pneumococcal Vaccine

This vaccine lowers your risk for pneumococcal pneumonia and its complications. People who have COPD are at higher risk for pneumonia than people who don't have COPD. Talk with your doctor about whether you should get this vaccine.

Pulmonary Rehabilitation

Pulmonary rehabilitation (rehab) is a broad program that helps improve the well-being of people who have chronic (ongoing) breathing problems.

Rehab may include an exercise program, disease management training, and nutritional and psychological counseling. The program's goal is to help you stay active and carry out your daily activities.

Your rehab team may include doctors, nurses, physical therapists, respiratory therapists, exercise specialists, and dietitians. These health professionals will create a program that meets your needs.

Oxygen Therapy

If you have severe COPD and low levels of oxygen in your blood, oxygen therapy can help you breathe better. For this treatment, you're given oxygen through nasal prongs or a mask.

You may need extra oxygen all the time or only at certain times. For some people who have severe COPD, using extra oxygen for most of the day can help them:

- do tasks or activities, while having fewer symptoms
- protect their hearts and other organs from damage
- sleep more during the night and improve alertness during the day
- live longer

Surgery

Surgery may benefit some people who have COPD. Surgery usually is a last resort for people who have severe symptoms that have not improved from taking medicines.

Surgeries for people who have COPD that's mainly related to emphysema include bullectomy and lung volume reduction surgery (LVRS). A lung transplant might be an option for people who have very severe COPD.

- bullectomy

- lung volume reduction surgery

- lung transplant

Managing Complications

COPD symptoms usually worsen slowly over time. However, they can worsen suddenly. For instance, a cold, the flu, or a lung infection may cause your symptoms to quickly worsen. You may have a much harder time catching your breath. You also may have chest tightness, more coughing, changes in the color or amount of your sputum (spit), and a fever.

Call your doctor right away if your symptoms worsen suddenly. He or she may prescribe antibiotics to treat the infection and other medicines, such as bronchodilators and inhaled steroids, to help you breathe.

Some severe symptoms may require treatment in a hospital.

How Can COPD Be Prevented?

You can take steps to prevent COPD before it starts. If you already have COPD, you can take steps to prevent complications and slow the progress of the disease.

Prevent COPD Before It Starts

The best way to prevent COPD is to not start smoking or to quit smoking. Smoking is the leading cause of COPD. If you smoke, talk with your doctor about programs and products that can help you quit.

If you have trouble quitting smoking on your own, consider joining a support group. Many hospitals, workplaces, and community groups voffer classes to help people quit smoking. Ask your family members and friends to support you in your efforts to quit.

157

Also, try to avoid lung irritants that can contribute to COPD. Examples include secondhand smoke, air pollution, chemical fumes, and dust. (Secondhand smoke is smoke in the air from other people smoking.)

Prevent Complications and Slow the Progress of COPD

If you have COPD, the most important step you can take is to quit smoking. Quitting can help prevent complications and slow the progress of the disease. You also should avoid exposure to the lung irritants mentioned above.

Follow your treatments for COPD exactly as your doctor prescribes. They can help you breathe easier, stay more active, and avoid or manage severe symptoms.

Talk with your doctor about whether and when you should get flu (influenza) and pneumonia vaccines. These vaccines can lower your chances of getting these illnesses, which are major health risks for people who have COPD.

Living with COPD

COPD has no cure yet. However, you can take steps to manage your symptoms and slow the progress of the disease. You can:

- avoid lung irritants

- get ongoing care

- manage the disease and its symptoms

  - Do activities slowly.

  - Put items that you need often in one place that's easy to reach.

  - Find very simple ways to cook, clean, and do other chores. For example, you might want to use a small table or cart with wheels to move things around and a pole or tongs with long handles to reach things.

  - Ask for help moving things around in your house so that you won't need to climb stairs as often.

  - Keep your clothes loose, and wear clothes and shoes that are easy to put on and take off.

- prepare for emergencies

Emotional Issues and Support

Living with COPD may cause fear, anxiety, depression, and stress. Talk about how you feel with your healthcare team. Talking to a professional counselor also might help. If you're very depressed, your doctor may recommend medicines or other treatments that can improve your quality of life.

Joining a patient support group may help you adjust to living with COPD. You can see how other people who have the same symptoms have coped with them. Talk with your doctor about local support groups or check with an area medical center.

Support from family and friends also can help relieve stress and anxiety. Let your loved ones know how you feel and what they can do to help you.

Chapter 13

Colorectal Cancer

What Is Colorectal Cancer?

Colorectal cancer is cancer that occurs in the colon or rectum. Sometimes it is called *colon cancer,* for short. As the drawing shows, the colon is the large intestine or large bowel. The rectum is the passageway that connects the colon to the anus.

Sometimes abnormal growths, called *polyps,* form in the colon or rectum. Over time, some polyps may turn into cancer. Screening tests can find polyps so they can be removed before turning into cancer. Screening also helps find colorectal cancer at an early stage, when treatment often leads to a cure.

What Are the Risk Factors for Colorectal Cancer?

Your risk of getting colorectal cancer increases as you get older. More than 90% of cases occur in people who are 50 years old or older. Other risk factors include having—

- Inflammatory bowel disease such as Crohn's disease or ulcerative colitis.

- A personal or family history of colorectal cancer or colorectal polyps.

This chapter includes text excerpted from "Colorectal (Colon) Cancer," Centers for Disease Control and Prevention (CDC), May 26, 2016.

- A genetic syndrome such as familial adenomatous polyposis (FAP) or hereditary non-polyposis colorectal cancer (Lynch syndrome).

Lifestyle factors that may contribute to an increased risk of colorectal cancer include—

- lack of regular physical activity
- a diet low in fruit and vegetables
- a low-fiber and high-fat diet
- overweight and obesity
- alcohol consumption
- tobacco use

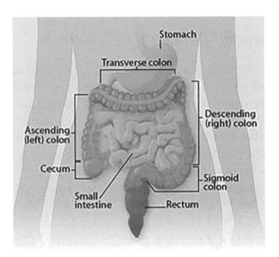

Figure 13.1. *Colon and Rectum*

What Can I Do to Reduce My Risk of Colorectal Cancer?

Almost all colorectal cancers begin as *precancerous polyps* (abnormal growths) in the colon or rectum. Such polyps can be present in the colon for years before invasive cancer develops. They may not cause any symptoms. Colorectal cancer screening can find precancerous polyps so they can be removed before they turn into cancer. In this way, colorectal cancer is prevented. Screening can also find colorectal cancer early, when there is a greater chance that treatment will be most effective and lead to a cure.

Research is underway to find out if changes to your diet can reduce your colorectal cancer risk. Medical experts don't agree on the role of diet in preventing colorectal cancer, but often recommend a diet low in animal fats and high in fruits, vegetables, and whole grains to reduce the risk of other chronic diseases, such as coronary artery disease and diabetes. This diet also may reduce the risk of colorectal cancer. Also, researchers are examining the role of certain medicines and supplements in preventing colorectal cancer.

The U.S. Preventive Services Task Force found that taking low-dose aspirin can help prevent cardiovascular disease and colorectal cancer in some adults, depending on age and risk factors.

What Are the Symptoms of Colorectal Cancer?

Colorectal polyps and colorectal cancer don't always cause symptoms, especially at first. Someone could have polyps or colorectal cancer and not know it. That is why getting screened regularly for colorectal cancer is so important.

If you have symptoms, they may include—

- blood in or on your stool (bowel movement)

- stomach pain, aches, or cramps that don't go away

- losing weight and you don't know why

If you have any of these symptoms, talk to your doctor. They may be caused by something other than cancer. The only way to know what is causing them is to see your doctor.

Chapter 14

Diabetes

What Is Diabetes?

Diabetes is a disease in which blood glucose levels are above normal. Most of the food we eat is turned into glucose, or sugar, for our bodies to use for energy. The pancreas, an organ that lies near the stomach, makes a hormone called insulin to help glucose get into the cells of our bodies. When you have diabetes, your body either doesn't make enough insulin or can't use its own insulin as well as it should. This causes sugar to build up in your blood.

Diabetes can cause serious health complications including heart disease, blindness, kidney failure, and lower-extremity amputations. Diabetes is the seventh leading cause of death in the United States.

What Are the Symptoms of Diabetes?

People who think they might have diabetes must visit a physician for diagnosis. They might have SOME or NONE of the following symptoms:

- frequent urination

- excessive thirst

- unexplained weight loss

This chapter includes text excerpted from "Basics about Diabetes," Centers for Disease Control and Prevention (CDC), March 31, 2015.

- extreme hunger

- sudden vision changes

- tingling or numbness in hands or feet

- feeling very tired much of the time

- very dry skin

- sores that are slow to heal

- more infections than usual

Nausea, vomiting, or stomach pains may accompany some of these symptoms in the abrupt onset of insulin-dependent diabetes, now called type 1 diabetes.

What Are the Types of Diabetes?

Type 1 diabetes, which was previously called insulin-dependent diabetes mellitus (IDDM) or juvenile-onset diabetes, may account for about 5% of all diagnosed cases of diabetes. **Type 2 diabetes**, which was previously called non-insulin-dependent diabetes mellitus (NIDDM) or adult-onset diabetes, may account for about 90% to 95% of all diagnosed cases of diabetes. **Other specific types of diabetes** resulting from specific genetic syndromes, surgery, drugs, malnutrition, infections, and other illnesses may account for 1% to 5% of all diagnosed cases of diabetes.

What Are the Risk Factors for Diabetes?

Risk factors for type 2 diabetes include older age, obesity, family history of diabetes, prior history of gestational diabetes, impaired glucose tolerance, physical inactivity, and race/ethnicity. African Americans, Hispanic/Latino Americans, American Indians, and some Asian Americans and Pacific Islanders are at particularly high risk for type 2 diabetes.

Risk factors are less well defined for type 1 diabetes than for type 2 diabetes, but autoimmune, genetic, and environmental factors are involved in developing this type of diabetes.

Gestational diabetes occurs more frequently in African Americans, Hispanic/Latino Americans, American Indians, and people with a family history of diabetes than in other groups. Obesity is also associated with higher risk.

Other specific types of diabetes, which may account for 1% to 5% of all diagnosed cases, result from specific genetic syndromes, surgery, drugs, malnutrition, infections, and other illnesses.

What Is the Treatment for Diabetes?

Healthy eating, physical activity, and insulin injections are the basic therapies for type 1 diabetes. The amount of insulin taken must be balanced with food intake and daily activities. Blood glucose levels must be closely monitored through frequent blood glucose testing.

Healthy eating, physical activity, and blood glucose testing are the basic therapies for type 2 diabetes. In addition, many people with type 2 diabetes require oral medication, insulin, or both to control their blood glucose levels.

People with diabetes must take responsibility for their day-to-day care, and keep blood glucose levels from going too low or too high.

People with diabetes should see a healthcare provider who will monitor their diabetes control and help them learn to manage their diabetes. In addition, people with diabetes may see endocrinologists, who may specialize in diabetes care; ophthalmologists for eye examinations; podiatrists for routine foot care; and dietitians and diabetes educators who teach the skills needed for daily diabetes management.

Can Diabetes Be Prevented?

Researchers are making progress in identifying the exact genetics and "triggers" that predispose some individuals to develop type 1 diabetes, but prevention remains elusive.

A number of studies have shown that regular physical activity can significantly reduce the risk of developing type 2 diabetes. Type 2 diabetes is associated with obesity.

Is There a Cure for Diabetes?

In response to the growing health burden of diabetes, the diabetes community has three choices: prevent diabetes; cure diabetes; and improve the quality of care of people with diabetes to prevent devastating complications. All three approaches are actively being pursued by the U.S. Department of Health and Human Services.

Both the National Institutes of Health (NIH) and the Centers for Disease Control and Prevention (CDC) are involved in prevention activities. The NIH is involved in research to cure both type 1 and type 2 diabetes, especially type 1. CDC focuses most of its programs on making sure that the proven science to prevent complications is put into daily practice for people with diabetes. The basic idea is that if all the important research and science are not applied meaningfully in the daily lives of people with diabetes, then the research is, in essence, wasted.

Several approaches to "cure" diabetes are currently under investigation:

- pancreas transplantation
- islet cell transplantation (islet cells produce insulin)
- artificial pancreas development
- genetic manipulation (fat or muscle cells that don't normally make insulin have a human insulin gene inserted—then these "pseudo" islet cells are transplanted into people with type 1 diabetes)

Each of these approaches still has a lot of challenges, such as preventing immune rejection; finding an adequate number of insulin cells; keeping cells alive; and others. But progress is being made in all areas.

Chapter 15

Heart Disease

Chapter Contents

Section 15.1—Congestive Heart Failure 170

Section 15.2—Coronary Artery Disease 179

Section 15.3—Heart Attack.. 189

Section 15.4—Taking Aspirin to Prevent Heart
              Attacks 199

Section 15.1

Congestive Heart Failure

This section includes text excerpted from "Heart Failure," National Heart, Lung, and Blood Institute (NHLBI), June 22, 2015.

What Is Heart Failure?

Heart failure is a condition in which the heart can't pump enough blood to meet the body's needs. In some cases, the heart can't fill with enough blood. In other cases, the heart can't pump blood to the rest of the body with enough force. Some people have both problems.

The term "heart failure" doesn't mean that your heart has stopped or is about to stop working. However, heart failure is a serious condition that requires medical care.

Other Names for Heart Failure

- Congestive heart failure.

- Left-side heart failure. This is when the heart can't pump enough oxygen-rich blood to the body.

- Right-side heart failure. This is when the heart can't fill with enough blood.

- Cor pulmonale. This term refers to right-side heart failure caused by high blood pressure in the pulmonary arteries and right ventricle (lower right heart chamber).

What Causes Heart Failure?

Conditions that damage or overwork the heart muscle can cause heart failure. Over time, the heart weakens. It isn't able to fill with and/or pump blood as well as it should. As the heart weakens, certain proteins and substances might be released into the blood. These substances have a toxic effect on the heart and blood flow, and they worsen heart failure.

Causes of heart failure include:

- coronary heart disease
- diabetes
- high blood pressure
- other heart conditions or diseases
  - arrhythmia
  - cardiomyopathy
  - congenital heart defects
  - heart valve disease
- other factors
  - alcohol abuse or cocaine and other illegal drug use
  - HIV/AIDS
  - thyroid disorders (having either too much or too little thyroid hormone in the body)
  - too much vitamin E
  - treatments for cancer, such as radiation and chemotherapy

Who Is at Risk for Heart Failure?

About 5.7 million people in the United States have heart failure. The number of people who have this condition is growing.

Heart failure is more common in:

- People who are age 65 or older
- Blacks are more likely to have heart failure than people of other races
- People who are overweight
- People who have had a heart attack

What Are the Signs and Symptoms of Heart Failure?

The most common signs and symptoms of heart failure are:

- shortness of breath or trouble breathing
- fatigue (tiredness)
- swelling in the ankles, feet, legs, abdomen, and veins in the neck

All of these symptoms are the result of fluid buildup in your body. When symptoms start, you may feel tired and short of breath after routine physical effort, like climbing stairs.

As your heart grows weaker, symptoms get worse. You may begin to feel tired and short of breath after getting dressed or walking across the room. Some people have shortness of breath while lying flat.

Fluid buildup from heart failure also causes weight gain, frequent urination, and a cough that's worse at night and when you're lying down. This cough may be a sign of acute pulmonary edema. This is a condition in which too much fluid builds up in your lungs. The condition requires emergency treatment.

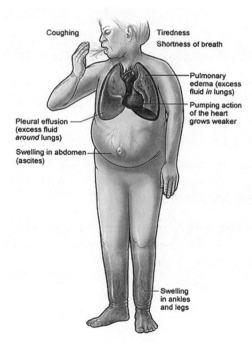

Figure 15.1. *Heart Failure Signs and Symptoms*

How Is Heart Failure Diagnosed?

Your doctor will diagnose heart failure based on your medical and family histories, a physical exam, and test results. The signs and symptoms of heart failure also are common in other conditions. Thus, your doctor will:

- Find out whether you have a disease or condition that can cause heart failure, such as coronary heart disease (CHD), high blood pressure, or diabetes.

- Rule out other causes of your symptoms.

- Find any damage to your heart and check how well your heart pumps blood.

Early diagnosis and treatment can help people who have heart failure live longer, more active lives.

Medical and Family Histories

Your doctor will ask whether you or others in your family have or have had a disease or condition that can cause heart failure.

Your doctor also will ask about your symptoms. He or she will want to know which symptoms you have, when they occur, how long you've had them, and how severe they are. Your answers will help show whether and how much your symptoms limit your daily routine.

Physical Exam

During the physical exam, your doctor will:

- Listen to your heart for sounds that aren't normal.

- Listen to your lungs for the sounds of extra fluid buildup.

- Look for swelling in your ankles, feet, legs, abdomen, and the veins in your neck.

Diagnostic Tests

No single test can diagnose heart failure. If you have signs and symptoms of heart failure, your doctor may recommend one or more tests.

Your doctor also may refer you to a cardiologist. A cardiologist is a doctor who specializes in diagnosing and treating heart diseases and conditions.

- EKG (Electrocardiogram)
- Chest X-ray
- BNP blood test
- echocardiography
- Doppler ultrasound
- Holter monitor

- nuclear heart scan
- cardiac catheterization
- coronary angiography
- stress test
- cardiac MRI
- thyroid function tests

How Is Heart Failure Treated?

Early diagnosis and treatment can help people who have heart failure live longer, more active lives. Treatment for heart failure depends on the type and severity of the heart failure.

The goals of treatment for all stages of heart failure include:

- Treating the condition's underlying cause, such as coronary heart disease, high blood pressure, or diabetes.

- Reducing symptoms.

- Stopping the heart failure from getting worse.

- Increasing your lifespan and improving your quality of life.

Treatments usually include heart-healthy lifestyle changes, medicines, and ongoing care. If you have severe heart failure, you also may need medical procedures or surgery.

Heart-Healthy Lifestyle Changes

Your doctor may recommend heart-healthy lifestyle changes if you have heart failure. Heart-healthy lifestyle changes include:

- Heart-healthy eating

- Aiming for a healthy weight

- Physical activity

- Quitting smoking

Medicines

Your doctor will prescribe medicines based on the type of heart failure you have, how severe it is, and your response to certain medicines. The following medicines are commonly used to treat heart failure:

- **ACE inhibitors** lower blood pressure and reduce strain on your heart. They also may reduce the risk of a future heart attack.

- **Aldosterone antagonists** trigger the body to remove excess sodium through urine. This lowers the volume of blood that the heart must pump.

- **Angiotensin receptor blockers** relax your blood vessels and lower blood pressure to decrease your heart's workload.

- **Beta blockers** slow your heart rate and lower your blood pressure to decrease your heart's workload.

- **Digoxin** makes the heart beat stronger and pump more blood.

- **Diuretics** (fluid pills) help reduce fluid buildup in your lungs and swelling in your feet and ankles.

- **Isosorbide dinitrate/Hydralazine hydrochloride** helps relax your blood vessels so your heart doesn't work as hard to pump blood. Studies have shown that this medicine can reduce the risk of death in blacks. More studies are needed to find out whether this medicine will benefit other racial groups.

Take all medicines regularly, as your doctor prescribes. Don't change the amount of your medicine or skip a dose unless your doctor tells you to. You should still follow a heart healthy lifestyle, even if you take medicines to treat your heart failure.

Ongoing Care

You should watch for signs that heart failure is getting worse. For example, weight gain may mean that fluids are building up in your body. Ask your doctor how often you should check your weight and when to report weight changes.

Getting medical care for other related conditions is important. If you have diabetes or high blood pressure, work with your healthcare team to control these conditions. Have your blood sugar level and blood pressure checked. Talk with your doctor about when you should have tests and how often to take measurements at home.

Try to avoid respiratory infections like the flu and pneumonia. Talk with your doctor or nurse about getting flu and pneumonia vaccines.

Many people who have severe heart failure may need treatment in a hospital from time to time. Your doctor may recommend oxygen therapy, which can be given in a hospital or at home.

Medical Procedures and Surgery

As heart failure worsens, lifestyle changes and medicines may no longer control your symptoms. You may need a medical procedure or surgery.

In heart failure, the right and left sides of the heart may no longer contract at the same time. This disrupts the heart's pumping. To correct this problem, your doctor might implant a cardiac resynchronization therapy device (a type of pacemaker) near your heart. This device helps both sides of your heart contract at the same time, which can decrease heart failure symptoms.

Some people who have heart failure have very rapid, irregular heartbeats. Without treatment, these heartbeats can cause sudden cardiac arrest. Your doctor might implant an implantable cardioverter defibrillator (ICD) near your heart to solve this problem. An ICD checks your heart rate and uses electrical pulses to correct irregular heart rhythms.

People who have severe heart failure symptoms at rest, despite other treatments, may need:

A mechanical heart pump, such as a left ventricular assist device. This device helps pump blood from the heart to the rest of the body. You may use a heart pump until you have surgery or as a long-term treatment.

Heart transplant. A heart transplant is an operation in which a person's diseased heart is replaced with a healthy heart from a deceased donor. Heart transplants are done as a life-saving measure for end-stage heart failure when medical treatment and less drastic surgery have failed.

How Can Heart Failure Be Prevented?

You can take steps to prevent heart failure. The sooner you start, the better your chances of preventing or delaying the condition.

For People Who Have Healthy Hearts

If you have a healthy heart, you can take action to prevent heart disease and heart failure. To reduce your risk of heart disease:

- Avoid using illegal drugs.
- Adopt heart-healthy lifestyle habits.

For People Who Are at High Risk for Heart Failure

Even if you're at high risk for heart failure, you can take steps to reduce your risk. People at high risk include those who have coronary heart disease, high blood pressure, or diabetes.

- Follow all of the steps listed above. Talk with your doctor about what types and amounts of physical activity are safe for you.
- Treat and control any conditions that can cause heart failure. Take medicines as your doctor prescribes.
- Avoid drinking alcohol.
- See your doctor for ongoing care.

For People Who Have Heart Damage but No Signs of Heart Failure

If you have heart damage but no signs of heart failure, you can still reduce your risk of developing the condition. In addition to the steps above, take your medicines as prescribed to reduce your heart's workload.

Living with Heart Failure

Currently, heart failure has no cure. You'll likely have to take medicine and follow a treatment plan for the rest of your life.

Despite treatment, symptoms may get worse over time. You may not be able to do many of the things that you did before you had heart failure. However, if you take all the steps your doctor recommends, you can stay healthier longer.

Researchers also might find new treatments that can help you in the future.

Follow Your Treatment Plan

Treatment can relieve your symptoms and make daily activities easier. It also can reduce the chance that you'll have to go to the hospital. Thus, it's important that you follow your treatment plan.

- Take your medicines as your doctor prescribes. If you have side effects from any of your medicines, tell your doctor. He or she might adjust the dose or type of medicine you take to relieve side effects.

- Make all of the lifestyle changes that your doctor recommends.

- Get advice from your doctor about how active you can and should be. This includes advice on daily activities, work, leisure time, sex, and exercise. Your level of activity will depend on the stage of your heart failure (how severe it is).

- Keep all of your medical appointments, including visits to the doctor and appointments to get tests and lab work. Your doctor needs the results of these tests to adjust your medicine doses and help you avoid harmful side effects.

Take Steps to Prevent Heart Failure from Getting Worse

Certain actions can worsen your heart failure, such as:

- Forgetting to take your medicines.

- Not following your diet (for example, eating salty foods).

- Drinking alcohol.

These actions can lead to a hospital stay. If you have trouble following your diet, talk with your doctor. He or she can help arrange for a dietitian to work with you. Avoid drinking alcohol.

People who have heart failure often have other serious conditions that require ongoing treatment. If you have other serious conditions, you're likely taking medicines for them as well as for heart failure.

Taking more than one medicine raises the risk of side effects and other problems. Make sure your doctors and your pharmacist have a complete list of all of the medicines and over-the-counter products that you're taking.

Tell your doctor right away about any problems with your medicines. Also, talk with your doctor before taking any new medicine prescribed by another doctor or any new over-the-counter medicines or herbal supplements.

Try to avoid respiratory infections like the flu and pneumonia. Ask your doctor or nurse about getting flu and pneumonia vaccines.

Plan Ahead

If you have heart failure, it's important to know:

- When to seek help. Ask your doctor when to make an office visit or get emergency care.

- Phone numbers for your doctor and hospital.

- Directions to your doctor's office and hospital and people who can take you there.

- A list of medicines you're taking.

Section 15.2

Coronary Artery Disease

This section includes text excerpted from " Coronary Heart Disease," National Heart, Lung, and Blood Institute (NHLBI), June 22, 2016.

What Is Coronary Heart Disease?

Coronary heart disease (CHD) is a disease in which a waxy substance called plaque builds up inside the coronary arteries. These arteries supply oxygen-rich blood to your heart muscle.

When plaque builds up in the arteries, the condition is called atherosclerosis. The buildup of plaque occurs over many years.

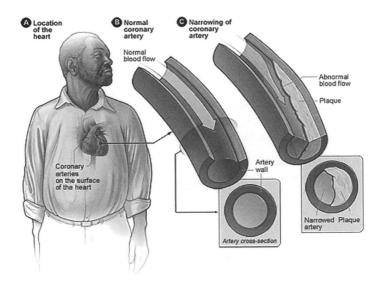

Figure 15.2. *Atherosclerosis*

Figure A shows the location of the heart in the body. Figure B shows a normal coronary artery with normal blood flow. The inset image shows a cross-section of a normal coronary artery. Figure C shows a coronary artery narrowed by plaque. The buildup of plaque limits the flow of oxygen-rich blood through the artery. The inset image shows a cross-section of the plaque-narrowed artery.

Over time, plaque can harden or rupture (break open). Hardened plaque narrows the coronary arteries and reduces the flow of oxygen-rich blood to the heart.

If the plaque ruptures, a blood clot can form on its surface. A large blood clot can mostly or completely block blood flow through a coronary artery. Over time, ruptured plaque also hardens and narrows the coronary arteries.

Other Names for Coronary Heart Disease

- Atherosclerosis
- Coronary artery disease
- Hardening of the arteries
- Heart disease
- Ischemic heart disease
- Narrowing of the arteries

What Causes Coronary Heart Disease?

Research suggests that coronary heart disease (CHD) starts when certain factors damage the inner layers of the coronary arteries. These factors include:

- smoking
- high levels of certain fats and cholesterol in the blood
- high blood pressure
- high levels of sugar in the blood due to insulin resistance or diabetes
- blood vessel inflammation

Plaque might begin to build up where the arteries are damaged. The buildup of plaque in the coronary arteries may start in childhood.

Over time, plaque can harden or rupture (break open). Hardened plaque narrows the coronary arteries and reduces the flow of oxygen-rich blood to the heart. This can cause angina (chest pain or discomfort).

If the plaque ruptures, blood cell fragments called platelets stick to the site of the injury. They may clump together to form blood clots.

Blood clots can further narrow the coronary arteries and worsen angina. If a clot becomes large enough, it can mostly or completely block a coronary artery and cause a heart attack.

Who Is at Risk for Coronary Heart Disease?

In the United States, coronary heart disease (CHD) is a leading cause of death for both men and women. Each year, about 370,000 Americans die from coronary heart disease.

Certain traits, conditions, or habits may raise your risk for CHD. The more risk factors you have, the more likely you are to develop the disease.

You can control many risk factors, which may help prevent or delay CHD.

Major Risk Factors

- unhealthy blood cholesterol levels
- high blood pressure
- smoking
- insulin resistance
- diabetes
- overweight or obesity
- metabolic syndrome
- lack of physical activity
- unhealthy diet
- older age
- a family history of early coronary heart disease

Although older age and a family history of early heart disease are risk factors, it doesn't mean that you'll develop CHD if you have one or both. Controlling other risk factors often can lessen genetic influences and help prevent CHD, even in older adults.

Emerging Risk Factors

Researchers continue to study other possible risk factors for CHD.

High levels of a protein called C-reactive protein (CRP) in the blood may raise the risk of CHD and heart attack. High levels of CRP are a sign of inflammation in the body.

Inflammation is the body's response to injury or infection. Damage to the arteries' inner walls may trigger inflammation and help plaque grow.

Research is under way to find out whether reducing inflammation and lowering CRP levels also can reduce the risk of CHD and heart attack.

High levels of triglycerides in the blood also may raise the risk of CHD Triglycerides are a type of fat.

Other Risks Related to Coronary Heart Disease

Other conditions and factors also may contribute to CHD, including:

- sleep apnea
- alcohol
- stress
- preeclampsia

What Are the Signs and Symptoms of Coronary Heart Disease?

A common symptom of coronary heart disease (CHD) is angina. Angina is chest pain or discomfort that occurs if an area of your heart muscle doesn't get enough oxygen-rich blood.

Angina may feel like pressure or squeezing in your chest. You also may feel it in your shoulders, arms, neck, jaw, or back. Angina pain may even feel like indigestion. The pain tends to get worse with activity and go away with rest. Emotional stress also can trigger the pain.

Another common symptom of CHD is shortness of breath. This symptom occurs if CHD causes heart failure. When you have heart failure, your heart can't pump enough blood to meet your body's needs. Fluid builds up in your lungs, making it hard to breathe.

The severity of these symptoms varies. They may get more severe as the buildup of plaque continues to narrow the coronary arteries.

Signs and Symptoms of Heart Problems Related to Coronary Heart Disease

Some people who have CHD have no signs or symptoms—a condition called silent CHD. The disease might not be diagnosed until a person has signs or symptoms of a heart attack, heart failure, or an arrhythmia (an irregular heartbeat).

Heart Attack

A heart attack occurs if the flow of oxygen-rich blood to a section of heart muscle is cut off. This can happen if an area of plaque in a coronary artery ruptures (breaks open).

Blood cell fragments called platelets stick to the site of the injury and may clump together to form blood clots. If a clot becomes large enough, it can mostly or completely block blood flow through a coronary artery.

If the blockage isn't treated quickly, the portion of heart muscle fed by the artery begins to die. Healthy heart tissue is replaced with scar tissue. This heart damage may not be obvious, or it may cause severe or long-lasting problems.

The most common heart attack symptom is chest pain or discomfort. Most heart attacks involve discomfort in the center or left side of the chest that often lasts for more than a few minutes or goes away and comes back.

The discomfort can feel like uncomfortable pressure, squeezing, fullness, or pain. The feeling can be mild or severe. Heart attack pain sometimes feels like indigestion or heartburn.

The symptoms of angina can be similar to the symptoms of a heart attack. Angina pain usually lasts for only a few minutes and goes away with rest.

Chest pain or discomfort that doesn't go away or changes from its usual pattern (for example, occurs more often or while you're resting) might be a sign of a heart attack. If you don't know whether your chest pain is angina or a heart attack, call 9–1–1.

All chest pain should be checked by a doctor.

Other common signs and symptoms of a heart attack include:

- Upper body discomfort in one or both arms, the back, neck, jaw, or upper part of the stomach.

- Shortness of breath, which may occur with or before chest discomfort.

- Nausea (feeling sick to your stomach), vomiting, light-headedness or fainting, or breaking out in a cold sweat.

- Sleep problems, fatigue (tiredness), or lack of energy.

Heart Failure

Heart failure is a condition in which your heart can't pump enough blood to meet your body's needs. Heart failure doesn't mean that your heart has stopped or is about to stop working.

The most common signs and symptoms of heart failure are shortness of breath or trouble breathing; fatigue; and swelling in the ankles, feet, legs, stomach, and veins in the neck.

All of these symptoms are the result of fluid buildup in your body. When symptoms start, you may feel tired and short of breath after routine physical effort, like climbing stairs.

Arrhythmia

An arrhythmia is a problem with the rate or rhythm of the heartbeat. When you have an arrhythmia, you may notice that your heart is skipping beats or beating too fast.

Some people describe arrhythmias as a fluttering feeling in the chest. These feelings are called palpitations.

Some arrhythmias can cause your heart to suddenly stop beating. This condition is called sudden cardiac arrest (SCA). SCA usually causes death if it's not treated within minutes.

How Is Coronary Heart Disease Diagnosed?

Your doctor will diagnose coronary heart disease (CHD) based on your medical and family histories, your risk factors for CHD, a physical exam, and the results from tests and procedures.

No single test can diagnose CHD. If your doctor thinks you have CHD, he or she may recommend one or more of the following tests.

- EKG (Electrocardiogram)

- stress testing

- echocardiography

- chest X-ray

- blood tests

- coronary angiography and cardiac catheterization

How Is Coronary Heart Disease Treated?

Treatments for coronary heart disease include heart-healthy lifestyle changes, medicines, medical procedures and surgery, and cardiac rehabilitation. Treatment goals may include:

- Lowering the risk of blood clots forming (blood clots can cause a heart attack).

- Preventing complications of coronary heart disease.

- Reducing risk factors in an effort to slow, stop, or reverse the buildup of plaque.

- Relieving symptoms.
- Widening or bypassing clogged arteries.

Heart-Healthy Lifestyle Changes

Your doctor may recommend heart-healthy lifestyle changes if you have coronary heart disease. Heart-healthy lifestyle changes include:

- heart-healthy eating
- maintaining a healthy weight
- managing stress
- physical activity
- quitting smoking

Medicines

Sometimes lifestyle changes aren't enough to control your blood cholesterol levels. For example, you may need statin medications to control or lower your cholesterol. By lowering your cholesterol level, you can decrease your chance of having a heart attack or stroke. Doctors usually prescribe statins for people who have:

- coronary heart disease, peripheral artery disease, or had a stroke
- diabetes
- high LDL cholesterol levels

Doctors may discuss beginning statin treatment with those who have an elevated risk for developing heart disease or having a stroke. Your doctor also may prescribe other medications to:

- Decrease your chance of having a heart attack or dying suddenly.
- Lower your blood pressure.
- Prevent blood clots, which can lead to heart attack or stroke.
- Prevent or delay the need for a stent or percutaneous coronary intervention (PCI) or surgery, such as coronary artery bypass grafting (CABG).
- Reduce your heart's workload and relieve coronary heart disease symptoms.

185

Take all medicines regularly, as your doctor prescribes. Don't change the amount of your medicine or skip a dose unless your doctor tells you to. You should still follow a heart healthy lifestyle, even if you take medicines to treat your coronary heart disease.

Medical Procedures and Surgery

You may need a procedure or surgery to treat coronary heart disease. Both percutaneous coronary intervention (PCI) and coronary artery bypass grafting (CABG) are used to treat blocked coronary arteries. You and your doctor can discuss which treatment is right for you.

Cardiac Rehabilitation

Your doctor may prescribe cardiac rehabilitation (rehab) for angina or after CABG, angioplasty, or a heart attack. Nearly everyone who has coronary heart disease can benefit from cardiac rehab. Cardiac rehab is a medically supervised program that may help improve the health and well-being of people who have heart problems.

The cardiac rehab team may include doctors, nurses, exercise specialists, physical and occupational therapists, dietitians or nutritionists, and psychologists or other mental health specialists.

Rehab has two parts:

1. Education, counseling, and training. This part of rehab helps you understand your heart condition and find ways to reduce your risk for future heart problems. The rehab team will help you learn how to cope with the stress of adjusting to a new lifestyle and how to deal with your fears about the future.

2. Exercise training. This part helps you learn how to exercise safely, strengthen your muscles, and improve your stamina. Your exercise plan will be based on your personal abilities, needs, and interests.

How Can Coronary Heart Disease Be Prevented or Delayed?

You can prevent and control coronary heart disease (CHD) by taking action to control your risk factors with heart-healthy lifestyle changes and medicines. Examples of risk factors you can control include high blood cholesterol, high blood pressure, and overweight and obesity. Only a few risk factors—such as age, gender, and family history—can't be controlled.

Your risk for CHD increases with the number of risk factors you have. To reduce your risk of CHD and heart attack, try to control each risk factor you have by adopting the following heart-healthy lifestyles:

- Heart-healthy eating
- Maintaining a healthy weight
- Managing stress
- Physical activity
- Quitting smoking

Know your family history of health problems related to CHD. If you or someone in your family has CHD, be sure to tell your doctor. If lifestyle changes aren't enough, you also may need medicines to control your CHD risk factors.

Living with Coronary Heart Disease

Coronary heart disease (CHD) can cause serious complications. However, if you follow your doctor's advice and adopt healthy lifestyle habits, you can prevent or reduce the risk of:

- Dying suddenly from heart problems.
- Having a heart attack and damaging your heart muscle.
- Damaging your heart because of reduced oxygen supply.
- Having arrhythmias (irregular heartbeats).

Ongoing Care

Lifestyle changes and medicines can help control CHD. Lifestyle changes include following a healthy diet, being physically active, maintaining a healthy weight, quitting smoking, and managing stress.

Work closely with your doctor to control your blood pressure and manage your blood cholesterol and blood sugar levels.

A blood test called a lipoprotein panel will measure your cholesterol and triglyceride levels. A fasting blood glucose test will check your blood sugar level and show whether you're at risk for or have diabetes.

These tests show whether your risk factors are controlled, or whether your doctor needs to adjust your treatment for better results.

Talk with your doctor about how often you should schedule office visits or blood tests. Between those visits, call your doctor if you have any new symptoms or if your symptoms worsen.

Heart Attack Warning Signs

CHD raises your risk for a heart attack. Learn the signs and symptoms of a heart attack, and call 9–1–1 if you have any of these symptoms:

- Chest pain or discomfort. This involves uncomfortable pressure, squeezing, fullness, or pain in the center or left side of the chest that can be mild or strong. This pain or discomfort often lasts more than a few minutes or goes away and comes back.

- Upper body discomfort in one or both arms, the back, neck, jaw, or upper part of the stomach.

- Shortness of breath, which may occur with or before chest discomfort.

- Nausea (feeling sick to your stomach), vomiting, light-headedness or fainting, or breaking out in a cold sweat.

Symptoms also may include sleep problems, fatigue (tiredness), and lack of energy.

The symptoms of angina can be similar to the symptoms of a heart attack. Angina pain usually lasts for only a few minutes and goes away with rest.

Chest pain or discomfort that doesn't go away or changes from its usual pattern (for example, occurs more often or while you're resting) can be a sign of a heart attack. If you don't know whether your chest pain is angina or a heart attack, call 9–1–1.

Let the people you see regularly know you're at risk for a heart attack. They can seek emergency care for you if you suddenly faint, collapse, or have other severe symptoms.

Section 15.3

Heart Attack

This section includes text excerpted from "Heart Attack," National
Heart, Lung, and Blood Institute (NHLBI), June 22, 2015.

What Is a Heart Attack?

A heart attack happens when the flow of oxygen-rich blood to a
section of heart muscle suddenly becomes blocked and the heart can't
get oxygen. If blood flow isn't restored quickly, the section of heart
muscle begins to die.

Heart attack treatment works best when it's given right after symptoms occur. If you think you or someone else is having a heart attack,
even if you're not sure, **call 9–1–1 right away.**

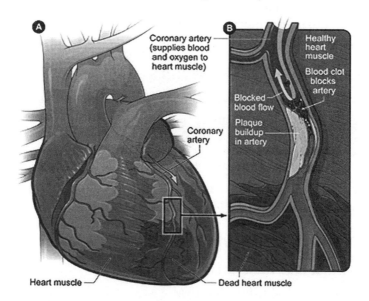

Figure 15.3. *Heart with Muscle Damage and a Blocked Artery*

*Figure A is an overview of a heart and coronary artery showing damage (dead heart
muscle) caused by a heart attack. Figure B is a cross-section of the coronary artery
with plaque buildup and a blood clot.*

A less common cause of heart attack is a severe spasm (tightening) of a coronary artery. The spasm cuts off blood flow through the artery. Spasms can occur in coronary arteries that aren't affected by atherosclerosis.

Heart attacks can be associated with or lead to severe health problems, such as heart failure and life-threatening arrhythmias.

Heart failure is a condition in which the heart can't pump enough blood to meet the body's needs. Arrhythmias are irregular heartbeats. Ventricular fibrillation is a life-threatening arrhythmia that can cause death if not treated right away.

Don't Wait—Get Help Quickly

Acting fast at the first sign of heart attack symptoms can save your life and limit damage to your heart. Treatment works best when it's given right after symptoms occur.

Many people aren't sure what's wrong when they are having symptoms of a heart attack.

Not all heart attacks begin with the sudden, crushing chest pain that often is shown on TV or in the movies, or other common symptoms such as chest discomfort. The symptoms of a heart attack can vary from person to person. Some people can have few symptoms and are surprised to learn they've had a heart attack. If you've already had a heart attack, your symptoms may not be the same for another one.

Quick Action Can Save Your Life: Call 9–1–1

If you think you or someone else may be having heart attack symptoms or a heart attack, don't ignore it or feel embarrassed to call for help. **Call 9–1–1 for emergency medical care.** Acting fast can save your life.

Do not drive to the hospital or let someone else drive you. Call an ambulance so that medical personnel can begin life-saving treatment on the way to the emergency room. Take a nitroglycerin pill if your doctor has prescribed this type of treatment.

Other Names for a Heart Attack

- Myocardial infarction (MI)
- Acute myocardial infarction (AMI)
- Acute coronary syndrome
- Coronary thrombosis
- Coronary occlusion

What Causes a Heart Attack?

Coronary Heart Disease

A heart attack happens if the flow of oxygen-rich blood to a section of heart muscle suddenly becomes blocked and the heart can't get oxygen. Most heart attacks occur as a result of coronary heart disease (CHD).

CHD is a condition in which a waxy substance called plaque builds up inside of the coronary arteries. These arteries supply oxygen-rich blood to your heart.

When plaque builds up in the arteries, the condition is called atherosclerosis. The buildup of plaque occurs over many years.

Eventually, an area of plaque can rupture (break open) inside of an artery. This causes a blood clot to form on the plaque's surface. If the clot becomes large enough, it can mostly or completely block blood flow through a coronary artery.

If the blockage isn't treated quickly, the portion of heart muscle fed by the artery begins to die. Healthy heart tissue is replaced with scar tissue. This heart damage may not be obvious, or it may cause severe or long-lasting problems.

Coronary Artery Spasm

A less common cause of heart attack is a severe spasm (tightening) of a coronary artery. The spasm cuts off blood flow through the artery. Spasms can occur in coronary arteries that aren't affected by atherosclerosis.

What causes a coronary artery to spasm isn't always clear. A spasm may be related to:

- Taking certain drugs, such as cocaine

- Emotional stress or pain

- Exposure to extreme cold

- Cigarette smoking

Who Is at Risk for a Heart Attack?

Certain risk factors make it more likely that you'll develop coronary heart disease (CHD) and have a heart attack. You can control many of these risk factors.

Risk Factors You Can Control

The major risk factors for a heart attack that you can control include:

- smoking

- high blood pressure

- high blood cholesterol

- overweight and obesity

- an unhealthy diet (for example, a diet high in saturated fat, trans fat, cholesterol, and sodium)

- lack of routine physical activity

- high blood sugar due to insulin resistance or diabetes

Some of these risk factors—such as obesity, high blood pressure, and high blood sugar—tend to occur together. When they do, it's called metabolic syndrome.

In general, a person who has metabolic syndrome is twice as likely to develop heart disease and five times as likely to develop diabetes as someone who doesn't have metabolic syndrome.

Risk Factors You Can't Control

Risk factors that you can't control include:

- age

- family history of early heart disease

- preeclampsia

What Are the Symptoms of a Heart Attack?

Not all heart attacks begin with the sudden, crushing chest pain that often is shown on TV or in the movies. In one study, for example, one-third of the patients who had heart attacks had no chest pain. These patients were more likely to be older, female, or diabetic.

The symptoms of a heart attack can vary from person to person. Some people can have few symptoms and are surprised to learn they've had a heart attack. If you've already had a heart attack, your symptoms may not be the same for another one.

It is important for you to know the most common symptoms of a heart attack and also remember these facts:

- Heart attacks can start slowly and cause only mild pain or discomfort. Symptoms can be mild or more intense and sudden. Symptoms also may come and go over several hours.

- People who have high blood sugar (diabetes) may have no symptoms or very mild ones.

- The most common symptom, in both men and women, is chest pain or discomfort.

Some people don't have symptoms at all. Heart attacks that occur without any symptoms or with very mild symptoms are called silent heart attacks.

Most Common Symptoms

The most common warning symptoms of a heart attack for both men and women are:

- chest pain or discomfort
- upper body discomfort
- shortness of breath

The symptoms of angina can be similar to the symptoms of a heart attack. Angina is chest pain that occurs in people who have coronary heart disease, usually when they're active. Angina pain usually lasts for only a few minutes and goes away with rest.

Chest pain or discomfort that doesn't go away or changes from its usual pattern (for example, occurs more often or while you're resting) can be a sign of a heart attack.

All chest pain should be checked by a doctor.

Other Common Signs and Symptoms

Pay attention to these other possible symptoms of a heart attack:

- Breaking out in a cold sweat.

- Feeling unusually tired for no reason, sometimes for days (especially if you are a woman).

- Nausea (feeling sick to the stomach) and vomiting.

- Light-headedness or sudden dizziness.
- Any sudden, new symptoms or a change in the pattern of symptoms you already have (for example, if your symptoms become stronger or last longer than usual).

Not everyone having a heart attack has typical symptoms. If you've already had a heart attack, your symptoms may not be the same for another one. However, some people may have a pattern of symptoms that recur.

The more signs and symptoms you have, the more likely it is that you're having a heart attack.

How Is a Heart Attack Diagnosed?

Your doctor will diagnose a heart attack based on your signs and symptoms, your medical and family histories, and test results.

Diagnostic Tests

- EKG (Electrocardiogram)
- blood tests
- coronary angiography

How Is a Heart Attack Treated?

Early treatment for a heart attack can prevent or limit damage to the heart muscle. Acting fast, by calling 9–1–1 at the first symptoms of a heart attack, can save your life. Medical personnel can begin diagnosis and treatment even before you get to the hospital.

Immediate Treatment

Certain treatments usually are started right away if a heart attack is suspected, even before the diagnosis is confirmed. These include:

- Aspirin to prevent further blood clotting
- Nitroglycerin to reduce your heart's workload and improve blood flow through the coronary arteries
- Oxygen therapy
- Treatment for chest pain

Once the diagnosis of a heart attack is confirmed or strongly suspected, doctors start treatments promptly to try to restore blood flow through the blood vessels supplying the heart. The two main treatments are clot-busting medicines and percutaneous coronary intervention, also known as coronary angioplasty, a procedure used to open blocked coronary arteries.

Clot-Busting Medicines

Thrombolytic medicines, also called clot busters, are used to dissolve blood clots that are blocking the coronary arteries. To work best, these medicines must be given within several hours of the start of heart attack symptoms. Ideally, the medicine should be given as soon as possible.

Percutaneous Coronary Intervention

Percutaneous coronary intervention is a nonsurgical procedure that opens blocked or narrowed coronary arteries. A thin, flexible tube (catheter) with a balloon or other device on the end is threaded through a blood vessel, usually in the groin (upper thigh), to the narrowed or blocked coronary artery. Once in place, the balloon located at the tip of the catheter is inflated to compress the plaque and related clot against the wall of the artery. This restores blood flow through the artery. During the procedure, the doctor may put a small mesh tube called a stent in the artery. The stent helps to keep the blood vessel open to prevent blockages in the artery in the months or years after the procedure.

Other Treatments for Heart Attack

Other treatments for heart attack include:

Medicines

Your doctor may prescribe one or more of the following medicines.

- ACE inhibitors
- Anticlotting medicines
- Anticoagulants
- Beta blockers
- Statin medicines

You also may be given medicines to relieve pain and anxiety, and treat arrhythmias. Take all medicines regularly, as your doctor prescribes. Don't change the amount of your medicine or skip a dose unless your doctor tells you to.

Medical procedures

Coronary artery bypass grafting also may be used to treat a heart attack. During coronary artery bypass grafting, a surgeon removes a healthy artery or vein from your body. The artery or vein is then connected, or grafted, to bypass the blocked section of the coronary artery. The grafted artery or vein bypasses (that is, goes around) the blocked portion of the coronary artery. This provides a new route for blood to flow to the heart muscle.

Heart-Healthy Lifestyle Changes

Treatment for a heart attack usually includes making heart-healthy lifestyle changes. Your doctor also may recommend:
Heart-healthy eating

- Aiming for healthy weight

- Managing stress

- Physical activity

- Quitting smoking

Taking these steps can lower your chances of having another heart attack.

How Can a Heart Attack Be Prevented?

Lowering your risk factors for coronary heart disease can help you prevent a heart attack. Even if you already have coronary heart disease, you still can take steps to lower your risk for a heart attack. These steps involve following a heart-healthy lifestyle and getting ongoing medical care.

Heart-Healthy Lifestyle

A heart-healthy lifestyle can help prevent a heart attack and includes heart-healthy eating, being physically active, quitting smoking, managing stress, and managing your weight.

Ongoing Care

Treat Related Conditions

Treating conditions that make a heart attack more likely also can help lower your risk for a heart attack. These conditions may include:

- diabetes (high blood sugar)
- high blood cholesterol
- high blood pressure

Have an Emergency Action Plan

Make sure that you have an emergency action plan in case you or someone in your family has a heart attack. This is very important if you're at high risk for, or have already had, a heart attack.

Write down a list of medicines you are taking, medicines you are allergic to, your healthcare provider's phone numbers (both during and after office hours), and contact information for a friend or relative. Keep the list in a handy place to share in a medical emergency.

Talk with your doctor about the signs and symptoms of a heart attack, when you should call 9–1–1, and steps you can take while waiting for medical help to arrive.

Life after a Heart Attack

Many people survive heart attacks and live active, full lives. If you get help quickly, treatment can limit damage to your heart muscle. Less heart damage improves your chances for a better quality of life after a heart attack.

Medical Followup

After a heart attack, you'll need treatment for coronary heart disease (CHD). This will help prevent another heart attack. Your doctor may recommend:

- Lifestyle changes, such as following a healthy diet, being physically active, maintaining a healthy weight, and quitting smoking.
- Medicines to control chest pain or discomfort, high blood cholesterol, high blood pressure, and your heart's workload.
- A cardiac rehabilitation program.

If you find it hard to get your medicines or take them, talk with your doctor. Don't stop taking medicines that can help you prevent another heart attack.

Returning to Normal Activities

After a heart attack, most people who don't have chest pain or discomfort or other problems can safely return to most of their normal activities within a few weeks. Most can begin walking right away.

Sexual activity also can begin within a few weeks for most patients. Talk with your doctor about a safe schedule for returning to your normal routine.

If allowed by State law, driving usually can begin within a week for most patients who don't have chest pain or discomfort or other problems. Each State has rules about driving a motor vehicle following a serious illness. People who have complications shouldn't drive until their symptoms have been stable for a few weeks.

Anxiety and Depression after a Heart Attack

After a heart attack, many people worry about having another heart attack. Sometimes they feel depressed and have trouble adjusting to new lifestyle changes.

Talk about how you feel with your healthcare team. Talking to a professional counselor also can help. If you're very depressed, your doctor may recommend medicines or other treatments that can improve your quality of life.

Joining a patient support group may help you adjust to life after a heart attack. You can see how other people who have the same symptoms have coped with them. Talk with your doctor about local support groups or check with an area medical center.

Support from family and friends also can help relieve stress and anxiety. Let your loved ones know how you feel and what they can do to help you.

Risk of a Repeat Heart Attack

Once you've had a heart attack, you're at higher risk for another one. Knowing the difference between angina and a heart attack is important. Angina is chest pain that occurs in people who have CHD.

The pain from angina usually occurs after physical exertion and goes away in a few minutes when you rest or take medicine as directed.

The pain from a heart attack usually is more severe than the pain from angina. Heart attack pain doesn't go away when you rest or take medicine.

If you don't know whether your chest pain is angina or a heart attack, call 9–1–1.

The symptoms of a second heart attack may not be the same as those of a first heart attack. Don't take a chance if you're in doubt. Always call 9–1–1 right away if you or someone else has heart attack symptoms.

Unfortunately, most heart attack victims wait 2 hours or more after their symptoms start before they seek medical help. This delay can result in lasting heart damage or death.

Section 15.4

Taking Aspirin to Prevent Heart Attacks

This section includes text excerpted from "Can an Aspirin a Day Help Prevent a Heart Attack?" U.S. Food and Drug Administration (FDA), May 5, 2014.

Can an Aspirin a Day Help Prevent a Heart Attack

Scientific evidence shows that taking an aspirin daily can help prevent a heart attack or stroke in some people, but not in everyone. It also can cause unwanted side effects.

According to Robert Temple, M.D., deputy director for clinical science at the U.S. Food and Drug Administration (FDA), one thing is certain: You should use daily aspirin therapy only after first talking to your healthcare professional, who can weigh the benefits and risks.

Who Can Benefit?

"Since the 1990s, clinical data have shown that in people who have experienced a heart attack, stroke or who have a disease of the blood vessels in the heart, a daily low dose of aspirin can help prevent a reoccurrence," Temple says. (A dose ranges from the 80 milligrams (mg) in a low-dose tablet to the 325 mg in a regular strength tablet.) This use is known as "secondary prevention."

However, after carefully examining scientific data from major studies, FDA has concluded that the data do not support the use of aspirin as a preventive medication by people who have not had a heart attack, stroke or cardiovascular problems, a use that is called "primary prevention." In such people, the benefit has not been established but risks—such as dangerous bleeding into the brain or stomach—are still present.

Caution Needed with Other Blood Thinners

When you have a heart attack, it's because one of the coronary arteries (which provide blood to the heart), has developed a clot that obstructs the flow of blood and oxygen to the heart. Aspirin works by interfering with your blood's clotting action.

Care is needed when using aspirin with other blood thinners, such as warfarin, dabigatran (Pradaxa), rivaroxaban (Xarelto) and apixiban (Eliquis).

What about people who have not had heart problems or a stroke but who, due to family history or showing other evidence of arterial disease are at increased risk? Is an aspirin a day a safe and effective strategy for them?

Again, Temple emphasizes, the clinical data do not show a benefit in such people.

He adds, however, that there are a number of ongoing, large-scale clinical studies continuing to investigate the use of aspirin in primary prevention of heart attack or stroke. FDA is monitoring these studies and will continue to examine the evidence as it emerges.

In the Meantime

The bottom line is that in people who have had a heart attack, stroke or cardiovascular problems, daily aspirin therapy is worth considering. And if you're thinking of using aspirin therapy, you should first talk to your healthcare professional to get an informed opinion, Temple says.

Finally, how much aspirin you take matters. It's important to your health and safety that the dose you use and how often you take it is right for you. Your healthcare professional can tell you the dose and frequency that will provide the greatest benefit with the least side effects.

If your healthcare professional recommends daily aspirin to lower the risk of a heart attack and clot-related stroke, read the labels carefully to make sure you have the right product. Some drugs combine aspirin with other pain relievers or other ingredients, and should not be used for long-term aspirin therapy.

Chapter 16

HIV and AIDS

What Is HIV/AIDS?

Human Immunodeficiency Virus (HIV)

HIV stands for human immunodeficiency virus. If left untreated, HIV can lead to the disease AIDS (acquired immunodeficiency syndrome).

Unlike some other viruses, the human body can't get rid of HIV completely. So once you have HIV, you have it for life.

HIV attacks the body's immune system, specifically the CD4 cells (T cells), which help the immune system fight off infections. If left untreated, HIV reduces the number of CD4 cells (T cells) in the body, making the person more likely to get infections or infection-related cancers. Over time, HIV can destroy so many of these cells that the body can't fight off infections and disease. These opportunistic infections or cancers take advantage of a very weak immune system and signal that the person has AIDS, the last state of HIV infection.

No effective cure for HIV currently exists, but with proper treatment and medical care, HIV can be controlled. The medicine used to treat HIV is called antiretroviral therapy or ART. If taken the right way, every day, this medicine can dramatically prolong the lives of many people with HIV, keep them healthy, and greatly lower their chance of transmitting the virus to others. Today, a person who is

This chapter includes text excerpted from "What Is HIV/AIDS?" AIDS.gov, U.S. Department of Health and Human Services (HHS), July 14, 2016.

diagnosed with HIV, treated before the disease is far advanced, and stays on treatment can live a nearly as long as someone who does not have HIV.

The only way to know for sure if you have HIV is to get tested. Testing is relatively simple. You can ask your healthcare provider for an HIV test. Many medical clinics, substance abuse programs, community health centers, and hospitals offer them too. You can also buy a home testing kit at a pharmacy or online.

Acquired Immunodeficiency Syndrome (AIDS)

AIDS stands for acquired immunodeficiency syndrome. AIDS is the final stage of HIV infection, and not everyone who has HIV advances to this stage.

AIDS is the stage of infection that occurs when your immune system is badly damaged and you become vulnerable to opportunistic infections. When the number of your CD4 cells falls below 200 cells per cubic millimeter of blood (200 cells/mm^3), you are considered to have progressed to AIDS. (The CD4 count of an uninfected adult/adolescent who is generally in good health ranges from 500 cells/mm^3 to 1,600 cells/mm^3.) You can also be diagnosed with AIDS if you develop one or more opportunistic infections, regardless of your CD4 count.

Without treatment, people who are diagnosed with AIDS typically survive about 3 years. Once someone has a dangerous opportunistic illness, life expectancy without treatment falls to about 1 year. People with AIDS need medical treatment to prevent death.

How Do You Get HIV or AIDS?

How Is HIV Spread?

You can get or transmit HIV only through specific activities. Most commonly, people get or transmit HIV through sexual behaviors and needle or syringe use.

HIV is not spread easily. Only certain body fluids from a person who has HIV can transmit HIV:

- blood
- semen (cum)
- pre-seminal fluid (pre-cum)
- rectal fluids
- vaginal fluids
- breast milk

These body fluids must come into contact with a mucous membrane or damaged tissue or be directly injected into your bloodstream (by a needle or syringe) for transmission to occur. Mucous membranes are found inside the rectum, vagina, penis, and mouth.

If you think you may have been exposed to HIV, get tested. You can get tested at your healthcare provider's office, a clinic, and other locations. You can also get a HIV home test kit from your local pharmacy.

Ways HIV Is Transmitted

In the United States, HIV is spread mainly by:

- Having anal or vaginal sex with someone who has HIV without using a condom or taking medicines to prevent or treat HIV.
  - Anal sex is the highest-risk sexual behavior. For the HIV-negative partner, receptive anal sex ("bottoming") is riskier than insertive anal sex ("topping").
  - Vaginal sex is the second highest-risk sexual behavior.
- Sharing needles or syringes, rinse water, or other equipment ("works") used to prepare injection drugs with someone who has HIV.

Less commonly, HIV may be spread:

- From mother to child during pregnancy, birth, or breastfeeding.
- By being stuck with an HIV-contaminated needle or other sharp object.

In extremely rare cases, HIV has been transmitted by:

- Oral sex
- Receiving blood transfusions, blood products, or organ/tissue transplants that are contaminated with HIV.
- Eating food that has been pre-chewed by an HIV-infected person.
- Being bitten by a person with HIV.
- Contact between broken skin, wounds, or mucous membranes and HIV-infected blood or blood-contaminated body fluids.
- Deep, open-mouth kissing if the person with HIV has sores or bleeding gums and blood from the HIV-positive partner gets into the bloodstream of the HIV-negative partner.

HIV Is Not Spread by

HIV does not survive long outside the human body (such as on surfaces) and it cannot reproduce outside a human host. It **is not** spread by:

- air or water

- mosquitoes, ticks or other insects

- saliva, tears, or sweat that is not mixed with the blood of an HIV-positive person

- shaking hands, hugging, sharing toilets, sharing dishes/drinking glasses, or closed-mouth or "social" kissing with someone who is HIV-positive

- drinking fountains

- other sexual activities that don't involve the exchange of body fluids (for example, touching)

HIV Treatment Reduces Transmission Risk

People with HIV who are using antiretroviral therapy (ART) consistently and who have achieved viral suppression (having the virus reduced to an undetectable level in the body) are very unlikely to transmit the virus to their uninfected partners. However, there is still some risk of transmission, so even with an undetectable viral load, people with HIV and their partners should continue to take steps to reduce the risk of HIV transmission.

I Have HIV, Does That Mean I Have AIDS?

No. The terms "HIV" and "AIDS" can be confusing because both terms refer to the same disease. However, "HIV" refers to the virus itself, and "AIDS" refers to the late stage of HIV infection, when an HIV-infected person's immune system is severely damaged and has difficulty fighting diseases and certain cancers. Before the development of certain medications, people with HIV could progress to AIDS in just a few years. But today, most people who are HIV-positive do not progress to AIDS. That's because if you have HIV and you take ART consistently, you can keep the level of HIV in your body low. This will help keep your body strong and healthy and reduce the likelihood that you will ever progress to AIDS. It will also help lower your risk of transmitting HIV to others.

Symptoms of HIV

How Can I Tell If I Have HIV?

You cannot rely on symptoms to tell whether you have HIV. **The only way to know for sure if you have HIV is to get tested.** Knowing your status is important because it helps you make healthy decisions to prevent getting or transmitting HIV.

The symptoms of HIV vary, depending on the individual and what stage of the disease you are in: the early stage, the clinical latency stage, or AIDS (the late stage of HIV infection). Below are the symptoms that some individuals may experience in these three stages. Not all individuals will experience these symptoms.

Early Stage of HIV

Some people may experience a flu-like illness within 2–4 weeks after HIV infection. But some people may not feel sick during this stage.

Flu-like symptoms can include:

- fever
- chills
- rash
- night sweats
- muscle aches
- sore throat
- fatigue
- swollen lymph nodes
- mouth ulcers

These symptoms can last anywhere from a few days to several weeks. During this time, HIV infection may not show up on an HIV test, but people who have it are highly infectious and can spread the infection to others.

You should not assume you have HIV just because you have any of these symptoms. Each of these symptoms can be caused by other illnesses. And some people who have HIV do not show any symptoms at all for 10 years or more.

If you think you may have been exposed to HIV, get an HIV test. Most HIV tests detect antibodies (proteins your body makes as a reaction against the presence of HIV), not HIV itself. But it takes a few weeks for your body to produce these antibodies, so if you test too early, you might not get an accurate test result. A new HIV test is available that can detect HIV directly during this early stage of infection. So be sure to let your testing site know if you think you may have been *recently* infected with HIV.

After you get tested, it's important to find out the result of your test so you can talk to your healthcare provider about treatment options if you're HIV-positive or learn ways to prevent getting HIV if you're HIV-negative.

You are at high risk of transmitting HIV to others during the early stage of HIV infection, even if you have no symptoms. For this reason, it is very important to take steps to reduce your risk of transmission.

Clinical Latency Stage

After the early stage of HIV infection, the disease moves into a stage called the clinical latency stage (also called "chronic HIV infection"). During this stage, HIV is still active but reproduces at very low levels. People with chronic HIV infection may not have any HIV-related symptoms, or only mild ones.

For people who aren't taking medicine to treat HIV (called antiretroviral therapy or ART), this period can last a decade or longer, but some may progress through this phase faster. People who are taking medicine to treat HIV the right way, every day may be in this stage for several decades because treatment helps keep the virus in check.

It's important to remember that people can still transmit HIV to others during this phase even if they have no symptoms, although people who are on ART and stay virally suppressed (having a very low level of virus in their blood) are much less likely to transmit HIV than those who are not virally suppressed.

Progression to AIDS

If you have HIV and you are not on ART, eventually the virus will weaken your body's immune system and you will progress to AIDS, the late stage of HIV infection.

Symptoms can include:

- rapid weight loss

- recurring fever or profuse night sweats

- extreme and unexplained tiredness

- prolonged swelling of the lymph glands in the armpits, groin, or neck

- diarrhea that lasts for more than a week

- sores of the mouth, anus, or genitals

- pneumonia

- red, brown, pink, or purplish blotches on or under the skin or inside the mouth, nose, or eyelids

- memory loss, depression, and other neurologic disorders

Each of these symptoms can also be related to other illnesses. So the only way to know for sure if you have HIV is to get tested.

Many of the severe symptoms and illnesses of HIV disease come from the

opportunistic infections that occur because your body's immune system has been damaged.

Chapter 17

Homicide

Trends by Sex

According to FBI statistics, men are more than twice as likely as women to be both the victims and the perpetrators of homicides in the United States. The data also show that men are eight times more likely than women to murder another man and more than ten times more likely to murder a woman.

Table 17.1. Homicide Offenders and Victims, by Sex, 2014*

Sex of victim	Total	Sex of offender		
		Male	**Female**	**Unknown**
Male	3,949	3,448	421	80
Female	1,691	1,523	149	19
Unknown sex	63	41	13	9

*The most recent full year for which statistics were available.

Murder Circumstance of Victims

From Table 17.2, it can be observed that 77.3 percent of murder victims were men, and compared to female victims, males were:

- 8 times more likely to be killed during robberies.

"Homicide," © 2017 Omnigraphics. Reviewed August 2016.

- 12 times more likely to be murdered during narcotics offenses.

- 20 times more likely to die in gangland killings, and 15 times more likely in juvenile gang killings.

Only rape offenses were reported to have a larger number of female murder victims. than male, while crimes such as arson, prostitution, and commercialized vice saw about the same number of male and female victims.

Table 17.2. Murder Circumstances by Sex of Victim, 2014

Circumstances	Total murder victims	Male	Female	Unknown
Total	**11,961**	**9,246**	**2,681**	**34**
Felony type total:	1,789	1,434	349	6
Rape	23	3	20	0
Robbery	565	502	63	0
Burglary	77	58	19	0
Larceny-theft	21	15	5	1
Motor vehicle theft	25	16	8	1
Arson	22	11	11	0
Prostitution and commercialized vice	19	10	9	0
Other sex offenses	3	2	1	0
Narcotic drug laws	371	341	29	1
Gambling	10	10	0	0
Other-not specified	653	466	184	3
Suspected felony type	83	58	25	0
Other than felony type total:	5,583	4,126	1,444	13
Romantic triangle	85	62	23	0
Child killed by babysitter	37	22	15	0
Brawl due to influence of alcohol	71	58	13	0
Brawl due to influence of narcotics	61	46	15	0
Argument over money or property	144	116	28	0
Other arguments	2,786	2,009	773	4
Gangland killings	145	138	7	0

Table 17.2. Continued

Circumstances	Total murder victims	Male	Female	Unknown
Juvenile gang killings	570	534	35	1
Institutional killings	18	16	2	0
Sniper attack	3	2	1	0
Other-not specified	1,663	1,123	532	8
Unknown	4,506	3,628	863	15

Homicide Trends by Age

Among the 11,961 murders reported in 2014, nearly 6 percent of the victims were men under the age of 18, while about 71 percent of male victims were over 18.

Table 17.3. Murder Victims by Age and Sex, 2014

Age	Total	Sex		
		Male	Female	Unknown
Total	**11,961**	**9,246**	**2,681**	**34**
Percent distribution[1]	100	77.3	22.4	0.3
Under 18[2]	1,085	692	388	5
18 and over[2]	10,773	8,493	2,268	12

Because of rounding, the percentages may not add to 100.0. [2] *Does not include unknown ages.*

Trends by Race and Ethnicity

As illustrated in Table 17.4:

- Nearly half the murder victims in 2014 were reported to be black, and the homicide victimization rate for black men was nearly 6 times more than for black women.

- About 45 percent victims were white, and 69 of those them were men.

- More than 12 percent of male murder victims were Hispanic or Latino, compared to about 3 percent of the women victims.

Table 17.4. Murder Victims by Race, Ethnicity, and Sex, 2014

Race	Total	Sex		
		Male	Female	Unknown
Total	**11,961**	**9,246**	**2,681**	**34**
White	5,397	3,733	1,664	0
Black	6,095	5,209	881	5
Other race	309	208	100	1
Unknown race	160	96	36	28
Hispanic or Latino[1]	1,871	1,510	361	0
Not Hispanic or Latino[1]	6,764	5,145	1,616	3
Unknown[1]	1,913	1,475	420	18

[1] *The ethnicity totals represent those agencies that provided ethnicity breakdowns. Not all agencies provide ethnicity data; therefore, the race and ethnicity totals will not equal.*

Reference

"Offenses Known to Law Enforcement: Expanded Offense Data," Federal Bureau of Investigation (FBI), U.S. Department of Justice, December 14, 2015.

Chapter 18

Influenza and Pneumonia

Chapter Contents

Section 18.1—Influenza 216
Section 18.2—Pneumonia 219

Section 18.1

Influenza

This section includes text excerpted from "Influenza (Flu)," Centers for Disease Control and Prevention (CDC), July 26, 2016.

Seasonal Influenza: Flu Basics

Influenza (flu) is a contagious respiratory illness caused by influenza viruses. It can cause mild to severe illness. Serious outcomes of flu infection can result in hospitalization or death. Some people, such as older people, young children, and people with certain health conditions, are at high risk for serious flu complications. The best way to prevent the flu is by getting **vaccinated** each year.

The upcoming season's flu vaccine will protect against the influenza viruses that research indicates will be most common during the season. This includes an influenza A (H1N1) virus, an influenza A (H3N2) virus, and one or two influenza B viruses, depending on the flu vaccine.

Key Facts about Influenza (Flu)

What Is Influenza (Also Called Flu)?

The flu is a contagious respiratory illness caused by influenza viruses that infect the nose, throat, and lungs. It can cause mild to severe illness, and at times can lead to death. The best way to prevent the flu is by getting a flu **vaccine** each year.

Signs and Symptoms of Flu

People who have the flu often feel some or all of these signs and symptoms:

- fever* or feeling feverish/chills
- cough
- sore throat
- runny or stuffy nose

- muscle or body aches
- headaches
- fatigue (very tired)
- some people may have vomiting and diarrhea, though this is more common in children than adults

*It's important to note that not everyone with flu will have a fever.

How Flu Spreads

Most experts believe that flu viruses spread mainly by droplets made when people with flu cough, sneeze or talk. These droplets can land in the mouths or noses of people who are nearby. Less often, a person might also get flu by touching a surface or object that has flu virus on it and then touching their own mouth, eyes or possibly their nose.

Period of Contagiousness

You may be able to pass on the flu to someone else before you know you are sick, as well as while you are sick. Most healthy adults may be able to infect others beginning 1 day **before** symptoms develop and up to 5 to 7 days **after** becoming sick. Some people, especially young children and people with weakened immune systems, might be able to infect others for an even longer time.

Onset of Symptoms

The time from when a person is exposed to flu virus to when symptoms begin is about 1 to 4 days, with an average of about 2 days.

Complications of Flu

Complications of flu can include bacterial pneumonia, ear infections, sinus infections, dehydration, and worsening of chronic medical conditions, such as congestive heart failure, asthma, or diabetes.

Preventing Flu

The first and most important step in preventing flu is to get a flu vaccination each year. CDC also recommends everyday preventive actions (like staying away from people who are sick, covering coughs and sneezes and frequent handwashing) to help slow the spread of germs that cause respiratory (nose, throat, and lungs) illnesses, like flu.

Diagnosing Flu

It is very difficult to distinguish the flu from other viral or bacterial causes of respiratory illnesses on the basis of symptoms alone. There are tests available to diagnose flu.

Treating

There are influenza antiviral drugs that can be used to treat flu illness.

Flu Complications

Most people who get influenza will recover in several days to less than two weeks, but some people will develop complications as a result of the flu. A wide range of complications can be caused by influenza virus infection of the upper respiratory tract (nasal passages, throat) and lower respiratory tract (lungs). While anyone can get sick with flu and become severely ill, some people are more likely to experience severe flu illness. Young children, adults aged 65 years and older, pregnant women, and people with certain chronic medical conditions are among those groups of people who are at high risk of serious flu complications, possibly requiring hospitalization and sometimes resulting in death. For example, people with chronic lung disease are at higher risk of developing severe pneumonia.

Sinus and ear infections are examples of moderate complications from flu, while pneumonia is a serious flu complication that can result from either influenza virus infection alone or from co-infection of flu virus and bacteria. Other possible serious complications triggered by flu can include inflammation of the heart (myocarditis), brain (encephalitis) or muscle (myositis, rhabdomyolysis) tissues, and multi-organ failure (for example, respiratory and kidney failure). Flu virus infection of the respiratory tract can trigger an extreme inflammatory response in the body and can lead to sepsis, the body's life-threatening response to infection. Flu also can make chronic medical problems worse. For example, people with asthma may experience asthma attacks while they have the flu, and people with chronic heart disease may experience a worsening of this condition triggered by flu.

Section 18.2

Pneumonia

Pneumonia is a general term for lung infections that can be caused by a variety of germs (viruses, bacteria, fungi, and parasites). Most cases, though, are caused by viruses, including adenoviruses, rhinovirus, influenza virus (flu), respiratory syncytial virus (RSV), human metapneumovirus, and parainfluenza virus (which causes croup).

Often, pneumonia begins after an upper respiratory tract infection (an infection of the nose and throat), with symptoms starting after 2 or 3 days of a cold or sore throat. It then moves to the lungs. Fluid, white blood cells, and debris start to gather in the air spaces of the lungs and block the smooth passage of air, making it harder for the lungs to work well.

Signs and Symptoms

Symptoms vary depending on what caused the pneumonia, but can include:

- fever
- shaking chills
- cough
- stuffy nose
- very fast breathing (in some cases, this is the only symptom)
- breathing with grunting or wheezing sounds
- working hard to breathe; this can include flaring of the nostrils, belly breathing, or movement of the muscles between the ribs
- vomiting
- chest pain
- abdominal pain, which often happens because a child is coughing and working hard to breathe

- less activity
- loss of appetite (in older kids) or poor feeding (in infants), which may lead to dehydration
- in extreme cases, bluish or gray color of the lips and fingernails

Start of Symptoms

The length of time between exposure to the germ and when someone starts feeling sick varies, depending on which virus or bacteria is causing the pneumonia (for instance, 4 to 6 days for RSV, but just 18 to 72 hours for the flu).

Duration

With treatment, most types of bacterial pneumonia can be cured within 1 to 2 weeks, although walking pneumonia may take 4 to 6 weeks to go away completely. Viral pneumonia may last longer.

Contagiousness

The viruses and bacteria that cause pneumonia are contagious. They're usually found in fluid from the mouth or nose of someone who's infected, so that person can spread the illness by coughing or sneezing. Sharing drinking glasses and eating utensils, and touching the used tissues or handkerchiefs of an infected person also can spread pneumonia.

Prevention

Some types of pneumonia can be prevented by vaccines. Kids usually get routine immunizations against *Haemophilus influenzae* and whooping cough (pertussis) beginning at 2 months of age. Vaccines are now also given against the pneumococcus, a common cause of bacterial pneumonia.

If someone in your home has a respiratory infection or throat infection, keep his or her drinking glasses and eating utensils separate from those of other family members, and wash your hands often, especially if you are handling used tissues or dirty handkerchiefs.

Professional Treatment

Doctors usually make a pneumonia diagnosis after a physical examination. They'll check the patient's appearance, breathing pattern, and vital signs, and listen to the lungs for abnormal sounds. They might order a chest X-ray, blood tests, and (sometimes) bacterial cultures of mucus produced by coughing.

In most cases, pneumonia is treated with antibiotics taken by mouth at home. The type of antibiotic used depends on the type of pneumonia. In some cases, other members of the household might be treated with medication to prevent illness.

Patients might be treated in a hospital if the pneumonia is caused by whooping cough, if another kind of bacterial pneumonia is causing a high fever and breathing problems, or if they:

- need oxygen therapy

- have a lung infection that may have spread to the bloodstream

- have a chronic illness that affects the immune system

- are vomiting so much that they cannot take medicine by mouth

- have frequent episodes of pneumonia

Hospital treatment can include intravenous (IV) antibiotics (given through a needle into a vein) and respiratory therapy (breathing treatments). More severe cases might be treated in the intensive care unit (ICU).

Home Care

Anyone with pneumonia needs to get plenty of rest and drink lots of fluids while the body works to fight the infection.

Chapter 19

Chronic Kidney Disease

Chronic Kidney Disease (CKD): The Basics

You have two kidneys, each about the size of your fist. Their main job is to filter wastes and excess water out of your blood to make urine. They also keep the body's chemical balance, help control blood pressure, and make hormones.

CKD means that your kidneys are damaged and can't filter blood like they should. This damage can cause wastes to build up in your body. It can also cause other problems that can harm your health.

CKD is often a "progressive" disease, which means it can get worse over time. CKD may lead to kidney failure. If your kidneys fail, you will need dialysis or a kidney transplant to maintain health.

You can take steps to keep your kidneys healthier longer:

- Choose foods with less salt (sodium).

- Keep your blood pressure at the level set by your healthcare provider.

- Keep your blood glucose in the target range, if you have diabetes.

This chapter includes text excerpted from "Chronic Kidney Disease (CKD) Basics," National Institute of Diabetes and Digestive and Kidney Diseases (NIDDK), August 6, 2014.

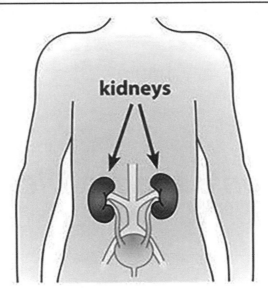

Figure 19.1. *Kidneys*

CKD and My Health

How Does My Healthcare Provider Know I Have CKD?

Chances are, you feel normal and were surprised to hear that you have CKD. It is called a "silent" disease, because many people don't have any symptoms until their kidneys are about to fail. The only way to know is to get your kidneys checked with blood and urine tests.

1. A blood test checks your GFR

2. A urine test checks for albumin

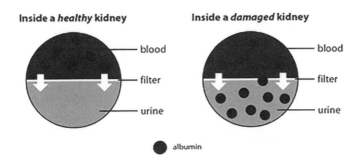

Figure 19.2. *Albumin Inside a Healthy Kidney and a Damaged Kidney*

These two tests are used to monitor CKD and make sure that treatment is working.

What Causes CKD?

Diabetes and high blood pressure are the most common causes of CKD.

Your provider will look at your health history and may do other tests. You need to know why you have CKD, so your treatment can address the cause of the CKD.

What Medicines Are Used to Treat CKD?

People with CKD often take medicines to lower blood pressure, control blood glucose, and lower blood cholesterol. Two types of blood pressure medicines—ACE inhibitors and ARBs—may slow CKD and delay kidney failure, even in people who don't have high blood pressure. Many people need to take two or more medicines for their blood pressure. They also may need to take a diuretic (water pill). The goal is to keep your blood pressure at the level set by your healthcare provider.

Do I Need to Change My Medicines?

Some medicines are not safe for people with CKD. Other medicines need to be taken in smaller doses. Tell your provider about all the medicines you take, including over-the-counter medicines (those you get without a prescription), vitamins, and supplements.

Can CKD Affect My Health in Other Ways?

People with CKD often have high blood pressure. They can also develop anemia (low number of red blood cells), bone disease, malnutrition, and heart and blood vessel diseases.

What Tests Will Help Track My CKD?

The blood and urine tests used to check for CKD are also used to monitor CKD. You need to keep track of your test results to see how you're doing.

Track your blood pressure.

If you have diabetes, monitor your blood glucose and keep it in your target range. Like high blood pressure, high blood glucose can be harmful to your kidneys. See CKD: Tracking My Test Results.

Will I Have to Go on Dialysis?

Some people live with CKD for years without going on dialysis. Others progress quickly to kidney failure. You may delay dialysis if you follow your provider's advice on medicine, diet, and lifestyle changes.

If your kidneys fail, you will need dialysis or a kidney transplant to maintain health. Most people with kidney failure are treated with dialysis.

Will I Be Able to Get a Kidney Transplant Instead of Going on Dialysis?

Some people with kidney failure may be able to receive a kidney transplant. The donated kidney can come from someone you don't know who has recently died, or from a living person—a relative, spouse, or friend. A kidney transplant isn't for everyone. You may have a condition that makes the transplant surgery dangerous or not likely to succeed.

CKD and My Lifestyle

People with CKD can and should continue to live their lives in a normal way: working, enjoying friends and family, and staying active. They also need to make some changes as explained here.

Do I Need to Change What I Eat?

What you eat may help to slow down CKD and keep your body healthier. Some points to keep in mind:

- Choose and prepare foods with less salt (sodium). Use less salt at the table.

- Select the right kinds and smaller amounts of protein.

- Choose foods that are healthy for your heart, like lean cuts of meat, skinless chicken, fish, fruits, vegetables, and beans.

- Read the Nutrition Facts Label, especially for sodium, to help you pick the right foods and drinks.

Your provider may refer you to a dietitian. Your dietitian will teach you how to choose foods that are easier on your kidneys. You will also learn about the nutrients that matter for CKD.

Do I Need to Change What I Drink?

- **Water**—You don't need to drink more water unless you have kidney stones. Drink as much water as you normally do.

- **Soda and other drinks**—If you are told to limit phosphorus, choose light-colored soda (or pop), like lemon-lime, and homemade iced tea and lemonade. Dark-colored sodas, fruit punch, and some bottled and canned iced teas can have a lot of phosphorus.

- **Juice**—If you are told to limit potassium, drink apple, grape, or cranberry juice instead of orange juice.

- **Alcohol**—You may be able to drink small amounts of alcohol. Drinking too much can damage the liver, heart, and brain and cause serious health problems.

Is Smoking Cigarettes Bad for My Kidneys?

Cigarette smoking can make kidney damage worse. Take steps to quit smoking as soon as you can.

CKD: Tracking My Test Results

You are the most important person on your healthcare team. Know your test results and track them over time to see how your kidneys are doing.

GFR—The GFR tells you how well your kidneys are filtering blood. You can't raise your GFR. The goal is to keep your GFR from going down to prevent or delay kidney failure.

- A GFR of *60 or higher* is in the normal range.

- A GFR *below 60* may mean kidney disease.

- A GFR of *15 or lower* may mean kidney failure.

Urine albumin—Albumin is a protein in your blood that can pass into the urine when kidneys are damaged. You can't undo kidney damage, but you may be able to lower the amount of albumin in your urine with treatment. Lowering your urine albumin is good for your kidneys.

Blood pressure—The most important thing you can do to slow down CKD is keep your blood pressure at the level set by your healthcare provider. This can delay or prevent kidney failure.

A1C—A1C test is a lab test that shows your average blood glucose level over the last 3 months. Lowering your A1C can help you to stay healthy. (For people with diabetes only.)

Chapter 20

Liver Cancer

What Is the Liver?

The liver is the largest organ in the human body, located on the upper right side of the body, behind the lower ribs. The liver does many jobs, including—

- storing nutrients

- removing waste products and worn-out cells from the blood

- filtering and processing chemicals in food, alcohol, and medications

- producing bile, a solution that helps digest fats and eliminate waste products

What Causes Liver Cancer?

Many liver cancer cases are related to the hepatitis B virus or hepatitis C virus. More than 4 million people are living with chronic

This chapter contains text excerpted from the following sources: Text beginning with the heading "What Is the Liver?" is excerpted from "Liver Cancer," Centers for Disease Control and Prevention (CDC), March 9, 2016; Text beginning with the heading "Adult Primary Liver Cancer Is a Disease in Which Malignant (Cancer) Cells Form in the Tissues of the Liver" is excerpted from " Adult Primary Liver Cancer Treatment (PDQ®)–Patient Version," National Cancer Institute (NCI), July 6, 2016.

Hepatitis B or chronic Hepatitis C in the United States. Most people don't know they have the virus.

Other behaviors and conditions that increase risk for getting liver cancer are—

- heavy alcohol use
- cirrhosis (scarring of the liver, which can also be caused by hepatitis and alcohol use)
- obesity
- diabetes
- having hemochromatosis, a condition where the body takes up and stores more iron than it needs
- eating foods that have aflatoxin (a fungus that can grow on foods, such as grains and nuts that have not been stored properly)

What Are the Symptoms of Liver Cancer?

In its early stages, liver cancer may not have symptoms that can be seen or felt. However, as the cancer grows larger, people may notice one or more of these common symptoms. It's important to remember that these symptoms could also be caused by other health conditions. If you have any of these symptoms, talk to your doctor.

Liver cancer symptoms may include—

- discomfort in the upper abdomen on the right side
- a swollen abdomen
- a hard lump on the right side just below the rib cage
- pain near the right shoulder blade or in the back
- jaundice (yellowing of the skin and whites of the eyes)
- easy bruising or bleeding
- unusual tiredness
- nausea and vomiting
- loss of appetite
- weight loss for no known reason

How Can I Reduce My Risk for Liver Cancer?

You can lower your risk of getting liver cancer in the following ways—

- Get vaccinated against Hepatitis B infection. The Hepatitis B vaccine is recommended for all infants at birth and for adults who may be at increased risk.

- Get tested for Hepatitis C, and get treated if you have it.

- Avoid drinking too much alcohol.

Adult Primary Liver Cancer Is a Disease in Which Malignant (Cancer) Cells Form in the Tissues of the Liver

The liver is one of the largest organs in the body. It has four lobes and fills the upper right side of the abdomen inside the rib cage. Three of the many important functions of the liver are:

- To filter harmful substances from the blood so they can be passed from the body in stools and urine.

- To make bile to help digest fat that comes from food.

- To store glycogen (sugar), which the body uses for energy.

Types of Adult Primary Liver Cancer

The two types of adult primary liver cancer are:

- hepatocellular carcinoma

- cholangiocarcinoma (bile duct cancer)

The most common type of adult primary liver cancer is hepatocellular carcinoma. This type of liver cancer is the third leading cause of cancer-related deaths worldwide.

This summary is about the treatment of primary liver cancer (cancer that begins in the liver). Treatment of cancer that begins in other parts of the body and spreads to the liver is not covered in this summary.

Primary liver cancer can occur in both adults and children. However, treatment for children is different than treatment for adults.

Having Hepatitis or Cirrhosis Can Affect the Risk of Adult Primary Liver Cancer

Anything that increases your chance of getting a disease is called a risk factor. Having a risk factor does not mean that you will get cancer; not having risk factors doesn't mean that you will not get cancer. Talk with your doctor if you think you may be at risk.

The following are risk factors for adult primary liver cancer:

- having hepatitis B or hepatitis C. Having both hepatitis B and hepatitis C increases the risk even more

- having cirrhosis

  - hepatitis (especially hepatitis C); or

  - drinking large amounts of alcohol for many years or being an alcoholic

- having metabolic syndrome, a set of conditions that occur together, including extra fat around the abdomen, high blood sugar, high blood pressure, high levels of triglycerides and low levels of high-density lipoproteins in the blood

- having liver injury that is long-lasting, especially if it leads to cirrhosis

- having hemochromatosis, a condition in which the body takes up and stores more iron than it needs. The extra iron is stored in the liver, heart, and pancreas.

- eating foods tainted with aflatoxin (poison from a fungus that can grow on foods, such as grains and nuts, that have not been stored properly)

Signs and Symptoms of Adult Primary Liver Cancer Include a Lump or Pain on the Right Side

These and other signs and symptoms may be caused by adult primary liver cancer or by other conditions. Check with your doctor if you have any of the following:

- a hard lump on the right side just below the rib cage

- discomfort in the upper abdomen on the right side

- a swollen abdomen

- pain near the right shoulder blade or in the back

- jaundice (yellowing of the skin and whites of the eyes)
- easy bruising or bleeding
- unusual tiredness or weakness
- nausea and vomiting
- loss of appetite or feelings of fullness after eating a small meal
- weight loss for no known reason
- pale, chalky bowel movements and dark urine
- fever

Tests That Examine the Liver and the Blood Are Used to Detect (Find) and Diagnose Adult Primary Liver Cancer

The following tests and procedures may be used:

- physical exam and history
- serum tumor marker test
- liver function tests
- CT scan (CAT scan)
- MRI (magnetic resonance imaging)
- ultrasound exam
- biopsy

    - fine-needle aspiration biopsy
    - core needle biopsy
    - laparoscopy

Certain Factors Affect Prognosis (Chance of Recovery) and Treatment Options

The prognosis (chance of recovery) and treatment options depend on the following:

- The stage of the cancer (the size of the tumor, whether it affects part or all of the liver, or has spread to other places in the body).
- How well the liver is working.
- The patient's general health, including whether there is cirrhosis of the liver.

Stages of Adult Primary Liver Cancer

After Adult Primary Liver Cancer Has Been Diagnosed, Tests Are Done to Find out If Cancer Cells Have Spread within the Liver or to Other Parts of the Body

The process used to find out if cancer has spread within the liver or to other parts of the body is called staging. The information gathered from the staging process determines the stage of the disease. It is important to know the stage in order to plan treatment. The following tests and procedures may be used in the staging process:

- CT scan (CAT scan)

- MRI (magnetic resonance imaging)

- PET scan (positron emission tomography scan)

There Are Three Ways That Cancer Spreads in the Body

Cancer can spread through tissue, the lymph system, and the blood:

- tissue
- blood
- lymph system

Cancer May Spread from Where It Began to Other Parts of the Body

When cancer spreads to another part of the body, it is called metastasis. Cancer cells break away from where they began (the primary tumor) and travel through the lymph system or blood.

- lymph system

- blood

The metastatic tumor is the same type of cancer as the primary tumor. For example, if primary liver cancer spreads to the lung, the cancer cells in the lung are actually liver cancer cells. The disease is metastatic liver cancer, not lung cancer.

The Barcelona Clinic Liver Cancer Staging System May Be Used to Stage Adult Primary Liver Cancer

There are several staging systems for liver cancer. The Barcelona Clinic Liver Cancer (BCLC) Staging System is widely used. This system is used to predict the patient's chance of recovery and to plan treatment, based on the following:

- Whether the cancer has spread within the liver or to other parts of the body.
- How well the liver is working.
- The general health and wellness of the patient.
- The symptoms caused by the cancer.

The BCLC staging system has five stages:

- Stage 0: Very early
- Stage A: Early
- Stage B: Intermediate
- Stage C: Advanced
- Stage D: End-stage

The Following Groups Are Used to Plan Treatment

BCLC stages 0, A, and B

Treatment to cure the cancer is given for BCLC stages 0, A, and B.

BCLC stages C and D

Treatment to relieve the symptoms caused by liver cancer and improve the patient's quality of life is given for BCLC stages C and D. Treatments are not likely to cure the cancer.

Recurrent Adult Primary Liver Cancer

Recurrent adult primary liver cancer is cancer that has recurred (come back) after it has been treated. The cancer may come back in the liver or in other parts of the body.

There Are Different Types of Treatment for Patients with Adult Primary Liver Cancer

Different types of treatments are available for patients with adult primary liver cancer. Some treatments are standard (the currently used treatment), and some are being tested in clinical trials. A treatment clinical trial is a research study meant to help improve current treatments or obtain information on new treatments for patients with cancer. When clinical trials show that a new treatment is better than the standard treatment, the new treatment may become the standard treatment. Patients may want to think about taking part in a clinical trial. Some clinical trials are open only to patients who have not started treatment.

Seven Types of Standard Treatment Are Used

1. surveillance
2. surgery
3. liver transplant
4. ablation therapy
   - radiofrequency ablation
   - microwave therapy
   - percutaneous ethanol injection
   - cryoablation
   - electroporation therapy
5. embolization therapy
   - transarterial embolization (TAE)
   - transarterial chemoembolization (TACE)
6. targeted therapy
7. radiation therapy
   - external radiation therapy
   - conformal radiation therapy
   - stereotactic body radiation therapy
   - proton beam radiation therapy
   - internal radiation therapy

The way the radiation therapy is given depends on the type and stage of the cancer being treated. External radiation therapy is used to treat adult primary liver cancer.

Treatment Options for Adult Primary Liver Cancer

Stages 0, A, and B Adult Primary Liver Cancer

Treatment of stages 0, A, and B adult primary liver cancer may include the following:

- surveillance for lesions smaller than 1 centimeter

- partial hepatectomy

- total hepatectomy and livertransplant

- ablation of the tumor

  - radiofrequency ablation

  - microwave therapy

  - percutaneous ethanol injection

  - cryoablation

- a clinical trial of electroporation therapy

Stages C and D Adult Primary Liver Cancer

Treatment of stages C and D adult primary liver cancer may include the following:

- embolization therapy using one of the following methods:

  - transarterial embolization (TAE)

  - transarterial chemoembolization (TACE)

- targeted therapy

- radiation therapy

- a clinical trial of targeted therapy after chemoembolization or combined with chemotherapy

- a clinical trial of new targeted therapy drugs

- a clinical trial of targeted therapy with or without stereotactic body radiation therapy

- a clinical trial of stereotactic body radiation therapy or proton-beam radiation therapy

Treatment of Recurrent Adult Primary Liver Cancer

Treatment options for recurrent adult primary liver cancer may include the following:

- total hepatectomy and liver transplant
- partial hepatectomy
- ablation
- transarterial chemoembolization and targeted therapy with sorafenib, as palliative therapy to relieve symptoms and improve quality of life
- a clinical trial of a new treatment

Chapter 21

Lung Cancer

What Is Lung Cancer?

Cancer is a disease in which cells in the body grow out of control. When cancer starts in the lungs, it is called *lung cancer*.

Lung cancer begins in the lungs and may spread to lymph nodes or other organs in the body, such as the brain. Cancer from other organs also may spread to the lungs. When cancer cells spread from one organ to another, they are called *metastases*.

Lung cancers usually are grouped into two main types called small cell and non-small cell. These types of lung cancer grow differently and are treated differently. Non-small cell lung cancer is more common than small cell lung cancer.

What Are the Risk Factors for Lung Cancer?

Research has found several risk factors that may increase your chances of getting lung cancer.

Smoking

Cigarette smoking is the number one risk factor for lung cancer. In the United States, cigarette smoking is linked to about 80% to 90% of lung cancers. Using other tobacco products such as cigars or pipes

---

This chapter includes text excerpted from "Lung Cancer," Centers for Disease Control and Prevention (CDC), August 28, 2014.

also increases the risk for lung cancer. Tobacco smoke is a toxic mix of more than 7,000 chemicals. Many are poisons. At least 70 are known to cause cancer in people or animals.

People who smoke cigarettes are 15 to 30 times more likely to get lung cancer or die from lung cancer than people who do not smoke. Even smoking a few cigarettes a day or smoking occasionally increases the risk of lung cancer. The more years a person smokes and the more cigarettes smoked each day, the more risk goes up.

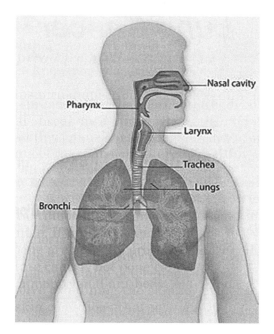

Figure 21.1. *Lung Cancer*

Secondhand Smoke

Smoke from other people's cigarettes, pipes, or cigars (secondhand smoke) also causes lung cancer. When a person breathes in second-hand smoke, it is like he or she is smoking. In the United States, two out of five adults who don't smoke and half of children are exposed to secondhand smoke, and about 7,300 people who never smoked die from lung cancer due to secondhand smoke every year.

Radon

Radon is a naturally occurring gas that comes from rocks and dirt and can get trapped in houses and buildings. It cannot be seen, tasted, or smelled. Nearly one out of every 15 homes in the United States is thought to have high radon levels. The EPA recommends testing homes for radon and using proven ways to lower high radon levels.

Other Substances

Examples of substances found at some workplaces that increase risk include asbestos, arsenic, diesel exhaust, and some forms of silica and chromium. For many of these substances, the risk of getting lung cancer is even higher for those who smoke.

Personal or Family History of Lung Cancer

If you are a lung cancer survivor, there is a risk that you may develop another lung cancer, especially if you smoke. Your risk of lung cancer may be higher if your parents, brothers or sisters, or children have had lung cancer. This could be true because they also smoke, or they live or work in the same place where they are exposed to radon and other substances that can cause lung cancer.

Radiation Therapy to the Chest

Cancer survivors who had radiation therapy to the chest are at higher risk of lung cancer.

Diet

Scientists are studying many different foods and dietary supplements to see whether they change the risk of getting lung cancer. There is much we still need to know. We do know that smokers who take beta-carotene supplements have increased risk of lung cancer.

What Are the Symptoms of Lung Cancer?

Different people have different symptoms for lung cancer. Some people have symptoms related to the lungs. Some people whose lung cancer has spread to other parts of the body (metastasized) have symptoms specific to that part of the body. Some people just have general symptoms of not feeling well. Most people with lung cancer don't have symptoms until the cancer is advanced. Lung cancer symptoms may include—

- coughing that gets worse or doesn't go away
- chest pain

- shortness of breath
- wheezing
- coughing up blood
- feeling very tired all the time
- weight loss with no known cause

Other changes that can sometimes occur with lung cancer may include repeated bouts of pneumonia and swollen or enlarged lymph nodes (glands) inside the chest in the area between the lungs.

These symptoms can happen with other illnesses, too. If you have some of these symptoms, talk to your doctor, who can help find the cause.

What Can I Do to Reduce My Risk of Lung Cancer?

You can help lower your risk of lung cancer in the following ways—

- don't smoke
- avoid secondhand smoke
- get your home tested for radon
- be careful at work

What Screening Tests Are There?

Screening means testing for a disease when there are no symptoms or history of that disease. Doctors recommend a screening test to find a disease early, when treatment may work better.

The only recommended screening test for lung cancer is low-dose computed tomography (also called a low-dose CT scan, or LDCT). In this test, an X-ray machine scans the body and uses low doses of radiation to make detailed pictures of the lungs.

Who Should Be Screened?

The U.S. Preventive Services Task Force recommends yearly lung cancer screening with LDCT for people who—

- have a history of heavy smoking, and
- smoke now or have quit within the past 15 years, and
- are between 55 and 80 years old

Heavy smoking means a smoking history of 30 pack years or more. A pack year is smoking an average of one pack of cigarettes per day for one year. For example, a person could have a 30 pack-year history by smoking one pack a day for 30 years or two packs a day for 15 years.

Risks of Screening

Lung cancer screening has at least three risks—

- A lung cancer screening test can suggest that a person has lung cancer when no cancer is present. This is called a false-positive result. False-positive results can lead to follow-up tests and surgeries that are not needed and may have more risks.

- A lung cancer screening test can find cases of cancer that may never have caused a problem for the patient. This is called overdiagnosis. Overdiagnosis can lead to treatment that is not needed.

- Radiation from repeated LDCT tests can cause cancer in otherwise healthy people.

That is why lung cancer screening is recommended only for adults who have no symptoms but who are at high risk for developing the disease because of their smoking history and age.

If you are thinking about getting screened, talk to your doctor. If lung cancer screening is right for you, your doctor can refer you to a high-quality treatment facility.

The best way to reduce your risk of lung cancer is to not smoke and to avoid secondhand smoke. Lung cancer screening is not a substitute for quitting smoking.

When Should Screening Stop?

The Task Force recommends that yearly lung cancer screening stop when the person being screened—

- turns 81 years old, or

- has not smoked in 15 years, or

- develops a health problem that makes him or her unwilling or unable to have surgery if lung cancer is found

How Is Lung Cancer Diagnosed and Treated?

Types of Lung Cancer

There two main types of lung cancer are small cell lung cancer and non-small cell lung cancer. These categories refer to what the cancer cells look like under a microscope. Non-small cell lung cancer is more common than small cell lung cancer.

Staging

If lung cancer is diagnosed, other tests are done to find out how far it has spread through the lungs, lymph nodes, and the rest of the body. This process is called staging. The type and stage of lung cancer tells doctors what kind of treatment you need.

Types of Treatment

Lung cancer is treated in several ways, depending on the type of lung cancer and how far it has spread. People with non-small cell lung cancer can be treated with surgery, chemotherapy, radiation therapy, targeted therapy, or a combination of these treatments. People with small cell lung cancer are usually treated with radiation therapy and chemotherapy.

- surgery
- chemotherapy
- radiation therapy
- targeted therapy

Doctors from different specialties often work together to treat lung cancer. Pulmonologists are doctors who are experts in diseases of the lungs. Surgeons are doctors who perform operations. Thoracic surgeons specialize in chest, heart, and lung surgery. Medical oncologists are doctors who treat cancer with medicines. Radiation oncologists are doctors who treat cancers with radiation.

Chapter 22

Motor Vehicle Accidents

Chapter Contents

Section 22.1—Aggressive Driving... 246

Section 22.2—Distracted Driving... 248

Section 22.3—Drowsy Driving 254

Section 22.4—Impaired Driving... 257

Section 22.5—Older Drivers.. 261

Section 22.1

Aggressive Driving

"Aggressive Driving," © 2017 Omnigraphics. Reviewed August 2016.

According to the National Highway Traffic Safety Administration (NHTSA), aggressive driving occurs when "an individual commits a combination of moving traffic offenses so as to endanger other persons or property." It can also be a single deliberate act that causes another driver to react defensively.

A related and more serious behavior, road rage, can be defined as an assault by the driver or passenger(s) of one motor vehicle on those in another vehicle using the vehicle itself or any dangerous weapon— that is triggered by an incident on the roadway. While aggressive driving is treated as a traffic violation, road rage is an intentional disregard for the safety of others and is considered to be a criminal offense.

It is estimated that more than 1,500 people are killed each year in the United States as a result of aggressive-driving incidents. And men—particularly young men between the ages of 18 and 26—are three times more likely to be aggressive drivers than women, making this behavior a significant men's health issue.

Signs of Aggressive Driving

Aggressive driving involves a range of unlawful driving behaviors such as:

- **Speeding**: This includes actions like driving too fast for current conditions, driving above the posted speed limit, and racing.

- **Frequent lane changes**: Cutting between vehicles to move ahead of traffic, changing lanes without warning, improper passing, or any similar action can put both the driver and other motorists in danger.

- **Running a red light or stop sign**: Ignoring a stop light, entering an intersection on yellow light, and not stopping at a stop sign are serious offenses that may cause injury to vehicle occupants and others.

- **Expressing frustration**: Condemning fellow motorists, either mentally or verbally, or making aggressive hand gestures to take out your frustration can result in violence or a crash.

- **Tailgating**: Following too closely to the vehicle ahead—especially in an aggressive manner—is one of the major causes of collisions and can result in serious injury or even death.

Other aggressive behaviors include driving recklessly; unnecessary use of the horn; excessive flashing of headlights at oncoming traffic; illegal driving on a sidewalk, median, road shoulder, or ditch; failing to yield right of way; and failing to obey traffic officers, traffic signs and control devices, or traffic laws concerning safety zones.

Avoiding Aggressive Driving

Avoid aggressive driving, as well as aggressive drivers, by following some simple measures, including:

- Drive within the posted speed limit.

- Make sure there's enough room when changing lanes or when entering traffic.

- Ensure a safe following distance between you and the vehicle ahead of you.

- Always signal before changing lanes or turning.

- To avoid traffic congestion, identify alternate routes.

- Opt for public transportation for some relief from sitting behind wheel.

- Pull over to get out of the way of an aggressive driver.

- Avoid conflict when possible. Be polite and avoid prolonged eye contact with an aggressive driver.

- Do not make offensive hand gestures, and ignore any made at you.

- Report dangerous aggressive drivers. If you are driving, either pull over to a safe spot to call the police or ask someone with you to make the call.

References

1. "Aggressive Driving," Arizona Department of Public Safety, n.d.

2. "Road Rage & Aggressive Driving," Washington State Patrol, n.d.

3. "Aggressive Driving," Insurance Information Institute, n.d.

4. "Aggressive Driving," National Highway Traffic Safety Administration, n.d.

5. Bierma, Paige. "Road Rage: When Stress Hits the Highway," HealthDay, January 20, 2016.

Section 22.2

Distracted Driving

This section includes text excerpted from "Distracted Driving at Work," National Institute for Occupational Safety and Health (NIOSH), March 23, 2016.

What Are the Main Types of Distractions?

Visual, Manual, and Cognitive Distractions

Visual: Taking your eyes off the road

- Reading a text message
- Programming the navigation system
- "Rubbernecking" at a crash site
- Looking at a map

Manual: Taking your hands off the wheel

- Reaching for things inside the vehicle
- Dialing the phone

- Adjusting the radio
- Eating or drinking
- Applying makeup

Cognitive: Taking your mind off driving

- Talking on the phone
- Arguing with a passenger
- Thinking about your next appointment

Why Are Phones So Distracting?

Talking and texting on a phone are driving distractions. Texting while driving is especially dangerous because it combines all three types of distractions.

Hands-free phones are not necessarily safer than hand-held devices. Your brain has limited capability to perform two cognitive tasks, such as driving and talking on the phone at the same time. You may think you are successfully doing two tasks at once; in reality, your brain is constantly switching between these tasks. When driving becomes the secondary task, you pay less attention to driving and surrounding roadway hazards.

Fatal Crashes Involving Distracted Driving

New research suggests that some type of distraction is present during 52% of normal driving. The most common distractions are interacting with an adult or teen passenger (15%), using a cell phone (6%), and using systems such as climate control and radio (4%). This information comes from a national "naturalistic driving" study which collected data on the normal driving behaviors of 3,500 volunteer participants over a three-year period. Researchers reported that drivers were at twice the risk of having a crash involving injury or property damage while distracted, compared to times they were not distracted. The same study found that distraction was present in 68% of crashes that involved injury or property damage, and estimated that 36% of all motor vehicle crashes in the United States could be avoided if no distractions were present.

The National Highway Traffic Safety Administration reports that in 2013:

- 16% of all motor vehicle crashes in the U.S. involved a distracted driver

- 3,154 people died in crashes involving a distracted driver

- 424,000 people were injured in motor vehicle crashes involving a distracted driver

- 480 non-occupants, such as pedestrians and cyclists, died in a crash that involved a distracted driver

Fatal distracted-driving crashes by age

The chart below shows that, for all drivers (occupational and non-occupational) and all age groups, persons 20 to 29 years old were most often:

- involved in a fatal crash;

- the driver in a fatal crash involving distracted driving; and,

- the driver in a fatal crash involving the use of a cell phone specifically.

Drivers ages 30 to 39 had the second highest proportions of fatal crashes in all three of these categories.

Although younger drivers might feel more comfortable and confident with using cell phones and other technologies, they account for more fatal distracted-driving crashes, including those involving cell phones, than any other age group. Employers with younger drivers should be especially aware of the need for policies and education to prevent distracted driving.

What Is the Role of Distraction in Motor Vehicle Crashes?

Fatal Crashes Involving Distracted Driving

New research suggests that some type of distraction is present during 52% of normal driving. The most common distractions are interacting with an adult or teen passenger (15%), using a cell phone (6%), and using systems such as climate control and radio (4%). This information comes from a national "naturalistic driving" study which collected data on the normal driving behaviors of 3,500 volunteer participants over a three-year period. Researchers reported that drivers were at twice the risk of having a crash involving injury or property damage while distracted, compared to times they were not distracted. The same study found that distraction was present in 68% of crashes that involved injury or property damage, and estimated that 36% of all motor vehicle crashes in the United States could be avoided if no distractions were present.

The National Highway Traffic Safety Administration reports that in 2013:

- 16% of all motor vehicle crashes in the United States involved a distracted driver.

- 3,154 people died in crashes involving a distracted driver.

- 424,000 people were injured in motor vehicle crashes involving a distracted driver.

- 480 non-occupants, such as pedestrians and cyclists, died in a crash that involved a distracted driver.

Fatal distracted-driving crashes by age

The chart below shows that, for all drivers (occupational and non-occupational) and all age groups, persons 20 to 29 years old were most often:

- involved in a fatal crash;

- the driver in a fatal crash involving distracted driving; and

- the driver in a fatal crash involving the use of a cell phone specifically.

Drivers ages 30 to 39 had the second highest proportions of fatal crashes in all three of these categories.

Although younger drivers might feel more comfortable and confident with using cell phones and other technologies, they account for more fatal distracted-driving crashes, including those involving cell phones, than any other age group. Employers with younger drivers should be especially aware of the need for policies and education to prevent distracted driving.

Why Is It Important to Prevent Distracted Driving at Work?

What the Research Says

Workers in a wide range of industries and occupations spend substantial portions of their workdays on the road. The National Highway Traffic Safety Administration estimates that at any given time in 2014,

2.2% of all drivers on the road were texting or visibly manipulating a hand-held device. This is a statistically significant increase from 1.7% in 2013.

While the number of distraction-related crashes and injuries that are work-related is unknown, research suggests that distracted driving is as likely to happen at work as during other types of driving.

One study showed that drivers were more likely to be in a hurry to reach their destination, think about work, be tired, or use a cell phone when they were driving for work. In another study conducted in a driving simulator, researchers engaged some participants in conversations about contentious social issues such as capital punishment, same-sex marriage, and the war in Iraq. Researchers engaged other participants in simple conversations about non-controversial topics such as music preferences and hobbies. Participants who were involved in emotionally intense conversations drove significantly worse than those involved in simple everyday conversations.

A worker who is driving a motor vehicle while negotiating a complex or contentious business deal over the phone at the same time is at greater risk of being in a crash. In this situation, neither task–driving a vehicle or doing business–gets the attention it deserves.

Laws and Regulations

State laws on texing and cell phones

- Most U.S. states now ban texting while driving, and a growing number of states have also banned the use of hand-held electronic devices.

Federal regulations for commercial drivers

- Drivers of commercial motor vehicles (large trucks and buses) are not permitted to send or read texts while driving, or to use a hand-held cell phone while driving.

How Can You Prevent Distracted Driving at Work?

Recommendations for Employers and Workers
For employers:

- Create a policy that includes these elements:
  - If you are driving a company vehicle: No sending or responding to texts or talking on a hand-held device.

- If you are driving a personal vehicle and using a company-issued cell phone: No sending or responding to texts or talking on the cell phone.

- Consider banning the use of hands-free phones.

- Before implementing these policies, prepare workers in advance by clearly communicating:

  - How distracted driving puts them at risk of a crash.

  - That driving requires their full attention while they are on the road.

  - What they need to do to comply with the policy.

  - What action you will take if they do not follow the policy.

- Consider having workers acknowledge that they have read and understand the policy.

- Consider using technology to block cell phone service while vehicles are in operation.

- Provide workers with information to help them talk to their family and friends about the dangers of distracted driving.

For workers:

- Before you drive...

  - Get enough sleep and stay well-rested.

  - Familiarize yourself with your vehicle's safety features.

  - Adjust controls such as mirrors, seat, radio, heat, or air conditioning.

  - Plan your route and travel schedule.

  - Record a voice mail greeting telling your callers that you are driving and will return their call as soon as you are able.

  - Program directions into your navigation system and enable the voice-activated function.

  - Turn off your phone when you get in your vehicle. Turn it back on when you are done driving.

  - If you spend a lot of time on the road, organize your route and schedule so you can make phone calls from the parking lot of one location before driving to the next one.

- While you drive...

  - Do not text or use a hand-held phone. It is not necessarily safer to use hands-free and voice recognition devices while driving—even if your employer allows them. Pull over in a safe location if you must text or make a call.

  - Do not program a navigation system while you are driving.

  - Do not reach to pick up items from the floor, open the glove box, or try to catch falling objects in the vehicle.

  - Avoid emotional conversations with passengers that cause anger or stress, or pull over in a safe location to continue the conversation. For normal conversation, passengers in the vehicle can often help lower crash risk for adult drivers.

  - Focus on the driving environment—the vehicles around you, pedestrians, cyclists, and objects or events that may mean you need to act quickly to control or stop your vehicle.

Section 22.3

Drowsy Driving

This section includes text excerpted from "Drowsy Driving," Center for Disease Control and Prevention (CDC), February 18, 2016.

Drive Alert and Stay Unhurt.

Learn the Risks of Drowsy Driving and How to Protect Yourself.

Drowsy driving is a major problem in the United States. The risk, danger, and sometimes tragic results of drowsy driving are alarming. Drowsy driving is the dangerous combination of driving and sleepiness or fatigue. This usually happens when a driver has not slept enough, but it can also happen due to untreated sleep disorders, medications, drinking alcohol, and shift work.

What is Drowsy Driving?

Operating a motor vehicle while fatigued or sleepy is commonly referred to as "drowsy driving."

The Impact of Drowsy Driving

Drowsy driving poses a serious risk not only for one's own health and safety, but also for the other people on the road.

The National Highway Traffic Safety Administration estimates that between 2005 and 2009 drowsy driving was responsible for an annual average of:

- 83,000 crashes

- 37,000 injury crashes

- 886 fatal crashes (846 fatalities in 2014)

These estimates are conservative, though, and up to 6,000 fatal crashes each year may be caused by drowsy drivers.

How Often Do Americans Fall Asleep While Driving?

- Approximately 1 out of 25 adults aged 18 years and older surveyed reported that they had fallen asleep while driving in the past 30 days.

- Individuals who snored or slept 6 hours or less per day were more likely to fall asleep while driving.

How Does Sleepiness Affect Driving?

Falling asleep at the wheel is very dangerous, but being sleepy affects your ability to drive safely even if you don't fall asleep. Drowsiness—

- makes drivers less attentive

- slows reaction time

- affects a driver's ability to make decisions

The Warning Signs of Drowsy Driving

- yawning or blinking frequently

- difficulty remembering the past few miles driven

- missing your exit
- drifting from your lane
- hitting a rumble strip

Who Is More Likely to Drive Drowsy?

- Drivers who do not get enough sleep.
- Commercial drivers who operate vehicles such as tow trucks, tractor trailers, and buses.
- Shift workers (work the night shift or long shifts).
- Drivers with untreated sleep disorders such as one where breathing repeatedly stops and starts (sleep apnea).
- Drivers who use medications that make them sleepy.

How to Prevent Drowsy Driving

There are four things you should do before taking the wheel to prevent driving while drowsy.

1. Get enough sleep! Most adults need at least 7 hours of sleep a day, while adolescents need at least 8 hours.8–9

2. Develop good sleeping habits such as sticking to a sleep schedule.

3. If you have a sleep disorder or have symptoms of a sleep disorder such as snoring or feeling sleepy during the day, talk to your physician about treatment options.

4. Avoid drinking alcohol or taking medications that make you sleepy. Be sure to check the label on any medications or talk to your pharmacist.

Drowsy Driving Is Similar to Drunk Driving

Your body needs adequate sleep on a daily basis. The more hours of sleep you miss, the harder it is for you to think and perform as well as you would like. Lack of sleep can make you less alert and affect your coordination, judgement, and reaction time while driving. This is known as cognitive impairment.

Studies have shown that going too long without sleep can impair your ability to drive the same way as drinking too much alcohol.

- Being awake for at least 18 hours is the same as someonc having a blood content (BAC) of 0.05%.

- Being awake for at least 24 hours is equal to having a blood alcohol content of 0.10%. This is higher than the legal limit (0.08% BAC) in all states.

Additionally, drowsiness increases the effect of even low amounts of alcohol.

Section 22.4

Impaired Driving

This section includes text excerpted from "Impaired Driving: Get the Facts," Centers for Disease Control and Prevention (CDC), April 15, 2016.

Every day, 28 people in the United States die in motor vehicle crashes that involve an alcohol-impaired driver. This amounts to one death every 53 minutes. The annual cost of alcohol-related crashes totals more than $44 billion.

Thankfully, there are effective measures that can help prevent injuries and deaths from alcohol-impaired driving.

How Big Is the Problem?

In 2014, 9,967 people were killed in alcohol-impaired driving crashes, accounting for nearly one-third (31%) of all traffic-related deaths in the United States.

Of the 1,070 traffic deaths among children ages 0 to 14 years in 2014, 209 (19%) involved an alcohol-impaired driver.

Of the 209 child passengers ages 14 and younger who died in alcohol-impaired driving crashes in 2014, over half (116) were riding in the vehicle with the alcohol-impaired driver.

In 2014, over 1.1 million drivers were arrested for driving under the influence of alcohol or narcotics.3 That's one percent of the 121 million self-reported episodes of alcohol-impaired driving among U.S. adults each year.

Drugs other than alcohol (legal and illegal) are involved in about 16% of motor vehicle crashes.

Marijuana use is increasing6 and 13% of nighttime, weekend drivers have marijuana in their system.

Marijuana users were about 25% more likely to be involved in a crash than drivers with no evidence of marijuana use, however other factors —such as age and gender—may account for the increased crash risk among marijuana users.

Who Is Most at Risk?

Young people:

At all levels of blood alcohol concentration (BAC), the risk of being involved in a crash is greater for young people than for older people.

Among drivers with BAC levels of 0.08% or higher involved in fatal crashes in 2014, three out of every 10 were between 21 and 24 years of age (30%). The next two largest groups were ages 25 to 34 (29%) and 35 to 44 (24%).

Motorcyclists:

Among motorcyclists killed in fatal crashes in 2014, 29% had BACs of 0.08% or greater.

Motorcyclists ages 40–49 have the highest percentage of deaths with BACs of 0.08% or greater (40% in 2013).

Drivers with prior driving while impaired (DWI) convictions: Drivers with a BAC of 0.08% or higher involved in fatal crashes were seven times more likely to have a prior conviction for DWI than were drivers with no alcohol in their system. (7% and 1%, respectively).

What Are the Effects of Blood Alcohol Concentration (BAC)?

Information in this table shows the blood alcohol concentration (BAC) level at which the effect usually is first observed.

Table 22.1. Effects of Blood Alcohol Concentration

Blood Alcohol Concentration (BAC)*	Typical Effects	Predictable Effects on Driving
.02% About 2 alcoholic drinks**	• Some loss of judgment • Relaxation • Slight body warmth • Altered mood	• Decline in visual functions (rapid tracking of a moving target) • Decline in ability to perform two tasks at the same time (divided attention)
.05% About 3 alcoholic drinks**	• Exaggerated behavior • May have loss of small-muscle control (e.g., focusing your eyes) • Impaired judgment • Usually good feeling • Lowered alertness • Release of inhibition	• Reduced coordination • Reduced ability to track moving objects • Difficulty steering • Reduced response to emergency driving situations
.08% About 4 alcoholic drinks**	• Muscle coordination becomes poor (e.g., balance, speech, vision, reaction time, and hearing) • Harder to detect danger • Judgment, self-control, reasoning, and memory are impaired	• Concentration • Short-term memory loss • Speed control • Reduced information processing capability (e.g., signal detection, visual search) • Impaired perception

Table 22.1. Continued

Blood Alcohol Concentration (BAC)*	Typical Effects	Predictable Effects on Driving
.10% About 5 alcoholic drinks**	• Clear deterioration of reaction time and control • Slurred speech, poor coordination, and slowed thinking	Reduced ability to maintain lane position and brake appropriately
.15% About 7 alcoholic drinks**	Far less muscle control than normal Vomiting may occur (unless this level is reached slowly or a person has developed a tolerance for alcohol) Major loss of balance	Substantial impairment in vehicle control, attention to driving task, and in necessary visual and auditory information processing

Blood Alcohol Concentration Measurement
The number of drinks listed represents the approximate amount of alcohol that a 160-pound man would need to drink in one hour to reach the listed BAC in each category.

**A Standard Drink Size in the United States*
A standard drink is equal to 14.0 grams (0.6 ounces) of pure alcohol. Generally, this amount of pure alcohol is found in

12-ounces of beer (5% alcohol content)

8-ounces of malt liquor (7% alcohol content)

5-ounces of wine (12% alcohol content)

1.5-ounces or a "shot" of 80-proof (40% alcohol content) distilled spirits or liquor (e.g., gin, rum, vodka, whiskey)

How Can Deaths and Injuries from Impaired Driving Be Prevented?

Effective measures include:

Actively enforcing existing 0.08% BAC laws, minimum legal drinking age laws, and zero tolerance laws for drivers younger than 21 years old in all states.

Requiring ignition interlocks for all offenders, including first-time offenders

Using sobriety checkpoints.

Putting health promotion efforts into practice that influence economic, organizational, policy, and school/community action.

Using community-based approaches to alcohol control and DWI prevention.

Requiring mandatory substance abuse assessment and treatment, if needed, for DWI offenders.

Raising the unit price of alcohol by increasing taxes.

Areas for continued research:

Reducing the illegal BAC threshold to 0.05%.

Mandatory blood alcohol testing when traffic crashes result in injury.

Does marijuana impair driving? How and at what level?

Does marijuana use increase the risk of motor vehicle crashes

What Safety Steps Can Individuals Take?

Whenever your social plans involve alcohol and/or drugs, make plans so that you don't have to drive while impaired. For example:

Before drinking, designate a non-drinking driver when with a group.

Don't let your friends drive impaired.

If you have been drinking or using drugs, get a ride home or call a taxi.

If you're hosting a party where alcohol will be served, remind your guests to plan ahead and designate their sober driver; offer alcohol-free beverages, and make sure all guests leave with a sober driver.

Section 22.5

Older Drivers

This section includes text excerpted from "Older Adult Drivers,"
Center for Disease Control and Prevention (CDC), May 27, 2015.

In 2012, there were almost 36 million licensed drivers ages 65 and older in the United States. Driving helps older adults stay mobile and independent. But the risk of being injured or killed in a motor vehicle crash increases as you age. An average of 586 older adults are injured every day in crashes. Thankfully, there are steps that older adults can take to stay safer on the roads.

How Big Is the Problem?

In 2012, more than 5,560 older adults were killed and more than 214,000 were injured in motor vehicle crashes. This amounts to 15 older adults killed and 586 injured in crashes on average every day.

There were almost 36 million licensed older drivers in 2012, which is a 34 percent increase from 1999.

Who Is Most at Risk?

Per mile traveled, fatal crash rates increase noticeably starting at ages 70–74 and are highest among drivers age 85 and older. This is largely due to increased susceptibility to injury and medical complications among older drivers rather than an increased tendency to get into crashes.

Age-related declines in vision and cognitive functioning (ability to reason and remember), as well as physical changes, may affect some older adults' driving abilities.

Across all age groups, males had substantially higher death rates than females.

How Can Older Driver Deaths and Injuries Be Prevented?

Existing protective factors that may help improve older drivers' safety include:

High incidence of seat belt use

More than three in every four (79%) older motor vehicle occupants (drivers and passengers) involved in fatal crashes were wearing seat belts at the time of the crash, compared to 66% for other adult occupants (18 to 64 years of age).

Tendency to drive when conditions are the safest

Older drivers tend to limit their driving during bad weather and at night and drive fewer miles than younger drivers.

Lower incidence of impaired driving

Older adult drivers are less likely to drink and drive than other adult drivers.8 Only 7% of older drivers involved in fatal crashes had a blood alcohol concentration (BAC) of 0.08 grams per deciliter (g/dL) or higher, compared to 24% of drivers between the ages of 21 and 64 years.

Older adults can take several steps to stay safe on the road, including:

- Exercising regularly to increase strength and flexibility.

- Asking your doctor or pharmacist to review medicines–both prescription and over-the counter–to reduce side effects and interactions.

- Having eyes checked by an eye doctor at least once a year. Wear glasses and corrective lenses as required.

- Driving during daylight and in good weather.

- Finding the safest route with well-lit streets, intersections with left turn arrows, and easy parking.

- Planning your route before you drive.

- Leaving a large following distance behind the car in front of you.

- Avoiding distractions in your car, such as listening to a loud radio, talking on your cell phone, texting, and eating.

- Considering potential alternatives to driving, such as riding with a friend or using public transit, that you can use to get around.

Chapter 23

Other Accidents and Injuries

Chapter Contents

Section 23.1—Falls 266

Section 23.2—Fire-Related Injuries.. 269

Section 23.3—Occupational Injuries... 275

Section 23.4—Poisoning 280

Section 23.5—Water-Related Accidents 284

Section 23.1

Falls

This section includes text excerpted from "Home and Recreational Safety," Centers for Disease Control and Prevention (CDC), September 21, 2015.

Important Facts about Falls

Each year, millions of older people—those 65 and older—fall. In fact, one out of three older people falls each year, but less than half tell their doctor. Falling once doubles your chances of falling again.

Falls Are Serious and Costly

- One out of five falls causes a serious injury such as broken bones or a head injury.

- Each year, 2.5 million older people are treated in emergency departments for fall injuries.

- Over 700,000 patients a year are hospitalized because of a fall injury, most often because of a head injury or hip fracture.

- Each year at least 250,000 older people are hospitalized for hip fractures.

- More than 95% of hip fractures are caused by falling, usually by falling sideways.

- Falls are the most common cause of traumatic brain injuries (TBI).

- Adjusted for inflation, the direct medical costs for fall injuries are $34 billion annually. Hospital costs account for two-thirds of the total.

What Can Happen after a Fall?

Many falls do not cause injuries. But one out of five falls does cause a serious injury such as a broken bone or a head injury. These injuries can make it hard for a person to get around, do everyday activities, or live on their own.

- Falls can cause broken bones, like wrist, arm, ankle, and hip fractures.

- Falls can cause head injuries. These can be very serious, especially if the person is taking certain medicines (like blood thinners). An older person who falls and hits their head should see their doctor right away to make sure they don't have a brain injury.

- Many people who fall, even if they're not injured, become afraid of falling. This fear may cause a person to cut down on their everyday activities. When a person is less active, they become weaker and this increases their chances of falling.

What Conditions Make You More Likely to Fall?

Research has identified many conditions that contribute to falling. These are called risk factors. Many risk factors can be changed or modified to help prevent falls. They include:

- lower body weakness

- vitamin D deficiency (that is, not enough vitamin D in your system)

- difficulties with walking and balance

- use of medicines, such as tranquilizers, sedatives, or antidepressants. Even some over-the-counter medicines can affect balance and how steady you are on your feet.

- vision problems

- foot pain or poor footwear

- home hazards or dangers such as

  - broken or uneven steps,

  - throw rugs or clutter that can be tripped over, and

  - no handrails along stairs or in the bathroom.

Most falls are caused by a combination of risk factors. The more risk factors a person has, the greater their chances of falling.

Healthcare providers can help cut down a person's risk by reducing the fall risk factors listed above.

What You Can Do to Prevent Falls

Falls can be prevented. These are some simple things you can do to keep yourself from falling.

Talk to Your Doctor

- Ask your doctor or healthcare provider to evaluate your risk for falling and talk with them about specific things you can do.
- Ask your doctor or pharmacist to review your medicines to see if any might make you dizzy or sleepy. This should include prescription medicines and over-the counter medicines.
- Ask your doctor or healthcare provider about taking vitamin D supplements with calcium.

Do Strength and Balance Exercises

Do exercises that make your legs stronger and improve your balance. Tai Chi is a good example of this kind of exercise.

Have Your Eyes Checked

Have your eyes checked by an eye doctor at least once a year, and be sure to update your eyeglasses if needed.

If you have bifocal or progressive lenses, you may want to get a pair of glasses with only your distance prescription for outdoor activities, such as walking. Sometimes these types of lenses can make things seem closer or farther away than they really are.

Make Your Home Safer

- get rid of things you could trip over
- add grab bars inside and outside your tub or shower and next to the toilet
- put railings on both sides of stairs
- make sure your home has lots of light by adding more or brighter light bulbs

Section 23.2

Fire-Related Injuries

This section includes text excerpted from "Civilian Fire
Injuries in Residential Buildings (2012–2014)," U.S.
Fire Administration (USFA), July 2016.

Fires can strike anywhere—in structures, buildings, automobiles
and the outdoors. Fires that affect our homes are often the most tragic
and the most preventable. While the loss of our possessions can be
upsetting, often far more devastating are the physical injuries and
psychological impact that fires can inflict on our lives. It is a sad fact
that each year, over 70 percent of all civilian fire injuries occurred as
a result of fires in residential buildings—our homes.

From 2012 to 2014, 78 percent of all civilian fire injuries occurred
in residential buildings. This topical fire report focuses on the characteristics of these injuries as reported to the National Fire Incident
Reporting System (NFIRS) from 2012 to 2014. NFIRS data is used for
the analyses presented throughout this report.

Civilian fire injuries by definition involve people not on active duty
with a firefighting organization who are injured as a result of a fire.
These injuries generally occur from activities of fire control, escaping
from the dangers of fire, or sleeping. Fires resulting in injuries are
those fires where one or more injuries occur.

Annually, from 2012 to 2014, an estimated 12,525 civilian fire
injuries resulted from an estimated 7,900 residential building fires
resulting in injuries and 377,900 total residential building fires. On
average, every 42 minutes someone is injured in a residential building fire.

For the purpose of this report, the term "residential building fires
resulting in injuries" is synonymous with "residential fires resulting in
injuries" and the term "residential building fires" is synonymous with
"residential fires." The term "residential fires resulting in injuries" is
used throughout the body of this report; the findings, tables, charts,
headings and endnotes reflect the full category, "residential building
fires resulting in injuries."

Civilian Injury Rates for Residential Building Fires

Not all fires produce injuries. When civilian fire injuries were averaged over all reported residential fires, the overall injury rate was nearly three civilian injuries per 100 residential fires. Residential fires that resulted in injuries, however, had 130 injuries for every 100 fires. Of the residential fires resulting in injuries, 82 percent resulted in one civilian injury, 13 percent resulted in two civilian injuries, and 6 percent resulted in three or more civilian injuries.

When Residential Building Fires Resulting in Injuries Occur

Residential fires resulting in injuries follow a daily pattern. In addition, unlike fatal residential fires, which occur more frequently in the late night and early morning hours, residential fires resulting in civilian injuries follow a pattern similar to that of all residential fires. Residential fires resulting in injuries occurred most frequently in the late afternoon and early evening hours, when many people are expected to be cooking dinner. The time period from 5 to 8 p.m. accounted for 17 percent of the residential fires resulting in injuries. Cooking, discussed later in the Causes of Residential Building Fires Resulting in Injuries section, was the primary cause (37 percent) for residential fires that resulted in injuries. In general, residential fires resulting in injuries decreased to the lowest point of the day, between 7 and 8 a.m., and then steadily increased during the daytime hours until reaching the daily peak.

Residential fires resulting in injuries also follow a yearly pattern similar to that of all residential fires. In addition, residential fires resulting in injuries tended to follow a seasonal trend, with more fires taking place during the colder months than the warmer months. January, at 10 percent, had the highest incidence of residential fires resulting in injuries. August and September had the least amount of residential fires resulting in injuries at 7 percent. This drop may be explained by a decrease in residential heating fires and their associated injuries during the warmer months. Similar to all fires in residential buildings, residential fires resulting in injuries occurred most often on Saturdays and Sundays.

Cause of Injury

The predominant cause of residential fire injuries, by far, involved exposure to fire products (80 percent), such as flame, heat, smoke or gas. The next two leading causes were exposure to toxic fumes other than smoke (8 percent) and other, unspecified causes (4 percent).

Primary Symptoms of Civilian Fire Injuries

Smoke inhalation and thermal burns were the primary symptoms of reported injuries, accounting for 78 percent of all injuries resulting from residential fires. Smoke inhalation alone accounted for 41 percent of residential fire injuries. Thermal burns (as opposed to scalds or chemical or electrical burns) accounted for another 24 percent, and burns combined with smoke inhalation accounted for an additional 13 percent. Breathing difficulty was reported for only 6 percent of injuries. Scalds (4 percent) and cuts or lacerations (3 percent) accounted for an even smaller proportion of the injuries.

Thermal burns are caused by contact with flames, hot liquids, hot surfaces, and other sources of high heat. Of the thermal burns to the body, 73 percent were to the upper and lower extremities (58 percent and 15 percent, respectively).

Of the smoke inhalation injuries, 70 percent were internal injuries, which are particularly critical, as they can lead to lung damage. The inflammation and damage caused by smoke inhalation to delicate breathing sacs in the lungs actually grow worse in the hours after the incident. A chest X-ray can look clear, and oxygen levels in the blood may appear normal in the first few hours after a fire. A day or two later, however, the victim can suddenly take a turn for the worse as the lungs become unable to properly exchange oxygen.

Based on the severity of the injury, 59 percent of the civilian fire injuries in residential fires were deemed minor. Only 14 percent of the injuries were considered serious or life-threatening.

Areas of the Body Affected

The body parts affected most by residential fire injuries included internal parts (32 percent) and the upper extremities (26 percent). As discussed, the types of injuries that affected most areas of the body consisted of smoke inhalation, thermal burns, or a combination of both.

Factors Contributing to Civilian Fire Injuries

The most notable factors contributing to civilian fire injuries (outside of "other (unspecified) factors") involved escape (27 percent), fire pattern (24 percent), and equipment-related factors (17 percent).

Escape factors include unfamiliarity with exits, excessive travel distance to the nearest clear exit, a choice of an inappropriate exit route, re-entering the building, and clothing catching fire while escaping. Fire pattern factors involve such situations as exits are blocked by smoke and flame, vision is blocked or impaired by smoke, and civilians are trapped above or below the fire. Equipment-related problems include such factors as the improper use of cooking or heating equipment and the use of unvented heating equipment.

Human Factors Contributing to Civilian Fire Injuries

Human factors also play an important role in residential fire injuries. Table 23.1 shows that the leading human factor contributing to injuries was being "asleep" (53 percent).

This is not unexpected, as the largest number of injuries occurred in bedrooms (33 percent). "Possibly impaired by alcohol" (16 percent) was the second leading human factor contributing to injuries. This was followed by "unattended or unsupervised" individuals (11 percent) and people with "physical disabilities" (also 11 percent).

Table 23.1. Human Factors Contributing to Civilian Fire Injuries in Residential Buildings (2012–2014)

Human Factors Contributing to Injury	Percent of Fire Injuries in Residential Buildings (Unknowns Apportioned)
Asleep	52.7
Possibly impaired by alcohol	16.4
Unattended or unsupervised	11.3
Physical disabilities	10.6
Possibly impaired by other drug or chemical	9
Possible intellectual disabilities	7.7
Unconscious	5.3
Physically restrained	0.8

Causes of Residential Building Fires Resulting in Injuries

"Cooking" (37 percent) was the leading reported cause of residential fires that resulted in injuries. "Open flame" (9 percent) and "other unintentional, careless" actions (8 percent) were the next leading causes. "Open flame" includes torches, candles, matches, lighters, embers and the like. "Other unintentional, careless" actions include misuse of material or product, abandoned or discarded materials or products, and heat source too close to combustibles. These two causes were followed by "appliances" (7 percent), "electrical malfunction" (7 percent) and "smoking" (also 7 percent).

Civilian Activity When Injured

Most civilian fire injuries occurred when the victim was attempting to control the fire (35 percent), followed by attempting to escape (26 percent) and sleeping (12 percent). U.S. Fire Administration (USFA) recommends leaving fighting a fire to trained firefighters and that efforts be focused on following a preset escape plan. To escape a fire, many civilians make the mistake of fleeing through the area where the fire is located. The area of a fire has tremendous heat, smoke and a toxic atmosphere that can render a person unconscious. As a result, it is imperative that an escape plan be prepared and practiced. With a well-thought out plan that includes multiple escape options, the chances of survival and escaping without injuries greatly increase. In addition, it has been demonstrated that people may not wake up from the smell of smoke while sleeping. Therefore, it is also vital that smoke alarms are installed in homes to alert sleeping people to the presence of fire.

Gender, Race, and Ethnicity of Civilian Fire Injuries

Males accounted for 53 percent and females accounted for 47 percent of residential fire injuries. Where racial information was provided, whites constituted 62 percent of the injuries, followed by blacks or African-Americans (30 percent); other, including multiracial (6 percent); Asians (2 percent); American Indians or Alaska Natives (less than 1 percent); and Native Hawaiians or other Pacific Islanders (also less than 1 percent).

The ethnicity element shows that 87 percent of the injuries occurred to non-Hispanics or non-Latinos, compared to Hispanics or Latinos (13 percent). Ethnicity was specified for 40 percent of reported injuries.

Age of Civilians Injured and Activity When Injured

Civilians between the ages of 20 and 49 accounted for 47 percent of injuries in residential fires. An additional 16 percent of those with injuries were less than 20 years old. Adults aged 50 and over accounted for the remaining 37 percent of those with injuries.

The first reaction of civilians of all ages is either to try to control or escape the fire. At the time of injury, for those aged 10 and over, trying to control the fire and escaping were the two leading activities that resulted in injuries. Those aged 10–69 primarily got injured trying to control the fire (38 percent), followed by trying to escape the fire (24 percent). Those aged 70 and over primarily got injured trying to escape the fire (34 percent), followed by trying to control the fire (22 percent).

For children aged 0–9, escaping and sleeping were the two leading activities that resulted in injuries. Those aged 0–9 primarily got injured when trying to escape the fire (40 percent), followed by sleeping (26 percent).

The young and the very old are less likely to be as mobile or ready to act in a fire situation. Infants, young children and older adults may require special provisions in a fire or emergency situation. Thus, it is not surprising that these individuals are less likely to attempt to control the fire.

Table 23.2. Leading Activities Resulting in Civilian Fire Injuries in Residential Buildings by Age Group (2012–2014)

Percent of Fire Injuries Where Age and Activity Reported (2012–2014)			
Age Group	**Fire Control**	**Escaping**	**Sleeping**
0–9	8.2	39.7	26.2
20–29	37.2	28.6	10.2
30–39	41.6	23.9	8.4
40–49	43.3	20.7	8.2
50–59	39.2	21	10.9
60–69	35.2	24	11.7
70–79	28.7	27.7	12.1
80–89	23.4	33.6	13.8
90+	15.1	30.2	14.2
Overall	21.2	34.5	11.9

Section 23.3

Occupational Injuries

This section includes text excerpted from "National Census
of Fatal Occupational Injuries in 2014," Bureau of Labor
Statistics (BLS), September 17, 2015.

Key preliminary findings of the 2014 Census of Fatal Occupational Injuries

- The number of fatal work injuries in private goods-producing industries in 2014 was 9 percent higher than the revised 2013 count but slightly lower in private service-providing industries. Fatal injuries were higher in mining (up 17 percent), agriculture (up 14 percent), manufacturing (up 9 percent), and construction (up 6 percent). Fatal work injuries for government workers were lower (down 12 percent).

- Falls, slips, and trips increased 10 percent to 793 in 2014 from 724 in 2013. This was driven largely by an increase in falls to a lower level to 647 in 2014 from 595 in 2013.

- Fatal work injuries involving workers 55 years of age and over rose 9 percent to 1,621 in 2014 up from 1,490 in 2013. The preliminary 2014 count for workers 55 and over is the highest total ever reported by CFOI.

- After a sharp decline in 2013, fatal work injuries among self-employed workers increased 10 percent in 2014 from 950 in 2013 to 1,047 in 2014.

- Fatal work injuries among Hispanic or Latino workers were lower in 2014, while fatal injuries among non-Hispanic white, black or African-American, and Asian workers were all higher.

- In 2014, 797 decedents were identified as contracted workers, 6 percent higher than the 749 fatally-injured contracted workers reported in 2013. Workers who were contracted at the time of their fatal injury accounted for 17 percent of all fatal work injury cases in 2014.

- The number of fatal work injuries among police officers and police supervisors was higher in 2014, rising from 88 in 2013 to 103 in 2014, an increase of 17 percent.

Worker Characteristics

Fatal injuries to self-employed workers rose 10 percent in 2014 to 1,047, up from 950 in 2013. Although higher than in 2013, the 2014 preliminary total for self-employed workers is about the same as the 10-year average for the series. Fatal injuries among wage and salary workers remained at about the same level as in 2013.

Fatal work injuries involving workers age 45 to 54 years, 55 to 64 years, and 65 years of age and over all increased in 2014 compared to 2013 totals. The number of workers 55 years and over who were fatally injured in 2014 increased 9 percent to 1,621, the highest annual total since the inception of the fatality census in 1992. Workers of a wide variety of ages are included in the 2014 CFOI counts–8 workers under the age of 16 are included as well as 8 workers age 90 and over. Fatal work injuries among men in 2014 were slightly higher than the previous year. Consistent with previous years, men accounted for 92 percent of all fatal occupational injuries. Fatal work injuries among Hispanic or Latino workers fell 3 percent to 789 in 2014, compared to 817 in 2013. Fatal work injuries were higher among non-Hispanic white, non-Hispanic black or African-American, and non-Hispanic Asian workers. Overall, there were 827 fatal work injuries involving foreign-born workers in 2014. These 827 foreign born workers came from over 80 different countries, of which the greatest share (334 or 40 percent) was born in Mexico. Of the 789 fatal work injuries incurred by Hispanic or Latino workers, 503 (64 percent) involved foreign-born workers. Of the 134 fatal work injuries incurred by non-Hispanic Asian workers, 116 (87 percent) involved foreign-born workers.

Type of Incident

In 2014, fatal work injuries due to transportation incidents were slightly higher–1,891, up from 1,865 in 2013. Overall, transportation incidents accounted for 40 percent of fatal workplace injuries in 2014. Within the transportation event category, roadway incidents consti-tuted 57 percent of the fatal work injury total in 2014. The second largest number of transportation fatalities in 2014 involved pedestrian vehicular incidents (17 percent). Fatalities resulting from pedestrian vehicular incidents were up 6 percent from last year's revised count

(313 in 2014 up from 294 in 2013). Rail vehicle incidents also increased in 2014, rising 34 percent to 55 fatal injuries from 41 in 2013. (Note that roadway incident counts presented in this release are expected to rise when updated 2014 data are released in the late spring of 2016 because key source documentation detailing specific transportation-related incidents has not yet been received.) Fatal work injuries due to violence and other injuries by persons or animals were lower in 2014, with 749 deaths in 2014 compared to 773 in 2013. The number of workplace homicides was about the same as the total in 2013, but workplace suicides decreased slightly in 2014, from 282 to 271. In workplace homicides involving men, robbers were the most common type of assailant (33 percent).

Fatal falls, slips, and trips were up 10 percent in 2014 from the previous year. Falls to lower level were up 9 percent to 647 from 595 in 2013, and falls on the same level increased 17 percent. In 532 of the 647 fatal falls to lower level, the height of the fall was known. Of those cases in which the height of fall was known, four-fifths involved falls of 30 feet or less (427) while about two-thirds (340) involved falls of 20 feet or less.

Work-related injury deaths due to contact with objects and equipment were down slightly from the revised 2013 number (721 to 708). The largest proportion of fatal injuries in this category (34 percent) occurred when workers were struck by falling objects or equipment. The next largest share (28 percent) involved injuries in which decedents were struck by powered vehicles in nontransport situations (e.g., struck by a rolling vehicle or by a vehicle that had tipped over while on jacks).

Fatal work injuries due to fires decreased 35 percent from 82 in 2013 to 53 in 2014. Fatal injuries resulting from explosions, however, increased 25 percent to 84 cases, led by an increase in explosions of pressure vessels, piping, or tires. A total of 372 workers were killed in 163 multiple fatality incidents (events where more than one worker was killed).

Occupation

Transportation and material moving occupations accounted for the largest share (28%) of fatal occupational injuries of any occupation group. Fatal work injuries in this group rose 3 percent to 1,289 in 2014, the highest total since 2008. Drivers/sales workers and truck drivers accounted for nearly 2 out of every 3 fatal injuries in this group (835 of the 1,289 fatal injuries in 2014). In this group, drivers/

sales workers increased 74 percent to 54 in 2014, and heavy and trac-tor-trailer drivers had their highest total since 2008 (725 fatalities in 2014).

Fatal work injuries in construction and extraction occupations increased 5 percent (40 cases) in 2014 to 885. This is the highest total for this occupation group since 2008. The fatal injury rate for workers in construction and extraction occupations was 11.8 per 100,000 FTE workers in 2014 and 12.2 per 100,000 FTE workers in 2013. Fatal injuries among construction trades workers increased 3 percent in 2014 to 611 fatalities, the highest count since 2009. Fatal work injuries to construction laborers, the occupation within construction trades workers with the highest number of fatalities, decreased by 14 cases in 2014 to 206. Conversely, the number of fatally-injured electricians increased by 14 cases in 2014 to 78.

The number of fatal work injuries among protective service occu-pations decreased 15 percent in 2014 to 211 fatalities, a series low for this occupation group. This was led by a drop in fatalities among firefighters and first-line supervisors of fire fighting and prevention workers, down 51 percent to 35 in 2014. Fatal injuries to police officers and first-line supervisors of police and detectives, however, increased 17 percent to 103 in 2014.

Fatalities among farming, fishing, and forestry occupations rose 9 percent to 253 in 2014. The increase was led by fatalities involving agricultural workers (up 12 percent to 143) and fatalities involving logging workers (up 31 percent to 77). Fatal injuries to resident mili-tary personnel declined to 55 from 71 in 2013.

Industry

In the private sector, a total of 4,251 fatal work injuries were recorded in 2014, 4 percent higher than the revised total of 4,101 in 2013. Goods-producing industries were up 9 percent in 2014. Totals were higher for private mining, quarrying, and oil and gas extraction (up 17 percent); agriculture, forestry, fishing and hunting (up 14 per-cent); manufacturing (up 9 percent); and construction (up 6 percent). Construction fatalities rose to 874 in 2014 from 828 in 2013. The num-ber of fatal work injuries in construction in 2014 was the highest reported total since 2008. The fatal injury rate for workers in the pri-vate construction industry was 9.5 per 100,000 FTE workers in 2014 and 9.7 per 100,000 FTE workers in 2013. Heavy and civil engineering construction recorded a series low of 138 fatal injuries in 2014, down from 165 in 2013.

Agriculture, forestry, fishing and hunting fatalities were 14 percent higher in 2014 at 568 compared to 500 in 2013. Fatal injuries in forestry and logging rose to 92 in 2014 from 81 in 2013 and the highest total since 2008. Agriculture, forestry, fishing and hunting recorded the highest fatal injury rate of any industry sector at 24.9 fatal work injuries per 100,000 FTE workers in 2014.

Fatal work injuries in the private mining, quarrying, and oil and gas extraction sector were 17 percent higher in 2014, rising to 181 from 155 in 2013, and the fatal injury rate also increased to 14.1 per 100,000 FTE workers in 2014 from 12.4 per 100,000 FTE workers in 2013. While coal mining recorded smaller numbers of fatal work injuries in 2014, the number of fatal work injury cases in oil and gas extraction industries were 27 percent higher in 2014, rising to 142 in 2014 from 112 in 2013. Oil and gas extraction industries include oil and gas extraction (North American Industry Classification System [NAICS] 21111), drilling oil and gas wells (NAICS 213111), and support activities for oil and gas operations (NAICS 213112).

Service-providing industries in the private sector decreased slightly from 2013. Fatal work injuries in transportation and warehousing accounted for 735 fatal work injuries in 2014, almost unchanged from the revised 2013 count of 733 fatalities. Financial activities rose 31 percent, while wholesale trade fell 11 percent.

Fatal occupational injuries among government workers fell 12 percent to a series low of 428 fatal work injuries in 2014, down from 484 in 2013. Federal government work fatalities, which fell 29 percent to 92 in 2014 from 129 in 2013, accounted for most of the decline.

Contracted workers

In 2014, the number of fatal occupational injuries incurred by contracted workers was 797, or 17 percent of all fatal injuries, compared to 749 (16 percent) reported in 2013. Falls to a lower level accounted for 33 percent of contracted worker deaths while struck by object or equipment (17 percent), pedestrian vehicular incidents (12 percent), and exposure to electricity (9 percent) incidents were also frequent events among contracted workers. These four types of incidents each constituted a greater share of fatalities among contracted workers than they did for all workers.

Fatally-injured contracted workers were most often contracted by a firm in the private construction industry sector (164 or 21 percent of all contracted workers). They were also frequently contracted by a government entity (148 or 19 percent) and by firms in the private financial activities (81 or 10 percent); private mining, quarrying, and oil and gas extraction (72 or 9 percent); and private manufacturing (70 or 9 percent) industry sectors.

Over half of all contracted workers (415 workers) were working in construction and extraction occupations when fatally injured. Decedents in this occupation group were most often employed as construction laborers (108); electricians (48); first-line supervisors of construction trades and extraction workers (44); roofers (42); and painters, construction and maintenance (25). Among contracted workers who were employed outside the construction and extraction occupation group, the largest number of fatal occupational injuries was incurred by heavy and tractor-trailer truck drivers (76 workers); landscaping and groundskeeping workers (21); security guards (17); tree trimmers and pruners (16); heating, air conditioning, and refrigeration mechanics and installers (15); and excavating and loading machine and dragline operators (13).

Section 23.4

Poisoning

This section includes text excerpted from "Tips to Prevent Poisonings," Centers for Disease Control and Prevention (CDC), November 24, 2015.

Poisoning Prevention

Every day, over 300 children in the United States ages 0 to 19 are treated in an emergency department, and two children die, as a result of being poisoned. It's not just chemicals in your home marked with clear warning labels that can be dangerous to children.

Everyday items in your home, such as household cleaners and medicines, can be poisonous to children as well. Medication dosing mistakes and unsupervised ingestions are common ways that children are poisoned. Active, curious children will often investigate—and sometimes try to eat or drink—anything that they can get into.

Thankfully, there are ways you can help poison-proof your home and protect the children you love.

Key Prevention Tips

Lock Them up and Away

Keep medicines and toxic products, such cleaning solutions and detergent pods, in their original packaging where children can't see or get them.

Know the Number

Put the nationwide poison control center phone number, 1-800-222-1222, on or near every telephone in your home and program it into your cell phone. Call the poison control center if you think a child has been poisoned but they are awake and alert; they can be reached 24 hours a day, seven days a week. Call 911 if you have a poison emergency and your child has collapsed or is not breathing.

Read the label

Follow label directions carefully and read all warnings when giving medicines to children.

Don't Keep It If You Don't Need It

Safely dispose of unused, unneeded, or expired prescription drugs and over the counter drugs, vitamins, and supplements. To dispose of medicines, mix them with coffee grounds or kitty litter and throw them away. You can also turn them in at a local take-back program or during National Drug Take-Back events.

Tips to Prevent Poisonings

Safety Tips for You, Your Family, and Friends

Unless noted, the safety tips below were adapted from the American Association of Poison Control Centers' poison prevention tips for children and adults.

Drugs and Medicines

- Only take prescription medications that are prescribed to you by a healthcare professional. Misusing or abusing prescription or over-the-counter medications is not a "safe" alternative to illicit substance abuse.

- Never take larger or more frequent doses of your medications, particularly prescription pain medications, to try to get faster or more powerful effects.

- Never share or sell your prescription drugs. Keep all prescription medicines (especially prescription painkillers, such as those containing methadone, hydrocodone, or oxycodone), over-the-counter medicines (including pain or fever relievers and cough and cold medicines), vitamins and herbals in a safe place that can only be reached by people who take or give them.

- Follow directions on the label when you give or take medicines. Read all warning labels. Some medicines cannot be taken safely when you take other medicines or drink alcohol.

- Turn on a light when you give or take medicines at night so that you know you have the correct amount of the right medicine.

- Keep medicines in their original bottles or containers.

- Monitor the use of medicines prescribed for children and teenagers, such as medicines for attention deficit hyperactivity disorder, or ADHD.

- Dispose of unused, unneeded, or expired prescription drugs

Household Chemicals and Carbon Monoxide

- Always read the label before using a product that may be poisonous.

- Keep chemical products in their original bottles or containers. Do not use food containers such as cups, bottles, or jars to store chemical products such as cleaning solutions or beauty products.

- Never mix household products together. For example, mixing bleach and ammonia can result in toxic gases.

- Wear protective clothing (gloves, long sleeves, long pants, socks, shoes) if you spray pesticides or other chemicals.

- Turn on the fan and open windows when using chemical products such as household cleaners.

Keep Young Children Safe from Poisoning

Be Prepared

Put the poison help number, 1-800-222-1222, on or near every home telephone and save it on your cell phone. The line is open 24 hours a day, 7 days a week.

Be Smart about Storage

- Store all medicines and household products up and away and out of sight in a cabinet where a child cannot reach them.

- When you are taking or giving medicines or are using household products:

  - Do not put your next dose on the counter or table where children can reach them—it only takes seconds for a child to get them.

  - If you have to do something else while taking medicine, such as answer the phone, take any young children with you.

  - Secure the child safety cap completely every time you use a medicine.

  - After using them, do not leave medicines or household products out. As soon as you are done with them, put them away and out of sight in a cabinet where a child cannot reach them.

  - Be aware of any legal or illegal drugs that guests may bring into your home. Ask guests to store drugs where children cannot find them. Children can easily get into pillboxes, purses, backpacks, or coat pockets.

Other Tips

- Do not call medicine "candy."

- Identify poisonous plants in your house and yard and place them out of reach of children or remove them.

What to Do If a Poisoning Occurs

- Remain calm.

- Call 911 if you have a poison emergency and the victim has collapsed or is not breathing. If the victim is awake and alert, dial 1-800-222-1222. Try to have this information ready:

283

- the victim's age and weight
- the container or bottle of the poison if available
- the time of the poison exposure
- the address where the poisoning occurred
- Stay on the phone and follow the instructions from the emergency operator or poison control center.

Section 23.5

Water-Related Accidents

This section includes text excerpted from "Home and Recreational Safety," Centers for Disease Control and Prevention (CDC), May 2, 2016.

Water-Related Injuries

Every day, about ten people die from unintentional drowning. Of these, two will be children aged 14 or younger. Drowning is the fifth leading cause of unintentional injury death for people of all ages, and the second leading cause of injury death for children ages 1 to 14 years.

In fact, more children 1–4 years die from drowning than any other cause of death except birth defects.

Unintentional Drowning: Get the Facts

Every day, about ten people die from unintentional drowning. Of these, two are children aged 14 or younger. Drowning ranks fifth among the leading causes of unintentional injury death in the United States.

How Big Is the Problem?

- From 2005–2014, there were an average of 3,536 fatal unintentional drownings (non-boating related) annually in the United

States—about ten deaths per day. An additional 332 people died each year from drowning in boating-related incidents.

- About one in five people who die from drowning are children 14 and younger. For every child who dies from drowning, another five receive emergency department care for nonfatal submersion injuries.

- More than 50% of drowning victims treated in emergency departments (EDs) require hospitalization or transfer for further care (compared with a hospitalization rate of about 6% for all unintentional injuries). These nonfatal drowning injuries can cause severe brain damage that may result in long-term disabilities such as memory problems, learning disabilities, and permanent loss of basic functioning (e.g., permanent vegetative state).

Who Is Most at Risk?

- **Males:** Nearly 80% of people who die from drowning are male.

- **Children:** Children ages 1 to 4 have the highest drowning rates. In 2014, among children 1 to 4 years old who died from an unintentional injury, one-third died from drowning. Among children ages 1 to 4, most drownings occur in home swimming pools. Drowning is responsible for more deaths among children 1–4 than any other cause except congenital anomalies (birth defects). Among those 1–14, fatal drowning remains the second-leading cause of unintentional injury-related death behind motor vehicle crashes.

- **Minorities:** Between 1999–2010, the fatal unintentional drowning rate for African Americans was significantly higher than that of whites across all ages. The disparity is widest among children 5–18 years old. The disparity is most pronounced in swimming pools; African American children 5–19 drown in swimming pools at rates 5.5 times higher than those of whites. This disparity is greatest among those 11–12 years where African Americans drown in swimming pools at rates 10 times those of whites.

- Factors such as access to swimming pools, the desire or lack of desire to learn how to swim, and choosing water-related recreational activities may contribute to the racial differences in drowning rates. Available rates are based on population, not

on participation. If rates could be determined by actual participation in water-related activities, the disparity in minorities'
drowning rates compared to whites would be much greater.

What Factors Influence Drowning Risk?

The main factors that affect drowning risk are lack of swimming
ability, lack of barriers to prevent unsupervised water access, lack of
close supervision while swimming, location, failure to wear life jackets,
alcohol use, and seizure disorders.

- **Lack of Swimming Ability:** Many adults and children report
  that they can't swim. Research has shown that participation in
  formal swimming lessons can reduce the risk of drowning among
  children aged 1 to 4 years.

- **Lack of Barriers:** Barriers, such as pool fencing, prevent young
  children from gaining access to the pool area without caregivers'
  awareness. A four-sided isolation fence (separating the pool area
  from the house and yard) reduces a child's risk of drowning 83%
  compared to three-sided property-line fencing.

- **Lack of Close Supervision:** Drowning can happen quickly and
  quietly anywhere there is water (such as bathtubs, swimming
  pools, buckets), and even in the presence of lifeguards.

- **Location:** People of different ages drown in different locations.
  For example, most children ages 1–4 drown in home swimming
  pools. The percentage of drownings in natural water settings,
  including lakes, rivers and oceans, increases with age. More
  than half of fatal and nonfatal drownings among those 15 years
  and older (57% and 57% respectively) occurred in natural water
  settings.

- **Failure to Wear Life Jackets:** In 2010, the U.S. Coast Guard
  received reports for 4,604 boating incidents; 3,153 boaters were
  reported injured, and 672 died. Most (72%) boating deaths that
  occurred during 2010 were caused by drowning, with 88% of victims not wearing life jackets.

- **Alcohol Use:** Among adolescents and adults, alcohol use is
  involved in up to 70% of deaths associated with water recreation, almost a quarter of ED visits for drowning, and about one
  in five reported boating deaths. Alcohol influences balance, coordination, and judgment, and its effects are heightened by sun
  exposure and heat.

- **Seizure Disorders:** For persons with seizure disorders, drowning is the most common cause of unintentional injury death, with the bathtub as the site of highest drowning risk.

What Has Research Found?

- **Swimming skills help.** Taking part in in formal swimming lessons reduces the risk of drowning among children aged 1 to 4 years.However, many people don't have basic swimming skills. A CDC study about self-reported swimming ability found that:

  - Younger adults reported greater swimming ability than older adults.

  - Self-reported ability increased with level of education.

  - Among racial groups, African Americans reported the most limited swimming ability.

  - Men of all ages, races, and educational levels consistently reported greater swimming ability than women.

- **Seconds count—learn CPR.** CPR performed by bystanders has been shown to save lives and improve outcomes in drowning victims. The more quickly CPR is started, the better the chance of improved outcomes.

- **Life jackets can reduce risk.** Potentially, half of all boating deaths might be prevented with the use of life jackets.

Tips to Help You Stay Safe in the Water

- **Supervise When in or Around Water.** Designate a responsible adult to watch young children while in the bath and all children swimming or playing in or around water. Supervisors of preschool children should provide "touch supervision", be close enough to reach the child at all times. Because drowning occurs quickly and quietly, adults should not be involved in any other distracting activity (such as reading, playing cards, talking on the phone, or mowing the lawn) while supervising children, even if lifeguards are present.

- **Use the Buddy System.** Always swim with a buddy. Select swimming sites that have lifeguards when possible.

- **Seizure Disorder Safety.** If you or a family member has a seizure disorder, provide one-on-one supervision around water, including swimming pools. Consider taking showers rather than using a bath tub for bathing. Wear life jackets when boating.

- **Learn to Swim.** Formal swimming lessons can protect young children from drowning. However, even when children have had formal swimming lessons, constant, careful supervision when children are in the water, and barriers, such as pool fencing to prevent unsupervised access, are still important.

- **Learn Cardiopulmonary Resuscitation (CPR).** In the time it takes for paramedics to arrive, your CPR skills could save someone's life.

- **Air-Filled or Foam Toys are not safety devices.** Don't use air-filled or foam toys, such as "water wings," "noodles," or inner-tubes, instead of life jackets. These toys are not life jackets and are not designed to keep swimmers safe.

- **Avoid Alcohol.** Avoid drinking alcohol before or during swimming, boating, or water skiing. Do not drink alcohol while supervising children.

- **Don't let swimmers hyperventilate before swimming underwateror try to hold their breath for long periods of time.** This can cause them to pass out (sometimes called "hypoxic blackout" or "shallow water blackout") and drown.

- **Know how to prevent recreational water illnesses**

- **Know the local weather conditions and forecast before swimming or boating.** Strong winds and thunderstorms with lightning strikes are dangerous.

If you have a swimming pool at home:

- **Install Four-Sided Fencing.** Install a four-sided pool fence that completely separates the pool area from the house and yard. The fence should be at least 4 feet high. Use self-closing and self-latching gates that open outward with latches that are out of reach of children. Also, consider additional barriers such as automatic door locks and alarms to prevent access or alert you if someone enters the pool area.

- **Clear the Pool and Deck of Toys.** Remove floats, balls and other toys from the pool and surrounding area immediately after use so children are not tempted to enter the pool area unsupervised.

If you are in and around natural water settings:

- **Use U.S. Coast Guard approved life jackets.** This is important regardless of the distance to be traveled, the size of the boat, or the swimming ability of boaters; life jackets can reduce risk for weaker swimmers too.

- **Know the meaning of and obey warnings represented by colored beach flags.** These may vary from one beach to another.

- **Watch for dangerous waves and signs of rip currents.** Some examples are water that is discolored and choppy, foamy, or filled with debris and moving in a channel away from shore.

- **If you are caught in a rip current, swim parallel to shore.** Once free of the current, swim diagonally toward shore.

Chapter 24

Penile Cancer

The penis is a rod-shaped male reproductive organ that passes sperm and urine from the body. It contains two types of erectile tissue (spongy tissue with blood vessels that fill with blood to make an erection):

- Corpora cavernosa: The two columns of erectile tissue that form most of the penis.

- Corpus spongiosum: The single column of erectile tissue that forms a small portion of the penis. The corpus spongiosum surrounds the urethra (the tube through which urine and sperm pass from the body).

The erectile tissue is wrapped in connective tissue and covered with skin. The glans (head of the penis) is covered with loose skin called the foreskin.

Risk Factors

Anything that increases your chance of getting a disease is called a risk factor. Having a risk factor does not mean that you will get cancer; not having risk factors doesn't mean that you will not get cancer. Talk with your doctor if you think you may be at risk. Risk factors for penile cancer include the following:

Circumcision may help prevent infection with the human papillomavirus (HPV). A circumcision is an operation in which the doctor

This chapter includes text excerpted from "Penile Cancer Treatment (PDQ®)— Patient Version," National Cancer Institute (NCI), July 19, 2016.

removes part or all of the foreskin from the penis. Many boys are circumcised shortly after birth. Men who were not circumcised at birth may have a higher risk of developing penile cancer.

Other risk factors for penile cancer include the following:

- Being age 60 or older.

- Having phimosis (a condition in which the foreskin of the penis cannot be pulled back over the glans).

- Having poor personal hygiene.

- Having many sexual partners.

- Using tobacco products.

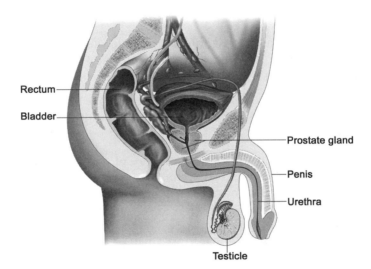

Figure 24.1. *Penile Anatomy*

Anatomy of the male reproductive and urinary systems showing the prostate, penis, testicles, bladder, and other organs.

Signs and Symptoms

These and other signs may be caused by penile cancer or by other conditions. Check with your doctor if you have any of the following:

- Redness, irritation, or a sore on the penis.

- A lump on the penis.

Diagnostic Tests

The following tests and procedures may be used:

- **Physical exam and history:** An exam of the body to check general signs of health, including checking the penis for signs of disease, such as lumps or anything else that seems unusual. A history of the patient's health habits and past illnesses and treatments will also be taken.

- **Biopsy:** The removal of cells or tissues so they can be viewed under a microscope by a pathologist to check for signs of cancer. The tissue sample is removed during one of the following procedures:

  - **Fine-needle aspiration (FNA) biopsy:** The removal of tissue or fluid using a thin needle.

  - **Incisional biopsy:** The removal of part of a lump or a sample of tissue that doesn't look normal.

  - **Excisional biopsy:** The removal of an entire lump or area of tissue that doesn't look normal.

Factors That Affect Prognosis and Treatment Options

The prognosis (chance of recovery) and treatment options depend on the following:

- The stage of the cancer.

- The location and size of the tumor.

- Whether the cancer has just been diagnosed or has recurred (come back).

Stages of Penile Cancer

After penile cancer has been diagnosed, tests are done to find out if cancer cells have spread within the penis or to other parts of the body.

The process used to find out if cancer has spread within the penis or to other parts of the body is called staging. The information gathered from the staging process determines the stage of the disease. It is important to know the stage in order to plan treatment.

The following tests and procedures may be used in the staging process:

CT scan (CAT scan): A procedure that makes a series of detailed pictures of areas inside the body, taken from different angles. The pictures are made by a computer linked to an X-ray machine. A dye may be injected into a vein or swallowed to help the organs or tissues show up more clearly. This procedure is also called computed tomography, computerized tomography, or computerized axial tomography.

MRI (magnetic resonance imaging): A procedure that uses a magnet, radio waves, and a computer to make a series of detailed pictures of areas inside the body. A substance called gadolinium is injected into a vein. The gadolinium collects around the cancer cells so they show up brighter in the picture. This procedure is also called nuclear magnetic resonance imaging (NMRI).

Ultrasound exam: A procedure in which high-energy sound waves (ultrasound) are bounced off internal tissues or organs and make echoes. The echoes form a picture of body tissues called a sonogram.

Chest X-ray: An X-ray of the organs and bones inside the chest. An X-ray is a type of energy beam that can go through the body and onto film, making a picture of areas inside the body.

Biopsy: The removal of cells or tissues so they can be viewed under a microscope by a pathologist to check for signs of cancer. The tissue sample is removed during one of the following procedures:

- **Sentinel lymph node biopsy:** The removal of the sentinel lymph node during surgery. The sentinel lymph node is the first lymph node to receive lymphatic drainage from a tumor. It is the first lymph node the cancer is likely to spread to from the tumor. A radioactive substance and/or blue dye is injected near the tumor. The substance or dye flows through the lymph ducts to the lymph nodes. The first lymph node to receive the substance or dye is removed. A pathologist views the tissue under a microscope to look for cancer cells. If cancer cells are not found, it may not be necessary to remove more lymph nodes.

- **Lymph node dissection:** A procedure to remove one or more lymph nodes during surgery. A sample of tissue is checked under a microscope for signs of cancer. This procedure is also called a lymphadenectomy.

There Are Three Ways That Cancer Spreads in the Body

Cancer can spread through tissue, the lymph system, and the blood:

1. Tissue. The cancer spreads from where it began by growing into nearby areas.

2. Lymph system. The cancer spreads from where it began by getting into the lymph system. The cancer travels through the lymph vessels to other parts of the body.

3. Blood. The cancer spreads from where it began by getting into the blood. The cancer travels through the blood vessels to other parts of the body.

Cancer May Spread from Where It Began to Other Parts of the Body

When cancer spreads to another part of the body, it is called metastasis. Cancer cells break away from where they began (the primary tumor) and travel through the lymph system or blood.

- Lymph system. The cancer gets into the lymph system, travels through the lymph vessels, and forms a tumor (metastatic tumor) in another part of the body.

- Blood. The cancer gets into the blood, travels through the blood vessels, and forms a tumor (metastatic tumor) in another part of the body.

The metastatic tumor is the same type of cancer as the primary tumor. For example, if penile cancer spreads to the lung, the cancer cells in the lung are actually penile cancer cells. The disease is metastatic penile cancer, not lung cancer.

The Following Stages Are Used for Penile Cancer:

Stage 0 (Carcinoma in Situ)

In stage 0, abnormal cells or growths that look like warts are found on the surface of the skin of the penis. These abnormal cells or growths may become cancer and spread into nearby normal tissue. Stage 0 is also called carcinoma in situ.

Stage I

In stage I, cancer has formed and spread to connective tissue just under the skin of the penis. Cancer has not spread to lymph vessels or blood vessels. The tumor cells look a lot like normal cells under a microscope.

Stage II

In stage II, cancer has spread:

- to connective tissue just under the skin of the penis. Also, cancer has spread to lymph vessels or blood vessels or the tumor cells may look very different from normal cells under a microscope; or

- through connective tissue to erectile tissue (spongy tissue that fills with blood to make an erection); or

- beyond erectile tissue to the urethra.

Stage III

Stage III is divided into stage IIIa and stage IIIb.

In stage IIIa, cancer has spread to one lymph node in the groin. Cancer has also spread:

- to connective tissue just under the skin of the penis. Also, cancer may have spread to lymph vessels or blood vessels or the tumor cells may look very different from normal cells under a microscope; or

- through connective tissue to erectile tissue (spongy tissue that fills with blood to make an erection); or

- beyond erectile tissue to the urethra.

In stage IIIb, cancer has spread to more than one lymph node on one side of the groin or to lymph nodes on both sides of the groin. Cancer has also spread:

- to connective tissue just under the skin of the penis. Also, cancer may have spread to lymph vessels or blood vessels or the tumor cells may look very different from normal cells under a microscope; or

- through connective tissue to erectile tissue (spongy tissue that fills with blood to make an erection); or

- beyond erectile tissue to the urethra.

Stage IV

In stage IV, cancer has spread:

- to tissues near the penis such as the prostate, and may have spread to lymph nodes in the groin or pelvis; or

- to one or more lymph nodes in the pelvis, or cancer has spread from the lymph nodes to the tissues around the lymph nodes; or

- to distant parts of the body.

Recurrent Penile Cancer

Recurrent penile cancer is cancer that has recurred (come back) after it has been treated. The cancer may come back in the penis or in other parts of the body.

Treatment Option Overview

Different types of treatments are available for patients with penile cancer. Some treatments are standard (the currently used treatment), and some are being tested in clinical trials. A treatment clinical trial is a research study meant to help improve current treatments or obtain information on new treatments for patients with cancer. When clinical trials show that a new treatment is better than the standard treatment, the new treatment may become the standard treatment. Patients may want to think about taking part in a clinical trial. Some clinical trials are open only to patients who have not started treatment.

Four types of standard treatment are used:

Surgery

Surgery is the most common treatment for all stages of penile cancer. A doctor may remove the cancer using one of the following operations:

- **Mohs microsurgery:** A procedure in which the tumor is cut from the skin in thin layers. During the surgery, the edges of the tumor and each layer of tumor removed are viewed through a microscope to check for cancer cells. Layers continue to be removed until no more cancer cells are seen. This type of surgery removes as little normal tissue as possible and is often used to remove cancer on the skin. It is also called Mohs surgery.

- **Laser surgery:** A surgical procedure that uses a laser beam (a narrow beam of intense light) as a knife to make bloodless cuts in tissue or to remove a surface lesion such as a tumor.

- **Cryosurgery:** A treatment that uses an instrument to freeze and destroy abnormal tissue. This type of treatment is also called cryotherapy.

- **Circumcision:** Surgery to remove part or all of the foreskin of the penis.

- **Wide local excision:** Surgery to remove only the cancer and some normal tissue around it.

- **Amputation of the penis:** Surgery to remove part or all of the penis. If part of the penis is removed, it is a partial penectomy. If all of the penis is removed, it is a total penectomy.

Lymph nodes in the groin may be taken out during surgery.

Even if the doctor removes all the cancer that can be seen at the time of the surgery, some patients may be given chemotherapy or radiation therapy after surgery to kill any cancer cells that are left. Treatment given after the surgery, to lower the risk that the cancer will come back, is called adjuvant therapy.

Radiation Therapy

Radiation therapy is a cancer treatment that uses high-energy X-rays or other types of radiation to kill cancer cells or keep them from growing. There are two types of radiation therapy:

- **External radiation therapy** uses a machine outside the body to send radiation toward the cancer.

- **Internal radiation therapy** uses a radioactive substance sealed in needles, seeds, wires, or catheters that are placed directly into or near the cancer.

The way the radiation therapy is given depends on the type and stage of the cancer being treated. External and internal radiation therapy are used to treat penile cancer.

Chemotherapy

Chemotherapy is a cancer treatment that uses drugs to stop the growth of cancer cells, either by killing the cells or by stopping them from dividing. When chemotherapy is taken by mouth or injected into a vein or muscle, the drugs enter the bloodstream and can reach cancer cells throughout the body (systemic chemotherapy). When chemotherapy is placed directly onto the skin (topical chemotherapy) or into the cerebrospinal fluid, an organ, or a body cavity such as the abdomen, the drugs mainly affect cancer cells in those areas (regional chemotherapy). The way the chemotherapy is given depends on the type and stage of the cancer being treated.

Topical chemotherapy may be used to treat stage 0 penile cancer.

Biologic Therapy

Biologic therapy is a treatment that uses the patient's immune system to fight cancer. Substances made by the body or made in a laboratory are used to boost, direct, or restore the body's natural defenses against cancer. This type of cancer treatment is also called biotherapy or immunotherapy. Topical biologic therapy with imiquimod may be used to treat stage 0 penile cancer.

New Types of Treatment Are Being Tested in Clinical Trials

Radiosensitizers

Radiosensitizers are drugs that make tumor cells more sensitive to radiation therapy. Combining radiation therapy with radiosensitizers helps kill more tumor cells.

Sentinel Lymph Node Biopsy Followed by Surgery

Sentinel lymph node biopsy is the removal of the sentinel lymph node during surgery. The sentinel lymph node is the first lymph node to receive lymphatic drainage from a tumor. It is the first lymph node the cancer is likely to spread to from the tumor. A radioactive substance and/or blue dye is injected near the tumor. The substance or dye flows through the lymph ducts to the lymph nodes. The first lymph node to receive the substance or dye is removed. A pathologist views the tissue under a microscope to look for cancer cells. If cancer cells are not found, it may not be necessary to remove more lymph nodes. After the sentinel lymph node biopsy, the surgeon removes the cancer.

Patients May Want to Think about Taking Part in a Clinical Trial

For some patients, taking part in a clinical trial may be the best treatment choice. Clinical trials are part of the cancer research process.

Clinical trials are done to find out if new cancer treatments are safe and effective or better than the standard treatment.

Many of today's standard treatments for cancer are based on earlier clinical trials. Patients who take part in a clinical trial may receive the standard treatment or be among the first to receive a new treatment.

Patients who take part in clinical trials also help improve the way cancer will be treated in the future. Even when clinical trials do not lead to effective new treatments, they often answer important questions and help move research forward.

Patients Can Enter Clinical Trials before, during, or after Starting Their Cancer Treatment

Some clinical trials only include patients who have not yet received treatment. Other trials test treatments for patients whose cancer has not gotten better. There are also clinical trials that test new ways to stop cancer from recurring (coming back) or reduce the side effects of cancer treatment.

Clinical trials are taking place in many parts of the country. See the Treatment Options section that follows for links to current treatment clinical trials. These have been retrieved from NCI's listing of clinical trials.

Follow-Up Tests May Be Needed

Some of the tests that were done to diagnose the cancer or to find out the stage of the cancer may be repeated. Some tests will be repeated in order to see how well the treatment is working. Decisions about whether to continue, change, or stop treatment may be based on the results of these tests.

Some of the tests will continue to be done from time to time after treatment has ended. The results of these tests can show if your condition has changed or if the cancer has recurred (come back). These tests are sometimes called follow-up tests or check-ups.

Treatment Options for Recurrent Penile Cancer

Treatment of recurrent penile cancer may include the following:

- Surgery (penectomy)
- Radiation therapy
- A clinical trial of biologic therapy
- A clinical trial of chemotherapy

Chapter 25

Prostate Cancer

Prostate Cancer Is a Disease in Which Malignant (Cancer) Cells Form in the Tissues of the Prostate

The prostate is a gland in the male reproductive system. It lies just below the bladder (the organ that collects and empties urine) and in front of the rectum (the lower part of the intestine). It is about the size of a walnut and surrounds part of the urethra (the tube that empties urine from the bladder). The prostate gland makes fluid that is part of the semen.

Prostate cancer is most common in older men. In the United States, about 1 out of 5 men will be diagnosed with prostate cancer.

Signs of Prostate Cancer Include a Weak Flow of Urine or Frequent Urination

These and other signs and symptoms may be caused by prostate cancer or by other conditions. Check with your doctor if you have any of the following:

- weak or interrupted ("stop-and-go") flow of urine

- sudden urge to urinate

- frequent urination (especially at night)

This chapter includes text excerpted from "Prostate Cancer Treatment (PDQ®)–Patient Version," National Cancer Institute (NCI), July 7, 2016.

- trouble starting the flow of urine
- trouble emptying the bladder completely
- pain or burning while urinating
- blood in the urine or semen
- a pain in the back, hips, or pelvis that doesn't go away
- shortness of breath, feeling very tired, fast heartbeat, dizziness, or pale skin caused by anemia

Other conditions may cause the same symptoms. As men age, the prostate may get bigger and block the urethra or bladder. This may cause trouble urinating or sexual problems. The condition is called benign prostatic hyperplasia (BPH), and although it is not cancer, surgery may be needed. The symptoms of benign prostatic hyperplasia or of other problems in the prostate may be like symptoms of prostate cancer.

Tests That Examine the Prostate and Blood Are Used to Detect (Find) and Diagnose Prostate Cancer

The following tests and procedures may be used:

- physical exam and history
- digital rectal exam (DRE)
- prostate-specific antigen (PSA) test
- transrectal ultrasound
- transrectal magnetic resonance imaging (MRI)
- biopsy

Certain Factors Affect Prognosis (Chance of Recovery) and Treatment Options

The prognosis (chance of recovery) and treatment options depend on the following:

- The stage of the cancer (level of PSA, Gleason score, grade of the tumor, how much of the prostate is affected by the cancer, and whether the cancer has spread to other places in the body).
- The patient's age.

- Whether the cancer has just been diagnosed or has recurred (come back).
  Treatment options also may depend on the following:

- Whether the patient has other health problems.

- The expected side effects of treatment.

- Past treatment for prostate cancer.

- The wishes of the patient.

Most men diagnosed with prostate cancer do not die of it.

Stages of Prostate Cancer

After Prostate Cancer Has Been Diagnosed, Tests Are Done to Find out If Cancer Cells Have Spread within the Prostate or to Other Parts of the Body

The process used to find out if cancer has spread within the prostate or to other parts of the body is called staging. The information gathered from the staging process determines the stage of the disease. It is important to know the stage in order to plan treatment. The results of the tests used to diagnose prostate cancer are often also used to stage the disease. In prostate cancer, staging tests may not be done unless the patient has symptoms or signs that the cancer has spread, such as bone pain, a high PSA level, or a high Gleason score.

The following tests and procedures also may be used in the staging process:

- bone scan

- MRI (magnetic resonance imaging)

- CT scan (CAT scan)

- pelvic lymphadenectomy

- seminal vesicle biopsy

- ProstaScint scan

The stage of the cancer is based on the results of the staging and diagnostic tests, including the prostate-specific antigen (PSA) test and the Gleason score. The tissue samples removed during the biopsy are used to find out the Gleason score. The Gleason score ranges from 2–10 and describes how different the cancer cells look from normal cells and how likely it is that the tumor will spread. The lower the number, the less likcly the tumor is to spread.

There Are Three Ways That Cancer Spreads in the Body

Cancer can spread through tissue, the lymph system, and the blood:

- tissue
- lymph system
- blood

Cancer May Spread from Where It Began to Other Parts of the Body

When cancer spreads to another part of the body, it is called metastasis. Cancer cells break away from where they began (the primary tumor) and travel through the lymph system or blood.

- lymph system
- blood

The metastatic tumor is the same type of cancer as the primary tumor. For example, if prostate cancer spreads to the bone, the cancer cells in the bone are actually prostate cancer cells. The disease is metastatic prostate cancer, not bone cancer.

Denosumab, a monoclonal antibody, may be used to prevent bone metastases.

The Following Stages Are Used for Prostate Cancer

Stage I

In stage I, cancer is found in the prostate only. The cancer:

- is found by needle biopsy (done for a high PSA level) or in a small amount of tissue during surgery for other reasons (such as benign prostatic hyperplasia). The PSA level is lower than 10 and the Gleason score is 6 or lower; or

- is found in one-half or less of one lobe of the prostate. The PSA level is lower than 10 and the Gleason score is 6 or lower; or

- cannot be felt during a digital rectal exam and cannot be seen in imaging tests. Cancer is found in one-half or less of one lobe of the prostate. The PSA level and the Gleason score are not known.

Stage II

In stage II, cancer is more advanced than in stage I, but has not spread outside the prostate. Stage II is divided into stages IIA and IIB.

In stage IIA, cancer:

- is found by needle biopsy (done for a high PSA level) or in a small amount of tissue during surgery for other reasons (such as benign prostatic hyperplasia). The PSA level is lower than 20 and the Gleason score is 7; or

- is found by needle biopsy (done for a high PSA level) or in a small amount of tissue during surgery for other reasons (such as benign prostatic hyperplasia). The PSA level is at least 10 but lower than 20 and the Gleason score is 6 or lower; or

- is found in one-half or less of one lobe of the prostate. The PSA level is at least 10 but lower than 20 and the Gleason score is 6 or lower; or

- is found in one-half or less of one lobe of the prostate. The PSA level is lower than 20 and the Gleason score is 7; or

- is found in more than one-half of one lobe of the prostate

In stage IIB, cancer:

- is found in opposite sides of the prostate. The PSA can be any level and the Gleason score can range from 2 to 10; or

- cannot be felt during a digital rectal exam and cannot be seen in imaging tests. The PSA level is 20 or higher and the Gleason score can range from 2 to 10; or

- cannot be felt during a digital rectal exam and cannot be seen in imaging tests. The PSA can be any level and the Gleason score is 8 or higher.

Stage III

In stage III, cancer has spread beyond the outer layer of the prostate and may have spread to the seminal vesicles. The PSA can be any level and the Gleason score can range from 2 to 10.

Stage IV

In stage IV, the PSA can be any level and the Gleason score can range from 2 to 10. Also, cancer:

- has spread beyond the seminal vesicles to nearby tissue or organs, such as the rectum, bladder, or pelvic wall; or

- may have spread to the seminal vesicles or to nearby tissue or organs, such as the rectum, bladder, or pelvic wall. Cancer has spread to nearby lymph nodes; or

- has spread to distant parts of the body, which may include lymph nodes or bones. Prostate cancer often spreads to the bones.

Recurrent Prostate Cancer

Recurrent prostate cancer is cancer that has recurred (come back) after it has been treated. The cancer may come back in the prostate or in other parts of the body.

Treatment Option Overview

There Are Different Types of Treatment for Patients with Prostate Cancer

Different types of treatment are available for patients with prostate cancer. Some treatments are standard (the currently used treatment), and some are being tested in clinical trials. A treatment clinical trial is a research study meant to help improve current treatments or obtain information on new treatments for patients with cancer. When clinical trials show that a new treatment is better than the standard treatment, the new treatment may become the standard treatment. Patients may want to think about taking part in a clinical trial. Some clinical trials are open only to patients who have not started treatment.

Seven Types of Standard Treatment Are Used

Watchful Waiting or Active Surveillance

Watchful waiting and active surveillance are treatments used for older men who do not have signs or symptoms or have other medical conditions and for men whose prostate cancer is found during a screening test.

Watchful waiting is closely monitoring a patient's condition without giving any treatment until signs or symptoms appear or change. Treatment is given to relieve symptoms and improve quality of life.

Active surveillance is closely following a patient's condition without giving any treatment unless there are changes in test results. It is used to find early signs that the condition is getting worse. In active surveillance, patients are given certain exams and tests, including digital rectal exam, PSA test, transrectal ultrasound, and transrectal needle biopsy, to check if the cancer is growing. When the cancer begins to grow, treatment is given to cure the cancer.

Other terms that are used to describe not giving treatment to cure prostate cancer right after diagnosis are observation, watch and wait, and expectant management.

Surgery

Patients in good health whose tumor is in the prostate gland only may be treated with surgery to remove the tumor. The following types of surgery are used:

- radical prostatectomy

  - retropubic prostatectomy

  - perineal prostatectomy

- pelvic lymphadenectomy

- transurethral resection of the prostate (TURP)

In some cases, nerve-sparing surgery can be done. This type of surgery may save the nerves that control erection. However, men with large tumors or tumors that are very close to the nerves may not be able to have this surgery.

Possible problems after prostate cancer surgery include the following:

- impotence

- leakage of urine from the bladder or stool from the rectum

- shortening of the penis (1 to 2 centimeters). The exact reason for this is not known

- inguinal hernia (bulging of fat or part of the small intestine through weak muscles into the groin). Inguinal hernia may occur more often in men treated with radical prostatectomy than in men who have some other types of prostate surgery, radiation therapy, or prostate biopsy alone. It is most likely to occur within the first 2 years after radical prostatectomy

Radiation Therapy and Radiopharmaceutical Therapy

Radiation therapy is a cancer treatment that uses high-energy X-rays or other types of radiation to kill cancer cells or keep them from growing. There are different types of radiation therapy:

- External radiation therapy uses a machine outside the body to send radiation toward the cancer. Conformal radiation is a type of external radiation therapy that uses a computer to make a 3-dimensional (3-D) picture of the tumor and shapes the radiation beams to fit the tumor. This allows a high dose of radiation to reach the tumor and causes less damage to nearby healthy tissue.

  Hypofractionated radiation therapy may be given because it has a more convenient treatment schedule. Hypofractionated radiation therapy is radiation treatment in which a larger than usual total dose of radiation is given once a day over a shorter period of time (fewer days) compared to standard radiation therapy. Hypofractionated radiation therapy may have worse side effects than standard radiation therapy, depending on the schedules used.

- Internal radiation therapy uses a radioactive substance sealed in needles, seeds, wires, or catheters that are placed directly into or near the cancer. In early-stage prostate cancer, the radioactive seeds are placed in the prostate using needles that are inserted through the skin between the scrotum and rectum. The placement of the radioactive seeds in the prostate is guided by images from transrectal ultrasound or computed tomography (CT). The needles are removed after the radioactive seeds are placed in the prostate.

- Radiopharmaceutical therapy uses a radioactivesubstance to treat cancer. Radiopharmaceutical therapy includes the following:

  - Alpha emitter radiation therapy uses a radioactive substance to treat prostate cancer that has spread to the bone. A radioactive substance called radium-223 is injected into a vein and travels through the bloodstream. The radium-223 collects in areas of bone with cancer and kills the cancer cells.

The way the radiation therapy is given depends on the type and stage of the cancer being treated. External radiation therapy, internal radiation therapy, and radiopharmaceutical therapy are used to treat prostate cancer.

Men treated with radiation therapy for prostate cancer have an increased risk of having bladder and/or gastrointestinal cancer.

Radiation therapy can cause impotence and urinary problems.

Hormone Therapy

Hormone therapy is a cancer treatment that removes hormones or blocks their action and stops cancer cells from growing. Hormones are substances made by glands in the body and circulated in the bloodstream. In prostate cancer, male sex hormones can cause prostate cancer to grow. Drugs, surgery, or other hormones are used to reduce the amount of male hormones or block them from working.

Hormone therapy for prostate cancer may include the following:

- Luteinizing hormone-releasing hormone agonists can stop the testicles from making testosterone. Examples are leuprolide, goserelin, and buserelin.

- Antiandrogens can block the action of androgens (hormones that promote male sex characteristics), such as testosterone. Examples are flutamide, bicalutamide, enzalutamide, and nilutamide.

- Drugs that can prevent the adrenal glands from making androgens include ketoconazole and aminoglutethimide.

- Orchiectomy is a surgical procedure to remove one or both testicles, the main source of male hormones, such as testosterone, to decrease the amount of hormone being made.

- Estrogens (hormones that promote female sex characteristics) can prevent the testicles from making testosterone. However, estrogens are seldom used today in the treatment of prostate cancer because of the risk of serious side effects.

Hot flashes, impaired sexual function, loss of desire for sex, and weakened bones may occur in men treated with hormone therapy. Other side effects include diarrhea, nausea, and itching.

Chemotherapy

Chemotherapy is a cancer treatment that uses drugs to stop the growth of cancer cells, either by killing the cells or by stopping them from dividing. When chemotherapy is taken by mouth or injected into a vein or muscle, the drugs enter the bloodstream and can reach cancer cells throughout the body (systemic chemotherapy). When chemotherapy is placed directly into the cerebrospinal fluid, an organ, or a body cavity such as the abdomen, the drugs mainly affect cancer cells in those areas (regional chemotherapy). The way the chemotherapy is given depends on the type and stage of the cancer being treated.

Biologic Therapy

Biologic therapy is a treatment that uses the patient's immune system to fight cancer. Substances made by the body or made in a laboratory are used to boost, direct, or restore the body's natural defenses against cancer. Sipuleucel-T is a type of biologic therapy used to treat prostate cancer that has metastasized (spread to other parts of the body).

Bisphosphonate Therapy

Bisphosphonate drugs, such as clodronate or zoledronate, reduce bone disease when cancer has spread to the bone. Men who are treated with antiandrogen therapy or orchiectomy are at an increased risk of bone loss. In these men, bisphosphonate drugs lessen the risk of bone fracture (breaks). The use of bisphosphonate drugs to prevent or slow the growth of bone metastases is being studied in clinical trials.

There Are Treatments for Bone Pain Caused by Bone Metastases or Hormone Therapy

Prostate cancer that has spread to the bone and certain types of hormone therapy can weaken bones and lead to bone pain. Treatments for bone pain include the following:

- pain medicine
- external radiation therapy
- strontium-89 (a radioisotope)
- targeted therapy with a monoclonal antibody, such as denosumab
- bisphosphonate therapy
- corticosteroids

New Types of Treatment Are Being Tested in Clinical Trials

This section describes treatments that are being studied in clinical trials. It may not mention every new treatment being studied.

Cryosurgery

Cryosurgery is a treatment that uses an instrument to freeze and destroy prostate cancer cells. Ultrasound is used to find the area that will be treated. This type of treatment is also called cryotherapy.

Cryosurgery can cause impotence and leakage of urine from the bladder or stool from the rectum.

High-Intensity–Focused Ultrasound Therapy

High-intensity–focused ultrasound therapy is a treatment that uses ultrasound (high-energy sound waves) to destroy cancer cells. To treat prostate cancer, an endorectal probe is used to make the sound waves.

Proton Beam Radiation Therapy

Proton beam radiation therapy is a type of high-energy, external radiation therapy that targets tumors with streams of protons (small, positively charged particles). This type of radiation therapy is being studied in the treatment of prostate cancer.

Patients May Want to Think about Taking Part in a Clinical Trial

For some patients, taking part in a clinical trial may be the best treatment choice. Clinical trials are part of the cancer research process. Clinical trials are done to find out if new cancer treatments are safe and effective or better than the standard treatment.

Many of today's standard treatments for cancer are based on earlier clinical trials. Patients who take part in a clinical trial may receive the standard treatment or be among the first to receive a new treatment.

Patients who take part in clinical trials also help improve the way cancer will be treated in the future. Even when clinical trials do not lead to effective new treatments, they often answer important questions and help move research forward.

Patients Can Enter Clinical Trials before, during, or after Starting Their Cancer Treatment

Some clinical trials only include patients who have not yet received treatment. Other trials test treatments for patients whose cancer has not gotten better. There are also clinical trials that test new ways to stop cancer from recurring (coming back) or reduce the side effects of cancer treatment.

Clinical trials are taking place in many parts of the country.

Follow-Up Tests May Be Needed

Some of the tests that were done to diagnose the cancer or to find out the stage of the cancer may be repeated. Some tests will be repeated in order to see how well the treatment is working. Decisions about whether to continue, change, or stop treatment may be based on the results of these tests.

Some of the tests will continue to be done from time to time after treatment has ended. The results of these tests can show if your condition has changed or if the cancer has recurred (come back). These tests are sometimes called follow-up tests or check-ups.

Treatment Options by Stage

Stage I Prostate Cancer

Standard treatment of stage I prostate cancer may include the following:

- watchful waiting

- active surveillance. If the cancer begins to grow, hormone therapy may be given

- radical prostatectomy, usually with pelvic lymphadenectomy. Radiation therapy may be given after surgery

- external radiation therapy. Hormone therapy may be given after radiation therapy

- internal radiation therapy with radioactive seeds

- a clinical trial of high-intensity–focused ultrasound therapy

- a clinical trial of cryosurgery

Stage II Prostate Cancer

Standard treatment of stage II prostate cancer may include the following:

- watchful waiting

- active surveillance. If the cancer begins to grow, hormone therapy may be given

- radical prostatectomy, usually with pelvic lymphadenectomy. Radiation therapy may be given after surgery

- external radiation therapy. Hormone therapy may be given after radiation therapy

- internal radiation therapy with radioactive seeds

- a clinical trial of cryosurgery

- a clinical trial of high-intensity–focused ultrasound therapy

- a clinical trial of proton beam radiation therapy

- clinical trials of new types of treatment, such as hormone therapy followed by radical prostatectomy

Stage III Prostate Cancer

Standard treatment of stage III prostate cancer may include the following:

- external radiation therapy. Hormone therapy may be given after radiation therapy

- hormone therapy

- radical prostatectomy. Radiation therapy may be given after surgery

- watchful waiting

- active surveillance. If the cancer begins to grow, hormone therapy may be given

Treatment to control cancer that is in the prostate and lessen urinary symptoms may include the following:

- external radiation therapy

- internal radiation therapy with radioactive seeds

313

- hormone therapy
- transurethral resection of the prostate (TURP)
- a clinical trial of new types of radiation therapy
- a clinical trial of cryosurgery

Stage IV Prostate Cancer

Standard treatment of stage IV prostate cancer may include the following:

- hormone therapy
- hormone therapy combined with chemotherapy
- bisphosphonate therapy
- external radiation therapy. Hormone therapy may be given after radiation therapy
- alpha emitter radiation therapy
- watchful waiting
- active surveillance. If the cancer begins to grow, hormone therapy may be given
- a clinical trial of radical prostatectomy with orchiectomy
  Treatment to control cancer that is in the prostate and lessen urinary symptoms may include the following:
- transurethral resection of the prostate (TURP)
- radiation therapy

Treatment Options for Recurrent Prostate Cancer

Standard treatment of recurrent prostate cancer may include the following:

- hormone therapy
- chemotherapy for patients already treated with hormone therapy
- biologic therapy with sipuleucel-T for patients already treated with hormone therapy
- external radiation therapy
- prostatectomy for patients already treated with radiation therapy
- alpha emitter radiation therapy

Chapter 26

Testicular Cancer

Overview

The testicles are 2 egg-shaped glands located inside the scrotum (a sac of loose skin that lies directly below the penis). The testicles are held within the scrotum by the spermatic cord, which also contains the vas deferens and vessels and nerves of the testicles.

The testicles are the male sex glands and produce testosterone and sperm. Germ cells within the testicles produce immature sperm that travel through a network of tubules (tiny tubes) and larger tubes into the epididymis (a long coiled tube next to the testicles) where the sperm mature and are stored.

Almost all testicular cancers start in the germ cells. The two main types of testicular germ cell tumors are seminomas and nonseminomas. These 2 types grow and spread differently and are treated differently. Nonseminomas tend to grow and spread more quickly than seminomas. Seminomas are more sensitive to radiation. A testicular tumor that contains both seminoma and nonseminoma cells is treated as a nonseminoma.

Testicular cancer is the most common cancer in men 20 to 35 years old.

Health history can affect the risk of testicular cancer.

Anything that increases the chance of getting a disease is called a risk factor. Having a risk factor does not mean that you will get cancer; not having risk factors doesn't mean that you will not get cancer.

This chapter includes text excerpted from "Testicular Cancer Treatment (PDQ®)–Patient Version," National Cancer Institute (NCI), July 7, 2016.

Talk with your doctor if you think you may be at risk. Risk factors for testicular cancer include:

- Having had an undescended testicle.
- Having had abnormal development of the testicles.
- Having a personal history of testicular cancer.
- Having a family history of testicular cancer (especially in a father or brother).
- Being white.

Signs and symptoms of testicular cancer include swelling or discomfort in the scrotum.

These and other signs and symptoms may be caused by testicular cancer or by other conditions. Check with your doctor if you have any of the following:

- A painless lump or swelling in either testicle.
- A change in how the testicle feels.
- A dull ache in the lower abdomen or the groin.
- A sudden build-up of fluid in the scrotum.
- Pain or discomfort in a testicle or in the scrotum.
- Tests that examine the testicles and blood are used to detect (find) and diagnose testicular cancer.

The following tests and procedures may be used:

- Physical exam and history
- Ultrasound exam
- Serum tumor marker test
  - Alpha-fetoprotein (AFP).
  - Beta-human chorionic gonadotropin (β-hCG).
- Inguinal orchiectomy

Certain factors affect prognosis (chance of recovery) and treatment options.

The prognosis (chance of recovery) and treatment options depend on the following:

- Stage of the cancer (whether it is in or near the testicle or has spread to other places in the body, and blood levels of AFP, β-hCG, and LDH).

- Type of cancer.

- Size of the tumor.

- Number and size of retroperitoneal lymph nodes.

Testicular cancer can usually be cured in patients who receive adjuvant chemotherapy or radiation therapy after their primary treatment.

Treatment for testicular cancer can cause infertility.

Certain treatments for testicular cancer can cause infertility that may be permanent. Patients who may wish to have children should consider sperm banking before having treatment. Sperm banking is the process of freezing sperm and storing it for later use.

Stages of Testicular Cancer

After testicular cancer has been diagnosed, tests are done to find out if cancer cells have spread within the testicles or to other parts of the body.

The process used to find out if cancer has spread within the testicles or to other parts of the body is called staging. The information gathered from the staging process determines the stage of the disease. It is important to know the stage in order to plan treatment.

The following tests and procedures may be used in the staging process:

- Chest X-ray

- CT scan (CAT scan)

- PET scan (positron emission tomography scan)

- MRI (magnetic resonance imaging)

- Abdominal lymph node dissection

- Serum tumor marker test

  - Alpha-fetoprotein (AFP)

  - Beta-human chorionic gonadotropin (β-hCG)

  - Lactate dehydrogenase (LDH)

There are three ways that cancer spreads in the body.

Cancer can spread through tissue, the lymph system, and the blood:

- Tissue

- Lymph system

- Blood

Cancer may spread from where it began to other parts of the body.

When cancer spreads to another part of the body, it is called metastasis. Cancer cells break away from where they began (the primary tumor) and travel through the lymph system or blood.

- Lymph system   • Blood

The metastatic tumor is the same type of cancer as the primary tumor. For example, if testicular cancer spreads to the lung, the cancer cells in the lung are actually testicular cancer cells. The disease is metastatic testicular cancer, not lung cancer.

The following stages are used for testicular cancer:

Stage 0 (Testicular Intraepithelial Neoplasia)

In stage 0, abnormal cells are found in the tiny tubules where the sperm cells begin to develop. These abnormal cells may become cancer and spread into nearby normal tissue. All tumor marker levels are normal. Stage 0 is also called testicular intraepithelial neoplasia and testicular intratubular germ cell neoplasia.

Stage I

In stage I, cancer has formed. Stage I is divided into stage IA, stage IB, and stage IS and is determined after an inguinal orchiectomy is done.

- In stage IA, cancer is in the testicle and epididymis and may have spread to the inner layer of the membrane surrounding the testicle. All tumor marker levels are normal.

- In stage IB, cancer:

  - is in the testicle and the epididymis and has spread to the blood vessels or lymph vessels in the testicle; or

  - has spread to the outer layer of the membrane surrounding the testicle; or

  - is in the spermatic cord or the scrotum and may be in the blood vessels or lymph vessels of the testicle.

- All tumor marker levels are normal.
- In stage IS, cancer is found anywhere within the testicle, spermatic cord, or the scrotum and either:
    - all tumor marker levels are slightly above normal; or
    - one or more tumor marker levels are moderately above normal or high.

Stage II

Stage II is divided into stage IIA, stage IIB, and stage IIC and is determined after an inguinal orchiectomy is done.

- In stage IIA, cancer:
    - is anywhere within the testicle, spermatic cord, or scrotum; and
    - has spread to up to 5 lymph nodes in the abdomen, none larger than 2 centimeters.
- All tumor marker levels are normal or slightly above normal.
- In stage IIB, cancer is anywhere within the testicle, spermatic cord, or scrotum; and either:
    - has spread to up to 5 lymph nodes in the abdomen; at least one of the lymph nodes is larger than 2 centimeters, but none are larger than 5 centimeters; or
    - has spread to more than 5 lymph nodes; the lymph nodes are not larger than 5 centimeters.
- All tumor marker levels are normal or slightly above normal.
- In stage IIC, cancer:
    - is anywhere within the testicle, spermatic cord, or scrotum; and
    - has spread to a lymph node in the abdomen that is larger than 5 centimeters.

All tumor marker levels are normal or slightly above normal.

Stage III

Stage III is divided into stage IIIA, stage IIIB, and stage IIIC and is determined after an inguinal orchiectomy is done.

In stage IIIA, cancer:

- is anywhere within the testicle, spermatic cord, or scrotum; and
- may have spread to one or more lymph nodes in the abdomen; and
- has spread to distant lymph nodes or to the lungs.

Tumor marker levels may range from normal to slightly above normal.

In stage IIIB, cancer:

- is anywhere within the testicle, spermatic cord, or scrotum; and
- may have spread to one or more lymph nodes in the abdomen, to distant lymph nodes, or to the lungs.

The level of one or more tumor markers is moderately above normal.

In stage IIIC, cancer:

- is anywhere within the testicle, spermatic cord, or scrotum; and
- may have spread to one or more lymph nodes in the abdomen, to distant lymph nodes, or to the lungs.

The level of one or more tumor markers is high.
or
Cancer:

- is anywhere within the testicle, spermatic cord, or scrotum; and
- may have spread to one or more lymph nodes in the abdomen; and
- has not spread to distant lymph nodes or the lung but has spread to other parts of the body.

Tumor marker levels may range from normal to high.

Treatment Option Overview

There are different types of treatment for patients with testicular cancer.

Different types of treatments are available for patients with testicular cancer. Some treatments are standard (the currently used treatment), and some are being tested in clinical trials. A treatment clinical trial is a research study meant to help improve current treatments or obtain information on new treatments for patients with cancer. When clinical trials show that a new treatment is better than the standard treatment, the new treatment may become the standard treatment. Patients may want to think about taking part in a clinical trial. Some clinical trials are open only to patients who have not started treatment.

Testicular tumors are divided into 3 groups, based on how well the tumors are expected to respond to treatment.

Good Prognosis

For nonseminoma, all of the following must be true:

- The tumor is found only in the testicle or in the retroperitoneum (area outside or behind the abdominal wall); and

- The tumor has not spread to organs other than the lungs; and

- The levels of all the tumor markers are slightly above normal.

For seminoma, all of the following must be true:

- The tumor has not spread to organs other than the lungs; and

- The level of alpha-fetoprotein (AFP) is normal. Beta-human chorionic gonadotropin (β-hCG) and lactate dehydrogenase (LDH) may be at any level.

Intermediate Prognosis

For nonseminoma, all of the following must be true:

- The tumor is found in one testicle only or in the retroperitoneum (area outside or behind the abdominal wall); and

- The tumor has not spread to organs other than the lungs; and

- The level of any one of the tumor markers is more than slightly above normal.

For seminoma, all of the following must be true:

- The tumor has spread to organs other than the lungs; and

- The level of AFP is normal. β-hCG and LDH may be at any level.

Poor Prognosis

For nonseminoma, at least one of the following must be true:

- The tumor is in the center of the chest between the lungs; or

- The tumor has spread to organs other than the lungs; or

- The level of any one of the tumor markers is high.

There is no poor prognosis grouping for seminoma testicular tumors.

Five types of standard treatment are used:

Surgery

Surgery to remove the testicle (inguinal orchiectomy) and some of the lymph nodes may be done at diagnosis and staging. (See the General Information and Stages sections of this summary.) Tumors that have spread to other places in the body may be partly or entirely removed by surgery.

Even if the doctor removes all the cancer that can be seen at the time of the surgery, some patients may be given chemotherapy or radiation therapy after surgery to kill any cancer cells that are left. Treatment given after the surgery, to lower the risk that the cancer will come back, is called adjuvant therapy.

Radiation therapy

Radiation therapy is a cancer treatment that uses high-energy X-rays or other types of radiation to kill cancer cells or keep them from growing. There are two types of radiation therapy:

- External radiation therapy uses a machine outside the body to send radiation toward the cancer.

- Internal radiation therapy uses a radioactive substance sealed in needles, seeds, wires, or catheters that are placed directly into or near the cancer.

The way the radiation therapy is given depends on the type and stage of the cancer being treated. External radiation therapy is used to treat testicular cancer.

Chemotherapy

Chemotherapy is a cancer treatment that uses drugs to stop the growth of cancer cells, either by killing the cells or by stopping the cells from dividing. When chemotherapy is taken by mouth or injected into a vein or muscle, the drugs enter the bloodstream and can reach cancer cells throughout the body (systemic chemotherapy). When chemotherapy is placed directly into the cerebrospinal fluid, an organ, or a body cavity such as the abdomen, the drugs mainly affect cancer cells in those areas (regional chemotherapy). The way the chemotherapy is given depends on the type and stage of the cancer being treated.

Surveillance

Surveillance is closely following a patient's condition without giving any treatment unless there are changes in test results. It is used to find early signs that the cancer has recurred (come back). In surveillance, patients are given certain exams and tests on a regular schedule.

High-dose chemotherapy with stem cell transplant

High-dose chemotherapy with stem cell transplant is a method of giving high doses of chemotherapy and replacing blood-forming cells destroyed by the cancer treatment. Stem cells (immature blood cells) are removed from the blood or bone marrow of the patient or a donor and are frozen and stored. After the chemotherapy is completed, the stored stem cells are thawed and given back to the patient through an infusion. These reinfused stem cells grow into (and restore) the body's blood cells.

New types of treatment are being tested in clinical trials.

Patients may want to think about taking part in a clinical trial.

For some patients, taking part in a clinical trial may be the best treatment choice. Clinical trials are part of the cancer research process. Clinical trials are done to find out if new cancer treatments are safe and effective or better than the standard treatment.

Many of today's standard treatments for cancer are based on earlier clinical trials. Patients who take part in a clinical trial may receive the standard treatment or be among the first to receive a new treatment.

Patients who take part in clinical trials also help improve the way cancer will be treated in the future. Even when clinical trials do not lead to effective new treatments, they often answer important questions and help move research forward.

Patients can enter clinical trials before, during, or after starting their cancer treatment.

Some clinical trials only include patients who have not yet received treatment. Other trials test treatments for patients whose cancer has not gotten better. There are also clinical trials that test new ways to stop cancer from recurring (coming back) or reduce the side effects of cancer treatment.

Clinical trials are taking place in many parts of the country.

Follow-up tests may be needed.

Some of the tests that were done to diagnose the cancer or to find out the stage of the cancer may be repeated. Some tests will be repeated in order to see how well the treatment is working. Decisions about whether to continue, change, or stop treatment may be based on the results of these tests.

Some of the tests will continue to be done from time to time after treatment has ended. The results of these tests can show if your condition has changed or if the cancer has recurred (come back). These tests are sometimes called follow-up tests or check-ups.

Men who have had testicular cancer have an increased risk of developing cancer in the other testicle. A patient is advised to regularly check the other testicle and report any unusual symptoms to a doctor right away.

Long-term clinical exams are very important. The patient will probably have check-ups frequently during the first year after surgery and less often after that.

Chapter 27

Stroke

What Is a Stroke?

A stroke occurs if the flow of oxygen-rich blood to a portion of the brain is blocked. Without oxygen, brain cells start to die after a few minutes. Sudden bleeding in the brain also can cause a stroke if it damages brain cells.

If brain cells die or are damaged because of a stroke, symptoms occur in the parts of the body that these brain cells control. Examples of stroke symptoms include sudden weakness; paralysis or numbness of the face, arms, or legs (paralysis is an inability to move); trouble speaking or understanding speech; and trouble seeing.

A stroke is a serious medical condition that requires emergency care. A stroke can cause lasting brain damage, long-term disability, or even death.

If you think you or someone else is having a stroke, call 9–1–1 right away. Do not drive to the hospital or let someone else drive you. Call an ambulance so that medical personnel can begin life-saving treatment on the way to the emergency room. During a stroke, every minute counts.

Overview

The two main types of stroke are ischemic and hemorrhagic. Ischemic is the more common type of stroke.

This chapter includes text excerpted from "Stroke," National Heart, Lung, and Blood Institute (NHLBI), June 22, 2016.

An ischemic stroke occurs if an artery that supplies oxygen-rich blood to the brain becomes blocked. Blood clots often cause the blockages that lead to ischemic strokes.

A hemorrhagic stroke occurs if an artery in the brain leaks blood or ruptures (breaks open). The pressure from the leaked blood damages brain cells. High blood pressure and aneurysms are examples of conditions that can cause hemorrhagic strokes. (Aneurysms are balloon-like bulges in an artery that can stretch and burst.)

Another condition that's similar to a stroke is a transient ischemic attack, also called a TIA or "mini-stroke." A TIA occurs if blood flow to a portion of the brain is blocked only for a short time. Thus, damage to the brain cells isn't permanent (lasting).

Like ischemic strokes, TIAs often are caused by blood clots. Although TIAs are not full-blown strokes, they greatly increase the risk of having a stroke. If you have a TIA, it's important for your doctor to find the cause so you can take steps to prevent a stroke.

Both strokes and TIAs require emergency care.

Outlook

Stroke is a leading cause of death in the United States. Many factors can raise your risk of having a stroke. Talk with your doctor about how you can control these risk factors and help prevent a stroke.

If you have a stroke, prompt treatment can reduce damage to your brain and help you avoid lasting disabilities. Prompt treatment also may help prevent another stroke.

Types of Stroke

Ischemic Stroke

An ischemic stroke occurs if an artery that supplies oxygen-rich blood to the brain becomes blocked. Blood clots often cause the blockages that lead to ischemic strokes.

The two types of ischemic stroke are thrombotic and embolic. In a thrombotic stroke, a blood clot (thrombus) forms in an artery that supplies blood to the brain.

In an embolic stroke, a blood clot or other substance (such as plaque, a fatty material) travels through the bloodstream to an artery in the brain. (A blood clot or piece of plaque that travels through the bloodstream is called an embolus.)

With both types of ischemic stroke, the blood clot or plaque blocks the flow of oxygen-rich blood to a portion of the brain.

Hemorrhagic Stroke

A hemorrhagic stroke occurs if an artery in the brain leaks blood or ruptures (breaks open). The pressure from the leaked blood damages brain cells.

Other Names for a Stroke

- Brain attack

- Cerebrovascular accident (CVA)

- Hemorrhagic stroke (includes intracerebral hemorrhage and subarachnoid hemorrhage)

- Ischemic stroke (includes thrombotic stroke and embolic stroke)

- A transient ischemic attack sometimes is called a TIA or mini-stroke. A TIA has the same symptoms as a stroke, and it increases your risk of having a stroke.

What Causes a Stroke?

Ischemic Stroke and Transient Ischemic Attack

An ischemic stroke or transient ischemic attack (TIA) occurs if an artery that supplies oxygen-rich blood to the brain becomes blocked. Many medical conditions can increase the risk of ischemic stroke or TIA.

For example, atherosclerosis is a disease in which a fatty substance called plaque builds up on the inner walls of the arteries. Plaque hardens and narrows the arteries, which limits the flow of blood to tissues and organs (such as the heart and brain).

Plaque in an artery can crack or rupture (break open). Blood platelets, which are disc-shaped cell fragments, stick to the site of the plaque injury and clump together to form blood clots. These clots can partly or fully block an artery.

Plaque can build up in any artery in the body, including arteries in the heart, brain, and neck. The two main arteries on each side of the neck are called the carotid arteries. These arteries supply oxygen-rich blood to the brain, face, scalp, and neck.

When plaque builds up in the carotid arteries, the condition is called carotid artery disease. Carotid artery disease causes many of the ischemic strokes and TIAs that occur in the United States.

An embolic stroke (a type of ischemic stroke) or TIA also can occur if a blood clot or piece of plaque breaks away from the wall of an artery.

The clot or plaque can travel through the bloodstream and get stuck in one of the brain's arteries. This stops blood flow through the artery and damages brain cells.

Heart conditions and blood disorders also can cause blood clots that can lead to a stroke or TIA. For example, atrial fibrillation, or AF, is a common cause of embolic stroke.

In AF, the upper chambers of the heart contract in a very fast and irregular way. As a result, some blood pools in the heart. The pooling increases the risk of blood clots forming in the heart chambers.

An ischemic stroke or TIA also can occur because of lesions caused by atherosclerosis. These lesions may form in the small arteries of the brain, and they can block blood flow to the brain.

Hemorrhagic Stroke

Sudden bleeding in the brain can cause a hemorrhagic stroke. The bleeding causes swelling of the brain and increased pressure in the skull. The swelling and pressure damage brain cells and tissues.

Examples of conditions that can cause a hemorrhagic stroke include high blood pressure, aneurysms, and arteriovenous malformations (AVMs).

"Blood pressure" is the force of blood pushing against the walls of the arteries as the heart pumps blood. If blood pressure rises and stays high over time, it can damage the body in many ways.

Aneurysms are balloon-like bulges in an artery that can stretch and burst. AVMs are tangles of faulty arteries and veins that can rupture within the brain. High blood pressure can increase the risk of hemorrhagic stroke in people who have aneurysms or AVMs.

What Are the Signs and Symptoms of a Stroke?

The signs and symptoms of a stroke often develop quickly. However, they can develop over hours or even days.

The type of symptoms depends on the type of stroke and the area of the brain that's affected. How long symptoms last and how severe they are vary among different people.

Signs and symptoms of a stroke may include:

- Sudden weakness

- Paralysis (an inability to move) or numbness of the face, arms, or legs, especially on one side of the body

- Confusion

- Trouble speaking or understanding speech

- Trouble seeing in one or both eyes

- Problems breathing

- Dizziness, trouble walking, loss of balance or coordination, and unexplained falls

- Loss of consciousness

- Sudden and severe headache

A transient ischemic attack (TIA) has the same signs and symptoms as a stroke. However, TIA symptoms usually last less than 1–2 hours (although they may last up to 24 hours). A TIA may occur only once in a person's lifetime or more often.

At first, it may not be possible to tell whether someone is having a TIA or stroke. All stroke-like symptoms require medical care.

If you think you or someone else is having a TIA or stroke, call 9–1–1 right away. Do not drive to the hospital or let someone else drive you. Call an ambulance so that medical personnel can begin life-saving treatment on the way to the emergency room. During a stroke, every minute counts.

Stroke Complications

After you've had a stroke, you may develop other complications, such as:

- Blood clots and muscle weakness. Being immobile (unable to move around) for a long time can raise your risk of developing blood clots in the deep veins of the legs. Being immobile also can lead to muscle weakness and decreased muscle flexibility.

- Problems swallowing and pneumonia. If a stroke affects the muscles used for swallowing, you may have a hard time eating or drinking. You also may be at risk of inhaling food or drink into your lungs. If this happens, you may develop pneumonia.

- Loss of bladder control. Some strokes affect the muscles used to urinate. You may need a urinary catheter (a tube placed into the bladder) until you can urinate on your own. Use of these catheters can lead to urinary tract infections. Loss of bowel control or constipation also may occur after a stroke.

How Is a Stroke Diagnosed?

Your doctor will diagnose a stroke based on your signs and symptoms, your medical history, a physical exam, and test results.

Your doctor will want to find out the type of stroke you've had, its cause, the part of the brain that's affected, and whether you have bleeding in the brain.

If your doctor thinks you've had a transient ischemic attack (TIA), he or she will look for its cause to help prevent a future stroke.

Medical History and Physical Exam

Your doctor will ask you or a family member about your risk factors for stroke. Examples of risk factors include high blood pressure, smoking, heart disease, and a personal or family history of stroke. Your doctor also will ask about your signs and symptoms and when they began.

During the physical exam, your doctor will check your mental alertness and your coordination and balance. He or she will check for numbness or weakness in your face, arms, and legs; confusion; and trouble speaking and seeing clearly.

Your doctor will look for signs of carotid artery disease, a common cause of ischemic stroke. He or she will listen to your carotid arteries with a stethoscope. A whooshing sound called a bruit may suggest changed or reduced blood flow due to plaque buildup in the carotid arteries.

Diagnostic Tests and Procedures

Your doctor may recommend one or more of the following tests to diagnose a stroke or TIA.

- brain computed tomography

- magnetic resonance imaging

- carotid ultrasound

- carotid angiography

- heart tests

  - EKG (Electrocardiogram)

  - echocardiography

How Is a Stroke Treated?

Treatment for a stroke depends on whether it is ischemic or hemorrhagic. Treatment for a transient ischemic attack (TIA) depends on its cause, how much time has passed since symptoms began, and whether you have other medical conditions.

Strokes and TIAs are medical emergencies. If you have stroke symptoms, call 9–1–1 right away. Do not drive to the hospital or let someone else drive you. Call an ambulance so that medical personnel can begin lifesaving treatment on the way to the emergency room. During a stroke, every minute counts.

Once you receive immediate treatment, your doctor will try to treat your stroke risk factors and prevent complications by recommending heart-healthy lifestyle changes.

Treating an Ischemic Stroke or Transient Ischemic Attack

An ischemic stroke or TIA occurs if an artery that supplies oxygen-rich blood to the brain becomes blocked. Often, blood clots cause the blockages that lead to ischemic strokes and TIAs. Treatment for an ischemic stroke or TIA may include medicines and medical procedures.

Medicines

If you have a stroke caused by a blood clot, you may be given a clot-dissolving, or clot-busting medication called tissue plasminogen activator (tPA). A doctor will inject tPA into a vein in your arm. This type of medication must be given within 4 hours of symptom onset. Ideally, it should be given as soon as possible. The sooner treatment begins, the better your chances of recovery. Thus, it's important to know the signs and symptoms of a stroke and to call 9–1–1 right away for emergency care.

If you can't have tPA for medical reasons, your doctor may give you antiplatelet medicine that helps stop platelets from clumping together to form blood clots or anticoagulant medicine (blood thinner) that keeps existing blood clots from getting larger. Two common medicines are aspirin and clopidogrel.

Medical Procedures

If you have carotid artery disease, your doctor may recommend a carotid endarterectomy or carotid artery angioplasty. Both procedures open blocked carotid arteries.

Researchers are testing other treatments for ischemic stroke, such as intra-arterial thrombolysis and mechanical clot removal in cerebral ischemia (MERCI).

In intra-arterial thrombolysis, a long flexible tube called a catheter is put into your groin (upper thigh) and threaded to the tiny arteries of the brain. Your doctor can deliver medicine through this catheter to break up a blood clot in the brain.

MERCI is a device that can remove blood clots from an artery. During the procedure, a catheter is threaded through a carotid artery to the affected artery in the brain. The device is then used to pull the blood clot out through the catheter.

Treating a Hemorrhagic Stroke

A hemorrhagic stroke occurs if an artery in the brain leaks blood or ruptures. The first steps in treating a hemorrhagic stroke are to find the cause of bleeding in the brain and then control it. Unlike ischemic strokes, hemorrhagic strokes aren't treated with antiplatelet medicines and blood thinners because these medicines can make bleeding worse.

If you're taking antiplatelet medicines or blood thinners and have a hemorrhagic stroke, you'll be taken off the medicine. If high blood pressure is the cause of bleeding in the brain, your doctor may prescribe medicines to lower your blood pressure. This can help prevent further bleeding.

Surgery also may be needed to treat a hemorrhagic stroke. The types of surgery used include aneurysm clipping, coil embolization, and arteriovenous malformation (AVM) repair.

Aneurysm Clipping and Coil Embolization

If an aneurysm (a balloon-like bulge in an artery) is the cause of a stroke, your doctor may recommend aneurysm clipping or coil embolization.

Aneurysm clipping is done to block off the aneurysm from the blood vessels in the brain. This surgery helps prevent further leaking of blood from the aneurysm. It also can help prevent the aneurysm from bursting again. During the procedure, a surgeon will make an incision (cut) in the brain and place a tiny clamp at the base of the aneurysm. You'll be given medicine to make you sleep during the surgery. After the surgery, you'll need to stay in the hospital's intensive care unit for a few days.

Coil embolization is a less complex procedure for treating an aneurysm. The surgeon will insert a tube called a catheter into an artery in the groin. He or she will thread the tube to the site of the aneurysm. Then, a tiny coil will be pushed through the tube and into the aneurysm. The coil will cause a blood clot to form, which will block blood flow through the aneurysm and prevent it from bursting again. Coil embolization is done in a hospital. You'll be given medicine to make you sleep during the surgery.

Arteriovenous Malformation Repair

If an AVM is the cause of a stroke, your doctor may recommend an AVM repair. (An AVM is a tangle of faulty arteries and veins that can rupture within the brain.) AVM repair helps prevent further bleeding in the brain.

Doctors use several methods to repair AVMs. These methods include:

- Injecting a substance into the blood vessels of the AVM to block blood flow

- Surgery to remove the AVM

- Using radiation to shrink the blood vessels of the AVM

Treating Stroke Risk Factors

After initial treatment for a stroke or TIA, your doctor will treat your risk factors. He or she may recommend heart-healthy lifestyle changes to help control your risk factors.

Heart-healthy lifestyle changes may include:

- Heart-healthy eating

- Aiming for a healthy weight

- Managing stress

- Physical activity

- Quitting smoking

If heart-healthy lifestyle changes aren't enough, you may need medicine to control your risk factors.

How Can a Stroke Be Prevented?

Taking action to control your risk factors can help prevent or delay a stroke. If you've already had a stroke, these actions can help prevent another one.

- Be physically active

- Don't smoke

- Aim for a healthy weight

- Make heart-healthy eating choices

- Manage stress

If you or someone in your family has had a stroke, be sure to tell your doctor. By knowing your family history of stroke, you may be able to lower your risk factors and prevent or delay a stroke. If you've had a transient ischemic attack (TIA), don't ignore it. TIAs are warnings, and it's important for your doctor to find the cause of the TIA so you can take steps to prevent a stroke.

Chapter 28

Suicide

Overview

Suicide is a serious public health problem that causes immeasurable pain, suffering, and loss to individuals, families, and communities nationwide. The causes of suicide are complex and determined by multiple combinations of factors, such as mental illness, substance abuse, painful losses, exposure to violence, and social isolation. Suicide prevention efforts seek to:

- Reduce factors that increase the risk for suicidal thoughts and behaviors

- Increase the factors that help strengthen, support, and protect individuals from suicide

Ideally, these efforts address individual, relationship, community, and societal factors while promoting hope, easing access into effective treatment, encouraging connectedness, and supporting recovery.

Nearly 40,000 people in the United States die from suicide annually, or 1 person every 13 minutes. This exceeds the rate of death from homicide and AIDS combined. More people die by suicide than from automobile accidents.

The suicide rate has been rising over the past decade, with much of the increase driven by suicides in mid-life, where the majority of

---

This chapter includes text excerpted from "Suicide Prevention," Substance Abuse and Mental Health Services Administration (SAMHSA), October 29, 2015.

all suicides in the United States now occur. From 1999 to 2013, the age-adjusted suicide rate for all ages in the United States increased (10.5% to 13.5%). Half of these deaths occur by use of a firearm.

Of all the death attributed to suicide in 2013, 78% of those are male. In 2013, the latest year for which data is available, the highest number of suicides among both men and women occurred among those aged 45 to 54. The highest rates of suicides (suicides per 100,000) occurred among men aged 75 and up and among women aged 45 to 54. Suicide was the second leading cause of death for young people ages 15 to 24 and for those aged 25 to 34.

Suicidal thoughts are also a significant concern. Having serious thoughts of suicide increases the risk of a person making an actual suicide attempt. There are more than 25 attempted suicides for each suicide death. In 2014, an estimated 9.4 million adults (3.9%) aged 18 or older had serious thoughts of suicide in the past year. A report on Suicidal Thoughts and Behaviors Among Adults from the 2014 NSDUH report showed that the percentage was highest among people aged 18 to 25, followed by people aged 26 to 49, then by people aged 50 or older. Among high school students, more than 17% (approximately 2.5 million ninth through twelfth graders) have seriously considered suicide, more than 13% have made a suicide plan, and more than 8% have attempted suicide.

The most critical risk factors for suicide are prior suicide attempts, mood disorders (such as depression), alcohol and drug use, and access to lethal means. In 2008, alcohol was a factor in approximately one-third of suicides reported in 16 states. According to SAMHSA's Drug Abuse Warning Network report on drug-related emergency department visits, in 2011, there was a 51% increase in drug-related suicide attempt visits to hospital emergency departments among people aged 12 and older.

Suicide touches all ages and backgrounds, all racial and ethnic groups, in all parts of the country. However, some populations are at higher risk for suicidal behavior. For example, the emotional toll of a person's suicide can put surviving family, friends, and other loved ones at greater risk of dying by suicide.

Fortunately, there is strong evidence that a comprehensive public health approach is effective in reducing suicide rates. Released by the U.S. Surgeon General and the National Action Alliance for Suicide Prevention in 2012, the National Strategy for Suicide Prevention is intended to guide suicide prevention actions in the United States over the next decade. The strategy provides guidance for schools, businesses, health systems, clinicians, and others, and emphasizes the role every American can play in protecting their friends, family members, and colleagues from suicide.

Warning Signs of Suicidal Behavior

These signs may mean that someone is at risk for suicide. Risk is greater if the behavior is new, or has increased, and if it seems related to a painful event, loss, or change:

- Talking about wanting to die or kill oneself.
- Looking for a way to kill oneself.
- Talking about feeling hopeless or having no reason to live.
- Talking about feeling trapped or being in unbearable pain.
- Talking about being a burden to others.
- Increasing the use of alcohol or drugs.
- Acting anxious or agitated; behaving recklessly.
- Sleeping too little or too much.
- Withdrawing or feeling isolated.
- Showing rage or talking about seeking revenge.
- Displaying extreme mood swings.

What You Can Do

If you believe someone may be thinking about suicide:

- Ask them if they are thinking about killing themselves. (This will not put the idea into their head or make it more likely that they will attempt suicide.)
- Listen without judging and show you care.
- Stay with the person (or make sure the person is in a private, secure place with another caring person) until you can get further help.
- Remove any objects that could be used in a suicide attempt.
- Call SAMHSA's National Suicide Prevention Lifeline at 1-800-273-TALK (8255) and follow their guidance.
- If danger for self-harm seems imminent, call 911.

Everyone has a role to play in preventing suicide. For instance, faith communities can work to prevent suicide simply by fostering cultures and norms that are life-preserving, providing perspective and social support to community members, and helping people navigate the struggles of life to find a sustainable sense of hope, meaning, and purpose.

Schools and Campus Suicide Prevention

SAMHSA's Garrett Lee Smith Campus Suicide Prevention Program provides funding to institutions of higher education to identify students who are at risk for suicide and suicide attempts, increase protective factors that promote mental health, reduce risk factors for suicide, and reduce suicides and suicide attempts.

Many of SAMHSA's Garrett Lee Smith Youth Suicide Prevention and Early Intervention grantees focus efforts on middle and high schools. SAMHSA also funded the development of Preventing Suicide: A Toolkit for High Schools–2012 to help high schools, school districts, and their partners design and implement strategies to prevent suicide and promote behavioral health among their students.

Now Is The Time—Prevention and Early Intervention

On January 16, 2013, President Barack Obama released the Now Is The Time plan, which outlines how the nation can better support the behavioral health needs of young people. Since then, SAMHSA has played a key role in supporting activities outlined in the plan, including developing and funding new grant programs.

Screening and Assessment Tools

Most people who die by suicide had seen a healthcare provider in the year prior to their suicide. Further, many people visited a healthcare provider in the month prior to their suicide. Screening and assessing for suicide risk is an important aspect of suicide prevention.

Suicide Attempt Survivors

Although prior suicide attempts is one of the strongest risk factors for suicide, the vast majority of people who attempt suicide (9 in 10) do not ultimately die by suicide. A growing number of people who have lived through suicidal experiences are writing and speaking about their experiences, connecting with one another, and sharing their pathways to wellness and recovery.

Loss Survivors

Losing a loved one to suicide can be profoundly painful for family members and friends. SAMHSA's Suicide Prevention Resource Center helps loss survivors find local and national organizations, websites, and other resources that provide support, healing, and a sense of community.

Part Three

Sexual and Reproductive Concerns

Chapter 29

Kidney and Urological Disorders

Chapter Contents

Section 29.1—Kidney Stones...344

Section 29.2—Urinary Incontinence in Men 351

Section 29.1

Kidney Stones

This section includes text excerpted from "Kidney Stones in Adults,"
National Institute of Diabetes and Digestive and Kidney Diseases
(NIDDK), February 2013. Reviewed August 2016.

What Is a Kidney Stone?

A kidney stone is a solid piece of material that forms in a kidney
when substances that are normally found in the urine become highly
concentrated. A stone may stay in the kidney or travel down the urinary
tract. Kidney stones vary in size. A small stone may pass on its own,
causing little or no pain. A larger stone may get stuck along the urinary
tract and can block the flow of urine, causing severe pain or bleeding.

Kidney stones are one of the most common disorders of the urinary
tract. Each year in the United States, people make more than a million visits to healthcare providers and more than 300,000 people go to
emergency rooms for kidney stone problems.

Urolithiasis is the medical term used to describe stones occurring in
the urinary tract. Other frequently used terms are urinary tract stone
disease and nephrolithiasis. Terms that describe the location of the
stone in the urinary tract are sometimes used. For example, a ureteral
stone—or ureterolithiasis—is a kidney stone found in the ureter.

Who Gets Kidney Stones?

Anyone can get a kidney stone, but some people are more likely to get
one. Men are affected more often than women, and kidney stones are more
common in non-Hispanic white people than in non-Hispanic black people
and Mexican Americans. Overweight and obese people are more likely to
get a kidney stone than people of normal weight. In the United States, 8.8
percent of the population, or one in 11 people, have had a kidney stone.

What Causes Kidney Stones?

Kidney stones can form when substances in the urine—such as calcium, oxalate, and phosphorus—become highly concentrated. Certain

foods may promote stone formation in people who are susceptible, but scientists do not believe that eating any specific food causes stones to form in people who are not susceptible. People who do not drink enough fluids may also be at higher risk, as their urine is more concentrated.

People who are at increased risk of kidney stones are those with

- hypercalciuria, a condition that runs in families in which urine contains unusually large amounts of calcium; this is the most common condition found in those who form calcium stones

- a family history of kidney stones

- cystic kidney diseases, which are disorders that cause fluid-filled sacs to form on the kidneys

- hyperparathyroidism, a condition in which the parathyroid glands, which are four pea-sized glands located in the neck, release too much hormone, causing extra calcium in the blood

- renal tubular acidosis, a disease that occurs when the kidneys fail to excrete acids into the urine, which causes a person's blood to remain too acidic

- cystinuria, a condition in which urine contains high levels of the amino acid cystine

- hyperoxaluria, a condition in which urine contains unusually large amounts of oxalate

- hyperuricosuria, a disorder of uric acid metabolism

- gout, a disorder that causes painful swelling of the joints

- blockage of the urinary tract

- chronic inflammation of the bowel

- a history of gastrointestinal (GI) tract surgery

Others at increased risk of kidney stones are people taking certain medications including

- diuretics—medications that help the kidneys remove fluid from the body

- calcium-based antacids

- the protease inhibitor indinavir (Crixivan), a medication used to treat HIV infection

- the anti-seizure medication topiramate (Topamax)

What Are the Types of Kidney Stones?

Four major types of kidney stones can form:

1. **Calcium stones** are the most common type of kidney stone and occur in two major forms: calcium oxalate and calcium phosphate. Calcium oxalate stones are more common. Calcium oxalate stone formation may be caused by high calcium and high oxalate excretion. Calcium phosphate stones are caused by the combination of high urine calcium and alkaline urine, meaning the urine has a high pH.

2. **Uric acid stones** form when the urine is persistently acidic. A diet rich in purines—substances found in animal protein such as meats, fish, and shellfish—may increase uric acid in urine. If uric acid becomes concentrated in the urine, it can settle and form a stone by itself or along with calcium.

3. **Struvite stones** result from kidney infections. Eliminating infected stones from the urinary tract and staying infection-free can prevent more struvite stones.

4. **Cystine stones** result from a genetic disorder that causes cystine to leak through the kidneys and into the urine, forming crystals that tend to accumulate into stones.

What Are the Symptoms of Kidney Stones?

People with kidney stones may have pain while urinating, see blood in the urine, or feel a sharp pain in the back or lower abdomen. The pain may last for a short or long time. People may experience nausea and vomiting with the pain. However, people who have small stones that pass easily through the urinary tract may not have symptoms at all.

How Are Kidney Stones Diagnosed?

To diagnose kidney stones, the healthcare provider will perform a physical exam and take a medical history. The medical history may include questions about family history of kidney stones, diet, GI problems, and other diseases and disorders. The healthcare provider may perform urine, blood, and imaging tests, such as an X-ray or computerized tomography (CT) scan to complete the diagnosis.

- urinalysis
- blood test

- abdominal X-ray
- CT scans

How Are Kidney Stones Treated?

Treatment for kidney stones usually depends on their size and what they are made of, as well as whether they are causing pain or obstructing the urinary tract. Kidney stones may be treated by a general practitioner or by a urologist—a doctor who specializes in the urinary tract. Small stones usually pass through the urinary tract without treatment. Still, the person may need pain medication and should drink lots of fluids to help move the stone along. Pain control may consist of oral or intravenous (IV) medication, depending on the duration and severity of the pain. IV fluids may be needed if the person becomes dehydrated from vomiting or an inability to drink. A person with a larger stone, or one that blocks urine flow and causes great pain, may need more urgent treatment, such as

- **Shock wave lithotripsy.** A machine called a lithotripter is used to crush the kidney stone. The procedure is performed by a urologist on an outpatient basis and anesthesia is used. In shock wave lithotripsy, the person lies on a table or, less commonly, in a tub of water above the lithotripter. The lithotripter generates shock waves that pass through the person's body to break the kidney stone into smaller pieces to pass more readily through the urinary tract.

- **Ureteroscopy.** A ureteroscope—a long, tubelike instrument with an eyepiece—is used to find and retrieve the stone with a small basket or to break the stone up with laser energy. The procedure is performed by a urologist in a hospital with anesthesia. The urologist inserts the ureteroscope into the person's urethra and slides the scope through the bladder and into the ureter. The urologist removes the stone or, if the stone is large, uses a flexible fiber attached to a laser generator to break the stone into smaller pieces that can pass out of the body in the urine. The person usually goes home the same day.

- **Percutaneous nephrolithotomy.** In this procedure, a wire-thin viewing instrument called a nephroscope is used to locate and remove the stone. The procedure is performed by a urologist in a hospital with anesthesia. During the procedure, a tube is inserted directly into the kidney through a small incision in the

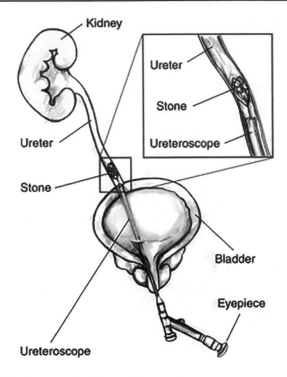

Figure 29.1. *Ureteroscopic Stone Removal*

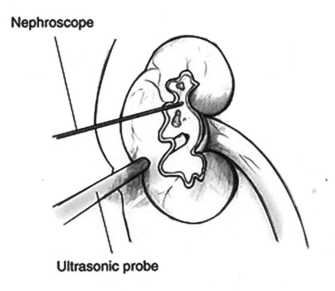

Figure 29.2. *Percutaneous Nephrolithotomy*

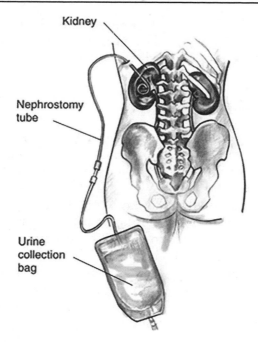

Figure 29.3. *Nephrostomy Tube*

person's back. For large stones, an ultrasonic probe that acts as a lithotripter may be needed to deliver shock waves that break the stone into small pieces that can be removed more easily. The person may have to stay in the hospital for several days after the procedure and may have a small tube called a nephrostomy tube inserted through the skin into the kidney. The nephrostomy tube drains urine and any residual stone fragments from the kidney into a urine collection bag. The tube is usually left in the kidney for 2 or 3 days while the person remains in the hospital.

How Are Kidney Stones Prevented?

The first step in preventing kidney stones is to understand what is causing the stones to form. The healthcare provider may ask the person to try to catch the kidney stone as it passes, so it can be sent to a lab for analysis. Stones that are retrieved surgically can also be sent to a lab for analysis.

The healthcare provider may ask the person to collect urine for 24 hours after a stone has passed or been removed to measure daily urine volume and mineral levels. Producing too little urine or having a mineral abnormality can make a person more likely to form stones. Kidney stones may be prevented through changes in eating, diet, and nutrition and medications.

Eating, Diet, and Nutrition

People can help prevent kidney stones by making changes in their fluid intake. Depending on the type of kidney stone a person has, changes in the amounts of sodium, animal protein, calcium, and oxalate consumed can also help.

Drinking enough fluids each day is the best way to help prevent most types of kidney stones. Healthcare providers recommend that a person drink 2 to 3 liters of fluid a day. People with cystine stones may need to drink even more. Though water is best, other fluids may also help prevent kidney stones, such as orange juice or lemonade. Talk with your healthcare provider if you can't drink the recommended amount due to other health problems, such as urinary incontinence, urinary frequency, or kidney failure.

Recommendations based on the specific type of kidney stone include the following:

Calcium Oxalate Stones

- reducing sodium
- reducing animal protein, such as meat, eggs, and fish
- getting enough calcium from food or taking calcium supplements with food
- avoiding foods high in oxalate, such as spinach, rhubarb, nuts, and wheat bran

Calcium Phosphate Stones

- reducing sodium
- reducing animal protein
- getting enough calcium from food or taking calcium supplements with food

Uric Acid Stones

limiting animal protein

Medications

The healthcare provider may prescribe certain medications to help prevent kidney stones based on the type of stone formed or conditions that make a person more prone to form stones:

- hyperuricosuria—allopurinol (Zyloprim), which decreases uric acid in the blood and urine

- hypercalciuria—diuretics, such as hydrochlorothiazide

- hyperoxaluria—potassium citrate to raise the citrate and pH of urine

- uric acid stones—allopurinol and potassium citrate

- cystine stones—mercaptopropionyl glycine, which decreases cystine in the urine, and potassium citrate

- struvite stones—antibiotics, which are bacteria-fighting medications, when needed to treat infections, or acetohydroxamic acid with long-term antibiotic medications to prevent infection

People with hyperparathyroidism sometimes develop calcium stones. Treatment in these cases is usually surgery to remove the parathyroid glands. In most cases, only one of the glands is enlarged. Removing the glands cures hyperparathyroidism and prevents kidney stones.

Section 29.2

Urinary Incontinence in Men

This section includes text excerpted from "Urinary Incontinence in Men," National Institute of Diabetes and Digestive and Kidney Diseases (NIDDK), November 2015.

What Is Urinary Incontinence (UI) in Men?

Urinary incontinence is the loss of bladder control, resulting in the accidental leakage of urine from the body. For example, a man may feel a strong, sudden need, or urgency, to urinate just before losing a large amount of urine, called urgency incontinence.

UI can be slightly bothersome or totally debilitating. For some men, the chance of embarrassment keeps them from enjoying many activities, including exercising, and causes emotional distress. When people are inactive, they increase their chances of developing other health problems, such as obesity and diabetes.

What Causes Urinary Incontinence in Men?

Urinary incontinence in men results when the brain does not properly signal the bladder, the sphincters do not squeeze strongly enough, or both. The bladder muscle may contract too much or not enough because of a problem with the muscle itself or the nerves controlling the bladder muscle. Damage to the sphincter muscles themselves or the nerves controlling these muscles can result in poor sphincter function. These problems can range from simple to complex.

A man may have factors that increase his chances of developing UI, including

- Birth defects

- A history of prostate cancer

UI is not a disease. Instead, it can be a symptom of certain conditions or the result of particular events during a man's life. Conditions or events that may increase a man's chance of developing UI include

- benign prostatic hyperplasia (BPH)

- chronic coughing

- neurological problems

- physical inactivity

- obesity

- older age

What Are the Types of Urinary Incontinence in Men?

The types of UI in men include

- urgency incontinence

- stress incontinence

- functional incontinence

- overflow incontinence
- transient incontinence

Urgency Incontinence

Urgency incontinence happens when a man urinates involuntarily after he has a strong desire, or urgency, to urinate. Involuntary bladder contractions are a common cause of urgency incontinence. Abnormal nerve signals might cause these bladder contractions.

Triggers for men with urgency incontinence include drinking a small amount of water, touching water, hearing running water, or being in a cold environment—even if for just a short while—such as reaching into the freezer at the grocery store. Anxiety or certain liquids, medications, or medical conditions can make urgency incontinence worse.

The following conditions can damage the spinal cord, brain, bladder nerves, or sphincter nerves, or can cause involuntary bladder contractions leading to urgency incontinence:

- Alzheimer disease
- Injury to the brain or spinal cord that interrupts nerve signals to and from the bladder
- Multiple sclerosis
- Parkinson disease
- Stroke

Urgency incontinence is a key sign of overactive bladder. Overactive bladder occurs when abnormal nerves send signals to the bladder at the wrong time, causing its muscles to squeeze without enough warning time to get to the toilet.

Stress Incontinence

Stress incontinence results from movements that put pressure on the bladder and cause urine leakage, such as coughing, sneezing, laughing, or physical activity. In men, stress incontinence may also occur

- after prostate surgery
- after neurologic injury to the brain or spinal cord
- after trauma, such as injury to the urinary tract
- during older age

Functional Incontinence

Functional incontinence occurs when physical disability, external obstacles, or problems in thinking or communicating keep a person from reaching a place to urinate in time. For example, a man with Alzheimer disease may not plan ahead for a timely trip to a toilet. A man in a wheelchair may have difficulty getting to a toilet in time. Arthritis—pain and swelling of the joints—can make it hard for a man to walk to the restroom quickly or open his pants in time.

Overflow Incontinence

When the bladder doesn't empty properly, urine spills over, causing overflow incontinence. Weak bladder muscles or a blocked urethra can cause this type of incontinence. Nerve damage from diabetes or other diseases can lead to weak bladder muscles; tumors and urinary stones can block the urethra. Men with overflow incontinence may have to urinate often, yet they release only small amounts of urine or constantly dribble urine.

Transient Incontinence

Transient incontinence is UI that lasts a short time. Transient incontinence is usually a side effect of certain medications, drugs, or temporary conditions, such as

- a urinary tract infection (UTI)
- caffeine or alcohol consumption
- chronic coughing
- constipation
- blood pressure medications
- short-term mental impairment
- short-term restricted mobility

How Common Is Urinary Incontinence in Men?

Urinary incontinence occurs in 11 to 34 percent of older men. Two to 11 percent of older men report daily UI. Although more women than men develop UI, the chances of a man developing UI increase with age because he is more likely to develop prostate problems as he ages. Men are also less likely to speak with a healthcare professional about UI, so UI in men is probably far more common than statistics show. Having a discussion with a healthcare professional about UI is the first step to fixing this treatable problem.

How Is Urinary Incontinence in Men Diagnosed?

Men should tell a healthcare professional, such as a family practice physician, a nurse, an internist, or a urologist—a doctor who specializes in urinary problems—they have UI, even if they feel embarrassed. To diagnose UI, the healthcare professional will

- take a medical history
- conduct a physical exam
- order diagnostic tests

Medical History

Taking a medical history can help a healthcare professional diagnose UI. He or she will ask the patient or caretaker to provide a medical history, a review of symptoms, a description of eating habits, and a list of prescription and over-the-counter medications the patient is taking. The healthcare professional will ask about current and past medical conditions.

The healthcare professional also will ask about the man's pattern of urination and urine leakage. To prepare for the visit with the healthcare professional, a man may want to keep a bladder diary for several days beforehand. Information that a man should record in a bladder diary includes

- the amount and type of liquid he drinks
- how many times he urinates each day and how much urine is released
- how often he has accidental leaks
- whether he felt a strong urge to go before leaking
- what he was doing when the leak occurred, for example, coughing or lifting
- how long the symptoms have been occurring

The healthcare professional also may ask about other lower urinary tract symptoms that may indicate a prostate problem, such as

- problems starting a urine stream

- problems emptying the bladder completely

- spraying urine

- dribbling urine

- weak stream

- recurrent UTIs

- painful urination

Physical Exam

A physical exam may help diagnose UI. The healthcare professional will perform a physical exam to look for signs of medical conditions that may cause UI. The healthcare professional may order further neurologic testing if necessary.

Digital rectal exam. The healthcare professional also may perform a digital rectal exam. A digital rectal exam is a physical exam of the prostate and rectum.

The healthcare professional may diagnose the type of UI based on the medical history and physical exam, or he or she may use the findings to determine if a man needs further diagnostic testing.

Diagnostic Tests

The healthcare professional may order one or more of the following diagnostic tests based on the results of the medical history and physical exam:

- urinalysis

- urine culture

- blood test

- urodynamic testing

  - Uroflowmetry, which measures how rapidly the bladder releases urine

  - Postvoid residual measurement, which evaluates how much urine remains in the bladder after urination

  - Reduced urine flow or residual urine in the bladder, which often suggests urine blockage due to BPH

How Is Urinary Incontinence in Men Treated?

Treatment depends on the type of UI.

Urgency Incontinence

As a first line of therapy for urgency incontinence, a healthcare professional may recommend the following techniques to treat a man's problem:

- behavioral and lifestyle changes
- bladder training
- pelvic floor exercises
- urgency suppression

If those treatments are not successful, the following additional measures may help urgency incontinence:

- medications
- electrical nerve stimulation
- bulking agents
- surgery

A healthcare professional may recommend other treatments for men with urgency incontinence caused by BPH.

Behavioral and lifestyle changes. Men with urgency incontinence may be able to reduce leaks by making behavioral and lifestyle changes:

- eating, diet, and nutrition
- engaging in physical activity
- losing weight
- preventing constipation

Bladder training. Bladder training is changing urination habits to decrease incidents of UI. The healthcare professional may suggest a man use the restroom at regular timed intervals, called timed voiding, based on the man's bladder diary. A man can gradually lengthen the time between trips to the restroom to help stretch the bladder so it can hold more urine.

Pelvic floor muscle exercises. Pelvic floor muscle, or Kegel, exercises involve strengthening pelvic floor muscles. Strong pelvic floor muscles hold in urine more effectively than weak muscles. A man does not need special equipment for Kegel exercises. The exercises involve tightening and relaxing the muscles that control urine flow. Pelvic floor exercises should not be performed during urination. A healthcare professional can help a man learn proper technique.

Men also may learn how to perform Kegel exercises properly by using biofeedback. Biofeedback uses special sensors to measure bodily functions, such as muscle contractions that control urination. A video monitor displays the measurements as graphs, and sounds indicate when the man is using the correct muscles. The healthcare professional uses the information to help the man change abnormal function of the pelvic floor muscles. At home, the man practices to improve muscle function. The man can perform the exercises while lying down, sitting at a desk, or standing up. Success with pelvic floor exercises depends on the cause of UI, its severity, and the man's ability to perform the exercises.

Urgency suppression. By using certain techniques, a man can suppress the urge to urinate, called urgency suppression. Urgency suppression is a way for a man to train his bladder to maintain control so he does not have to panic about finding a restroom. Some men use distraction techniques to take their mind off the urge to urinate. Other men find taking long, relaxing breaths and being still can help. Doing pelvic floor exercises also can help suppress the urge to urinate.

Medications. Healthcare professionals may prescribe medications that relax the bladder, decrease bladder spasms, or treat prostate enlargement to treat urgency incontinence in men.

- **Alpha-blockers.** Terazosin (Hytrin), doxazosin (Cardura), tamsulosin (Flomax), alfuzosin (Uroxatral), and silodosin (Rapaflo) are used to treat problems caused by prostate enlargement and bladder outlet obstruction. These medications relax the smooth muscle of the prostate and bladder neck, which lets urine flow normally and prevents abnormal bladder contractions that can lead to urgency incontinence.

- **Antimuscarinics.** Antimuscarinics can help relax bladder muscles and prevent bladder spasms. These medications include oxybutynin (Oxytrol), tolterodine (Detrol), darifenacin (Enablex), trospium (Sanctura), fesoterodine (Toviaz), and solifenacin (VESIcare). They are available in pill, liquid, and patch form.

- **Beta-3 agonists.** Mirabegron (Myrbetriq) is a beta-3 agonist a person takes by mouth to help prevent symptoms of urgency incontinence. Mirabegron suppresses involuntary bladder contractions.

- **Botox.** A healthcare professional may use onabotulinumtoxinA (Botox), also called botulinum toxin type A, to treat UI in men with neurological conditions such as spinal cord injury or multiple sclerosis. Injecting Botox into the bladder relaxes the bladder, increasing storage capacity and decreasing UI. A healthcare professional performs the procedure during an office visit. A man receives local anesthesia. The healthcare professional uses a cystoscope to guide the needle for injecting the Botox. Botox is effective for up to 10 months.

- **5-alpha reductase inhibitors.** Finasteride (Proscar) and dutasteride (Avodart) block the production of the male hormone dihydrotestosterone, which accumulates in the prostate and may cause prostate growth. These medications may help to relieve urgency incontinence problems by shrinking an enlarged prostate.

- **Tricyclic antidepressants.** Tricyclic antidepressants such as imipramine (Tofranil) can calm nerve signals, decreasing spasms in bladder muscles.

Electrical nerve stimulation. If behavioral and lifestyle changes and medications do not improve symptoms, a urologist may suggest electrical nerve stimulation as an option to prevent UI, urinary frequency—urination more often than normal—and other symptoms. Electrical nerve stimulation involves altering bladder reflexes using pulses of electricity. The two most common types of electrical nerve stimulation are percutaneous tibial nerve stimulation and sacral nerve stimulation.

- **Percutaneous tibial nerve stimulation** uses electrical stimulation of the tibial nerve, which is located in the ankle, on a weekly basis. The patient receives local anesthesia for the procedure. In an outpatient center, a urologist inserts a battery-operated stimulator beneath the skin near the tibial nerve. Electrical stimulation of the tibial nerve prevents bladder activity by interfering with the pathway between the bladder and the spinal cord or brain. Although researchers consider percutaneous tibial nerve stimulation safe, they continue to study the exact ways that it prevents symptoms and how long the treatment can last.

- **Sacral nerve stimulation** involves implanting a battery-operated stimulator beneath the skin in the lower back near the sacral nerve. The procedure takes place in an outpatient center using local anesthesia. Based on the patient's feedback, the healthcare professional can adjust the amount of stimulation so it works best for that individual. The electrical pulses enter the body for minutes to hours, two or more times a day, either through wires placed on the lower back or just above the pubic area—between the navel and the pubic hair. Sacral nerve stimulation may increase blood flow to the bladder, strengthen pelvic muscles that help control the bladder, and trigger the release of natural substances that block pain. The patient can turn the stimulator on or off at any time.

A patient may consider getting an implanted device that delivers regular impulses to the bladder. A urologist places a wire next to the tailbone and attaches it to a permanent stimulator under the skin.

Bulking agents. A urologist injects bulking agents, such as collagen and carbon spheres, near the urinary sphincter to treat incontinence. The bulking agent makes the tissues thicker and helps close the bladder opening. Before the procedure, the healthcare professional may perform a skin test to make sure the man doesn't have an allergic reaction to the bulking agent. A urologist performs the procedure during an office visit. The man receives local anesthesia. The urologist uses a cystoscope—a tubelike instrument used to look inside the urethra and bladder—to guide the needle for injection of the bulking agent. Over time, the body may slowly eliminate certain bulking agents, so a man may need to have injections again.

Surgery. As a last resort, surgery to treat urgency incontinence in men includes the artificial urinary sphincter (AUS) and the male sling. A healthcare professional performs the surgery in a hospital with regional or general anesthesia. Most men can leave the hospital the same day, although some may need to stay overnight.

Stress Incontinence

Men who have stress incontinence can use the same techniques for treating urgency incontinence.

Functional Incontinence

Men with functional incontinence may wear protective undergarments if they worry about reaching a restroom in time. These products include adult diapers or pads and are available from drugstores, grocery stores, and medical supply stores. Men who have functional incontinence should talk to a healthcare professional about its cause and how to prevent or treat functional incontinence.

Overflow Incontinence

A healthcare professional treats overflow incontinence caused by a blockage in the urinary tract with surgery to remove the obstruction. Men with overflow incontinence that is not caused by a blockage may need to use a catheter to empty the bladder. A catheter is a thin, flexible tube that is inserted through the urethra into the bladder to drain urine. A healthcare professional can teach a man how to use a catheter. A man may need to use a catheter once in a while, a few times a day, or all the time. Catheters that are used continuously drain urine from the bladder into a bag that is attached to the man's thigh with a strap. Men using a continuous catheter should watch for symptoms of an infection.

Transient Incontinence

A healthcare professional treats transient incontinence by addressing the underlying cause. For example, if a medication is causing increased urine production leading to UI, a healthcare professional may try lowering the dose or prescribing a different medication. A healthcare professional may prescribe bacteria-fighting medications called antibiotics to treat UTIs.

Chapter 30

Penile Concerns

Chapter Contents

Section 30.1—Circumcision 364

Section 30.2—Balanitis 367

Section 30.3—Penile Intraepithelial Neoplasia
(Erythroplasia of Queyrat) 370

Section 30.4—Penile Trauma 372

Section 30.5—Peyronie Disease 374

Section 30.6—Phimosis and Paraphimosis 381

Section 30.1

Circumcision

This section includes text excerpted from "Male
Circumcision," Centers for Disease Control and
Prevention (CDC), December 21, 2013. Reviewed August 2016.

What Is Male Circumcision?

Male circumcision is the surgical removal of some or all of the foreskin (or prepuce) from the penis.

Male Circumcision and Risk for HIV Acquisition by Heterosexual Men

Several types of research have documented that male circumcision significantly reduces the risk of men contracting HIV through
penile-vaginal sex.

Biologic Plausibility

Compared with the dry external skin surface of the glans penis
and penile shaft, the inner mucosa of the foreskin has less keratini-
zation (deposition of fibrous protein) and a higher density of target
cells for HIV infection. Some laboratory studies have shown the
foreskin is more susceptible to HIV infection than other penile tissue,
although others have failed to show any difference in the ability of
HIV to penetrate inner compared with outer foreskin surface. The
foreskin may also have greater susceptibility to traumatic epithelial
disruptions (tears) during intercourse, providing a portal of entry
for pathogens, including HIV. In addition, the microenvironment in
the preputial sac between the unretracted foreskin and the glans
penis may be conducive to viral survival. Finally, the presence of
other sexually transmitted diseases (STDs), which independently
may be more common in uncircumcised men, increase the risk for
HIV acquisition.

Male Circumcision and Other Health Conditions

Carcinogenic subtypes of human papillomavirus (HPV)—which are believed to cause 100 percent of cervical cancers, 90 percent of anal cancers, and 40 percent of cancers of the penis, vulva, and vagina—have also been associated with lack of circumcision in men. A Ugandan RCT found a lower prevalence of high-risk HPV subtypes among men in the circumcised group. In a South African trial, circumcision was also associated with a lower prevalence of high-risk HPV subtypes. These prevalence associations may result from an effect of circumcision on HPV acquisition by men, its persistence, or both. The Ugandan RCT also found incidence of high-risk HPV infection among women to be lower among those with circumcised male partners.

Risks Associated with Male Circumcision

In large studies of infant circumcision in the United States, reported inpatient complication rates are approximately 0.2 percent. The most common complications are bleeding and infection, which are usually minor and easily managed.

Minimizing pain is an important consideration for male circumcision. Appropriate use of analgesia is considered standard of care for the procedure at all ages and can substantially control pain. One study found that 93.5 percent of neonates circumcised in the first week of life using analgesia gave no indication of pain on an objective, standardized neonatal pain rating system.

Effects of Male Circumcision on Penile Sensation and Sexual Function

Well-designed studies of sexual sensation and function in relation to male circumcision are few, and the results present a mixed picture. Taken as a whole, the studies suggest that some decrease in sensitivity of the glans to fine touch can occur following circumcision. However, several studies conducted among men after adult circumcision suggest that few men report their sexual functioning is worse after circumcision; most report either improvement or no change.

HIV Infection and Male Circumcision in the United States

The United States has a much lower population prevalence of HIV infection (0.4%) than sub-Saharan Africa, and an epidemic that is concentrated among men who have sex with men, rather than men who have sex with women.

In one prospective study of heterosexual men attending an urban STD clinic, when other risk factors were controlled, uncircumcised men had a 3.5-fold higher risk for HIV infection than men who were circumcised. However, this association was not statistically significant due to small sample size. And in an analysis of clinic records for African American men attending an STD clinic, circumcision was not associated with HIV status overall, but among heterosexual men with known HIV exposure, circumcision was associated with a statistically significant 58 percent reduction in risk for HIV infection.

Considerations for the United States

The overall risk of HIV infection is considerably lower in the United States, changing risk-benefit and cost-effectiveness considerations. Also, studies to date have demonstrated efficacy only for penile-vaginal sex, the predominant mode of HIV transmission in Africa, whereas the predominant mode of sexual HIV transmission in the United States is by penile-anal sex among MSM. There are as yet no convincing data to help determine whether male circumcision will have any effect on HIV risk for men who engage in anal sex with either a female or male partner, as either the insertive or receptive partner. Receptive anal sex is associated with a substantially greater risk of HIV acquisition than is insertive anal sex. It is more biologically plausible that male circumcision would reduce HIV acquisition risk for the insertive partner rather than for the receptive partner, but relatively few MSM engage solely in insertive anal sex.

In addition, although the prevalence of circumcision may be somewhat lower in U.S. racial and ethnic groups with higher rates of HIV infection, most American men are already circumcised; and it is not known whether men at higher risk for HIV infection would be willing to be circumcised or whether parents would be willing to have their infants circumcised to reduce possible future HIV infection risk.

Section 30.2

Balanitis

Balanitis is a condition in which the head of the penis (glans) becomes inflamed. Although it rarely occurs among circumcised adult males, it affects approximately 3.3% of uncircumcised males at some point in their lives, as well as 4% of all boys under the age of 4. A related condition, posthitis, involves inflammation of the foreskin that covers the head of the penis in uncircumcised males. When both the glans and foreskin are affected, the condition is known as balanoposthitis.

Symptoms

The primary symptoms of balanitis include:

- swelling, redness, and tenderness of the glans
- skin irritation or rash on the end of the penis
- itching and discomfort
- thick, lumpy discharge under the foreskin
- unpleasant smell
- painful urination
- difficulty retracting the foreskin (phimosis)

Causes and Risk Factors

Balanitis has many possible causes, ranging from skin conditions and allergic reactions that affect the penis to sexually transmitted infections and poor hygiene. Men with phimosis—a condition in which the foreskin is tight and difficult to retract—are particularly susceptible to balanitis. Diabetes also increases the risk of developing balanitis because glucose in the urine can remain on the penis, creating a favorable environment for bacteria to grow. Some of the main causes of balanitis include the following:

- Skin conditions such as eczema, psoriasis, or lichen planus

- Dermatitis (inflammation of the skin) due to contact with an irritant or allergen, such as latex condoms, lubricants, spermicides, medicated ointments, detergents, fabric softeners, or perfumed bath products

- Irritation or minor trauma to the skin of the penis from friction, sexual intercourse, excessive washing with harsh soap, or vigorous drying with an abrasive towel

- Candida (also known as yeast infection or thrush)

- Sexually transmitted infections, such as genital herpes, chlamydia, or syphilis

- Bacterial infection from poor hygiene practices, such as infrequent washing of the glans or failure to dry the tissue beneath the foreskin after washing

Diagnosis and Treatment

To make a diagnosis of balanitis, a doctor merely needs to observe inflammation of the glans. In order to treat the condition effectively, however, the doctor must also determine the underlying cause. This process may involve examining the skin for evidence of eczema, psoriasis, or other skin conditions that may affect the penis. The doctor may also advise the patient to avoid potential skin irritants or allergens, such as lubricants or perfumed bath products, to see whether the balanitis resolves itself. Finally, the doctor may order diagnostic tests—such as blood tests, urine tests, or a swab of the glans—to see whether the patient has diabetes, a yeast infection, or a sexually transmitted infection.

If the balanitis appears to be related to a skin condition, the patient will likely be referred to a dermatologist for treatment. For balanitis caused by an allergic reaction, the patient may be prescribed a mild topical steroid cream, such as 1% hydrocortisone, to help relieve the swelling and other symptoms. If the cause is candida, the recommended treatment will include an antifungal cream—such as clotrimazole or miconazole—for both the patient and his sex partner. For balanitis caused by a bacterial infection, the patient will likely be prescribed an oral antibiotic, such as penicillin or erythromycin. If no infection or irritant can be identified, treatment may include astringent compresses with diluted vinegar or potassium permanganate. In rare cases, if the patient has phimosis and the balanitis recurs frequently, the doctor may recommend circumcision (surgery to remove the foreskin).

Prevention of Balanitis

Left untreated, chronic balanitis can lead to health complications, including:

- Phimosis (the foreskin cannot be retracted over the inflamed glans, which may require surgery to correct)
- Balanitis xerotica obliterans (chronic dermatitis affecting the glans and foreskin)
- Scarring and narrowing of the opening of the penis
- Reduction in blood supply to the tip of the penis
- Increased risk of penile cancer

Good hygiene is key to preventing the occurrence or recurrence of balanitis. Doctors recommend washing the penis daily with warm water, making sure to pull back the foreskin to expose the glans. Although regular soap may cause irritation, an aqueous cream or other non-soap cleanser may be used as long as it is completely rinsed off. It is important to dry the head of the penis thoroughly before replacing the foreskin, because moisture promotes the growth of bacteria. Men who tend to develop balanitis following sexual intercourse should wash the penis after sex. Finally, men who are prone to balanitis should avoid contact with potential irritants such as lubricants, detergents, or other chemicals.

References

1. Ngan, Vanessa. "Balanitis." DermNet NZ, 2016.

2. Nordqvist, Christian. "Balanitis: Causes, Symptoms, and Treatments." Medical News Today, September 28, 2015.

3. Sobol, Jennifer. "Balanitis." MedlinePlus, August 31, 2015.

Section 30.3

Penile Intraepithelial Neoplasia (Erythroplasia of Queyrat)

"Penile Intraepithelial Neoplasia," © 2017 Omnigraphics. Reviewed August 2016.

Penile intraepithelial neoplasia (PEIN) is pre-cancerous condition in which abnormal cell growth occurs in the outer layer of skin on the penis. Intraepithelial refers to the layer of cells that forms the surface or lining of an organ, while neoplasia refers to cystic lesions or tumors. Penile intraepithelial neoplasia is also known as erythroplasia of Queyrat, Bowen disease of the penis, squamous intraepithelial lesion, or squamous cell carcinoma in-situ of the penis. Although PEIN is not a form of cancer, up to 30% of cases may develop into penile cancer (invasive squamous cell carcinoma of the penis) if left untreated.

Risk Factors

Penile cancer is rare in the United States, with only about 2,000 new cases diagnosed each year. Some studies suggest that human papilloma virus (HPV) infection in the genital area, which also causes genital warts, is a significant risk factor in the development of penile intraepithelial cancer. As a result, many developed nations have instituted immunization programs aimed at vaccinating both boys and girls against HPV.

Studies have also shown that PEIN is most likely to affect uncircumcised males over the age of 50. Other risk factors include chronic skin diseases, such as lichen planus or lichen sclerosus; chronic irritation of the penis by friction, urine, allergens, or injury; suppression of the immune system by medications or disease; and smoking.

Symptoms and Diagnosis

The main symptom of PEIN is the presence of one or more lesions, growths, or tumors on the glans or foreskin of the penis. The surface of these lesions may appear smooth, velvety, crusty, scaly, or bumpy.

Men with PEIN may also experience inflammation, redness, itching, or pain in the area. In advanced stages, PEIN may cause bleeding, discharge, difficulty retracting the foreskin, or difficulty with urination.

Some of the symptoms of penile intraepithelial neoplasia may resemble other conditions, such as balanitis or dermatitis, so a skin biopsy should be performed to confirm the diagnosis and rule out invasive squamous cell carcinoma.

Treatment

Penile intraepithelial neoplasia can be treated with medications, surgery, or both. In addition to practicing good genital hygiene, men with PEIN may benefit from the use of topical medications such as 5-fluorouracil cream, which destroys abnormal skin cells, or imiquimod cream, which stimulates the immune system's response to abnormal cells. The lesions may also be removed using a variety of techniques, such as cryotherapy, curettage and cautery, excision, laser vaporization, Mohs micrographic surgery, photodynamic therapy, and radiotherapy. Since up to 10% of patients may experience a recurrence of PEIN following successful treatment, it is important to maintain a regular schedule of follow-up examinations.

Patients diagnosed with PEIN should undergo treatment promptly to prevent the pre-cancerous lesions from becoming cancerous. Although penile cancer is highly curable in its early stages, the prognosis declines sharply for more advanced stages. Finally, sexual partners of patients with penile intraepithelial neoplasia should be screened for related conditions—such as cervical, vulvar, and anal cancer—which can also be caused by the human papilloma virus.

References

1. Ngan, Vanessa. "Penile Intraepithelial Neoplasia." DermNet NZ, April 25, 2016.

2. "Penile Cancer Treatment." National Cancer Institute, February 18, 2016.

Section 30.4

Penile Trauma

Penile trauma can describe any sort of injury or wound that affects the penis. Since the penis contains no bone and is very flexible in its regular, flaccid state, penile injuries are rare compared to injuries affecting most other parts of the body. Trauma usually occurs when the penis is in its erect state, with between 30% and 50% of penile injuries resulting from sexual intercourse. Although most types of penile trauma will heal with appropriate treatment, many men resist seeking medical attention for penis injuries. Left untreated, however, penile trauma may result in pain, swelling, infection, sexual dysfunction, or permanent curvature of the penis (Peyronie disease).

Causes of Penile Trauma

Although most cases of penile trauma are related to sexual intercourse, injuries to the penis may result from a variety of other causes. Some of the most common types of injuries and associated causes include:

- Blunt force trauma

  Sports-related injuries—such as being hit in the groin by a ball, stick, foot, or knee—are a leading cause of blunt force trauma to the penis, which can result in pain, swelling, and bruising. Other common sources of blunt force trauma to the penis include automobile accidents and industrial accidents.

- Cuts, abrasions, and burns

  Penis abrasion can result from vigorous, repetitive exercise, chafing from coarse fabrics, or rug burns. Minor cuts and bruises to the penis may occur from being caught in a zipper or from using a penile pump or other stretching device in an effort to enlarge the penis. Burns to the penis can result from hot liquids being spilled or clothing catching on fire.

- Punctures

  Inserting objects into the tip of the penis can damage the urethra (the tube that carries urine and semen out of the penis). Bleeding from the penis or blood in the urine are indications of a serious injury to the urethra.

- Severe trauma or amputation

  Part or all of the penis may be damaged or severed as a result of gunshot wounds, automobile accidents, or industrial accidents. In addition, placing a rubber tube, metal ring, or other constricting device around the base of the penis can block blood flow and cause lasting damage to the organ.

- Penis "fracture"

  The most common form of penile trauma occurs when an erect penis is bent sharply, resulting in a tear or rupture in the tube-like structures (tunica albuginea) that carry blood to the penis. It usually occurs during sexual intercourse as a result of vigorous thrusting. Men who experience this type of injury typically feel a sharp pain and hear a popping or cracking sound. Discoloration and swelling usually occur as blood collects under the skin of the penis. Although urologists often refer to this particular injury as a penile fracture, the term is somewhat misleading since there is no bone in the penis.

Diagnosis and Treatment

To diagnose an injury to the penis, a urologist will discuss the patient's medical history and conduct a physical examination, checking the organ carefully for bruises, cuts, abrasions, dents, sensitive areas, or bleeding. The urologist may also order blood and urine tests as well as diagnostic tests, such as an ultrasound or magnetic resonance imaging (MRI) exam, to determine the extent of damage to the penis. Another diagnostic tool involves inserting a tiny fiber optic camera into the urethra. Finally, the urologist may perform a retrograde urethrogram—an X-ray study that is performed by injecting a special dye into the urethra and checking to see whether it leaks out.

Treatment of penile trauma varies depending on the type and extent of injury. Many minor injuries can be treated with rest and anti-inflammatory medications. The usual treatment for penile fracture is surgery to repair tears or ruptures in the tunica albuginea and remove any blood clots. Studies have shown that surgery offers the lowest rates of penile scarring, curvature, and sexual dysfunction. The typical procedure is performed under general anesthesia. It involves making an incision around the shaft near the head of the penis and retracting the skin to locate and repair tissue damage. Afterward, the area is bandaged and a catheter is placed in the urethra to drain urine from the bladder and allow the penis to heal. Most patients remain in the hospital under observation for one to two days and take antibiotics and pain relievers for one to two weeks after returning home.

Surgery is also the preferred option for patients with severe penile trauma or amputation. In cases where part or all of the penis has been severed, surgical reattachment may be possible for up to 16 hours if the organ is wrapped in gauze, placed in a plastic bag containing a sterile salt solution, and stored in a cooler of ice-cold water. Surgical reconstruction of the penis may also be possible following massive injuries, although the extent of the damage will determine how much function the organ retains afterward.

References

1. "What Is Penile Trauma?" Urology Care Foundation, 2016.

2. "Your Guide to Penis Pain and Injury." Herbal Love, 2016.

Section 30.5

Peyronie Disease

This section includes text excerpted from "Penile Curvature (Peyronie's Disease)," National Institute of Diabetes and Digestive and Kidney Diseases (NIDDK), July 2014.

What Is Peyronie Disease?

Peyronie disease is a disorder in which scar tissue, called a plaque, forms in the penis—the male organ used for urination and sex. The plaque builds up inside the tissues of a thick, elastic membrane called the tunica albuginea. The most common area for the plaque is on the top or bottom of the penis. As the plaque builds up, the penis will curve or bend, which can cause painful erections. Curves in the penis can make sexual intercourse painful, difficult, or impossible. Peyronie disease begins with inflammation, or swelling, which can become a hard scar.

The plaque that develops in Peyronie disease is not the same plaque that can develop in a person's arteries. The plaque seen in Peyronie disease is benign, or noncancerous, and is not a tumor. Peyronie disease is not contagious or caused by any known transmittable disease.

Early researchers thought Peyronie disease was a form of impotence, now called erectile dysfunction (ED). ED happens when a man is unable to achieve or keep an erection firm enough for sexual intercourse. Some men with Peyronie disease may have ED. Usually men with Peyronie disease are referred to a urologist—a doctor who specializes in sexual and urinary problems.

How Does an Erection Occur?

An erection occurs when blood flow increases into the penis, making it expand and become firm. Two long chambers inside the penis, called the corpora cavernosa, contain a spongy tissue that draws blood into the chambers. The spongy tissue contains smooth muscles, fibrous tissues, spaces, veins, and arteries. The tunica albuginea encases the corpora cavernosa. The urethra, which is the tube that carries urine and semen outside of the body, runs along the underside of the corpora cavernosa in the middle of a third chamber called the corpus spongiosum.

An erection requires a precise sequence of events:

- An erection begins with sensory or mental stimulation, or both. The stimulus may be physical contact or a sexual image or thought.

- When the brain senses a sexual urge, it sends impulses to local nerves in the penis that cause the muscles of the corpora cavernosa to relax. As a result, blood flows in through the arteries and fills the spaces in the corpora cavernosa like water filling a sponge.

- The blood creates pressure in the corpora cavernosa, making the penis expand.

- The tunica albuginea helps trap the blood in the corpora cavernosa, thereby sustaining the erection.

- The erection ends after climax or after the sexual urge has passed. The muscles in the penis contract to stop the inflow of blood. The veins open and the extra blood flows out of the penis and back into the body.

What Causes Peyronie Disease?

Medical experts do not know the exact cause of Peyronie disease. Many believe that Peyronie disease may be the result of

- acute injury to the penis

- chronic, or repeated, injury to the penis

- autoimmune disease—a disorder in which the body's immune system attacks the body's own cells and organs

How Common Is Peyronie Disease?

Researchers estimate that Peyronie disease may affect 1 to 23 percent of men between 40 and 70 years of age. However, the actual occurrence of Peyronie disease may be higher due to men's embarrassment and healthcare providers' limited reporting. The disease is rare in young men, although it has been reported in men in their 30s. The chance of developing Peyronie disease increases with age.

Who Is More Likely to Develop Peyronie Disease?

The following factors may increase a man's chance of developing Peyronie disease:

- vigorous sexual or nonsexual activities that cause microscopic injury to the penis

- certain connective tissue and autoimmune disorders

  - plantar fasciitis

  - scleroderma

  - systemic lupus erythematosus

  - Sjögren syndrome

  - Behcet syndrome

- a family history of Peyronie disease

- aging

What Are the Signs and Symptoms of Peyronie Disease?

The signs and symptoms of Peyronie disease may include

- hard lumps on one or more sides of the penis
- pain during sexual intercourse or during an erection
- a curve in the penis either with or without an erection
- narrowing or shortening of the penis
- ED

Symptoms of Peyronie disease range from mild to severe. Symptoms may develop slowly or appear quickly. In many cases, the pain decreases over time, although the curve in the penis may remain. In milder cases, symptoms may go away without causing a permanent curve.

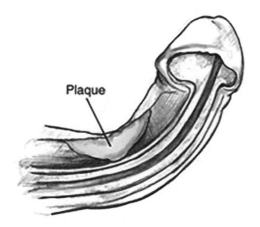

Plaque

Figure 30.1. *Cross Section of a Curved Penis during Erection*

What Are the Complications of Peyronie Disease?

Complications of Peyronie disease may include

- the inability to have sexual intercourse
- ED
- anxiety, or stress, about sexual abilities or the appearance of the penis

377

- stress on a relationship with a sexual partner
- problems fathering a child because intercourse is difficult

How Is Peyronie Disease Diagnosed?

A urologist diagnoses Peyronie disease based on

- a medical and family history
- a physical exam
- imaging tests

Medical and Family History

Taking a medical and family history is one of the first things a urologist may do to help diagnose Peyronie disease. He or she will ask the man to provide a medical and family history, which may include the following questions:

- What is the man's ability to have an erection?
- What are the problems with sexual intercourse?
- When did the symptoms begin?
- What is the family medical history?
- What medications is the man taking?
- What other symptoms is the man experiencing?
- What other medical conditions does the man have?

Physical Exam

A physical exam may help diagnose Peyronie disease. During a physical exam, a urologist usually examines the man's body, including the penis.

A urologist can usually feel the plaque in the penis with or without an erection. Sometimes the urologist will need to examine the penis during an erection. The urologist will give the man an injectable medication to cause an erection.

Imaging Tests

To help pinpoint the location of the plaque buildup inside the penis, a urologist may perform

- ultrasound of the penis

- an X-ray of the penis

How Is Peyronie Disease Treated?

A urologist may treat Peyronie disease with nonsurgical treatments or surgery.

The goal of treatment is to reduce pain and restore and maintain the ability to have intercourse. Men with small plaques, minimal penile curvature, no pain, and satisfactory sexual function may not need treatment until symptoms get worse. Peyronie disease often resolves on its own without treatment.

A urologist may recommend changes in a man's lifestyle to reduce the risk of ED associated with Peyronie disease.

Nonsurgical Treatments

Nonsurgical treatments include medications and medical therapies.

Medications. A urologist may prescribe medications aimed at decreasing a man's penile curvature, plaque size, and inflammation. A man may take prescribed medications to treat Peyronie disease orally—by mouth—or a urologist may inject medications directly into the plaque. Verapamil is one type of topical medication that a man may apply to the skin over the plaque.

- **Oral medications.** Oral medications may include

  - vitamin E

  - potassium para-aminobenzoate (Potaba)

  - tamoxifen

  - colchicine

  - acetyl-L-carnitine

  - pentoxifylline

- **Injections.** Medications injected directly into plaques may include

  - verapamil

  - interferon alpha 2b

  - steroids

  - collagenase (Xiaflex)

To date, collagenase is the first and only medication specifically approved for Peyronie disease.

Medical therapies. A urologist may use medical therapies to break up scar tissue and decrease plaque size and curvature. Therapies to break up scar tissue may include

- high-intensity, focused ultrasound directed at the plaque
- radiation therapy—high-energy rays, such as X-rays, aimed at the plaque
- shockwave therapy—focused, low-intensity electroshock waves directed at the plaque

A urologist may use iontophoresis—painless, low-level electric current that delivers medications through the skin over the plaque—to decrease plaque size and curvature.

A urologist may use mechanical traction and vacuum devices aimed at stretching or bending the penis to reduce curvature.

Surgery

A urologist may recommend surgery to remove plaque or help straighten the penis during an erection. Medical experts recommend surgery for long-term cases when

- symptoms have not improved
- erections, intercourse, or both are painful
- the curve or bend in the penis does not allow the man to have sexual intercourse

Some men may develop complications after surgery, and sometimes surgery does not correct the effects of Peyronie disease—such as shortening of the penis. Some surgical methods can cause shortening of the penis. Medical experts suggest waiting 1 year or more from the onset of symptoms before having surgery because the course of Peyronie disease is different in each man.

A urologist may recommend the following surgeries:

- grafting
- plication
- device implantation

A urologist performs these surgeries in a hospital.

Lifestyle Changes

A man can make healthy lifestyle changes to reduce the chance of ED associated with Peyronie disease by

- quitting smoking

- reducing alcohol consumption

- exercising regularly

- avoiding illegal drugs

Section 30.6

Phimosis and Paraphimosis

What Is Phimosis?

Phimosis is a condition in which the foreskin (prepuce) of an uncircumcised male cannot be retracted over the head (glans) of the penis. It often appears to be a tight ring around the tip of the penis.

Causes

Phimosis can either be physiologic or pathologic.

- Physiologic phimosis occurs when a child is born with a tight foreskin. The condition generally corrects itself without intervention some time between late childhood and early adolescence. In the United States, about 10 percent of boys are born with phimosis.

- Pathologic phimosis occurs in older boys and adult men, often due to poor hygiene, infection, inflammation, or other medical conditions. Forceful retraction of the foreskin can lead to scarring and repeated swelling of the foreskin and glans.

Symptoms

Symptoms of phimosis include:

- ballooning of the foreskin during urination
- difficulty or pain during urination
- urinary tract infections
- painful erection
- paraphimosis

Diagnosis

Phimosis is diagnosed by a physical examination, in which the doctor can observe the symptoms, and does not usually require additional tests.

Treatment

Treatment depends on such factors as the age of the individual, type of symptoms, and the severity of the condition. Phimosis may be treated by gently retracting the foreskin manually and applying topical corticosteroid ointment. Steroid ointment softens the foreskin, and full retraction may be possible in 4–6 weeks, following which this treatment is discontinued. In rare cases—such as unsuccessful steroid treatment, recurrent or severe inflammation, paraphimosis, or recurrent urinary tract infections—circumcision might be required.

What Is Paraphimosis?

Paraphimosis is a condition in which the retracted foreskin cannot be returned to its normal position. This leads to decreased blood flow to the glans penis, which then becomes a urologic emergency.

Causes

Paraphimosis is most often observed in children and the elderly. It can be caused by an injury to the area, failure to return the foreskin to its original position after retraction, or infection that may occur when the area is not washed properly. It commonly occurs in hospitals and nursing homes when the foreskin is retracted by a healthcare professional to prepare a patient for a medical procedure, such as the insertion of a Foley catheter.

Symptoms

When a retracted foreskin stays behind the glans penis for too long, it causes the glans and the foreskin to become swollen. This swelling often aggravates the restriction, forming a tight tissue ring around the head of the penis. This in turn worsens the swelling and causes considerable pain.

Diagnosis

Paraphimosis is diagnosed by a physical examination, in which a "doughnut" is usually observed close to the head of the penis.

Treatment

The first option is to reduce the swelling manually by pushing the foreskin forward while simultaneously pressing on the glans penis. The application of ice to the swollen area can also help. To reduce discomfort, the person may be given pain medication or a local anesthetic or anesthetic cream, applied to the penis. Another effective option, used to decrease swelling, is a local injection of hyaluronidase.

In circumstances in which none of these options are successful, or if a faster reduction is required, the doctor may make a small surgical incision on the back (dorsal) side of the constricting ring. If this procedure is followed, circumcision must be done at a later time to prevent recurrence.

References

1. Balentine, Jerry R. "Phimosis and Paraphimosis (Penis Disorders)," MedicineNet, Inc., March 23, 2016.

2. "Phimosis," Department of Urology, University of California, San Francisco, n.d.

3. Zieve, David. "Paraphimosis," A.D.A.M., Inc., January 21, 2015.

Chapter 31

Disorders of the Scrotum and Testicles

Chapter Contents

Section 31.1—Epididymitis 386

Section 31.2—Hydrocele 390

Section 31.3—Inguinal Hernia... 393

Section 31.4—Spermatocele 401

Section 31.5—Testicular Torsion 403

Section 31.6—Perineal Injury in Males..................................... 407

Section 31.7—Undescended Testicle... 414

Section 31.8—Varicocele... 416

Section 31.1

Epididymitis

This section includes text excerpted from "Epididymitis," Centers for
Disease Control and Prevention (CDC), June 4, 2015.

Acute epididymitis is a clinical syndrome consisting of pain, swelling, and inflammation of the epididymis that lasts <6 weeks. Sometimes the testis is also involved—a condition referred to as epididymo-orchitis. A high index of suspicion for spermatic cord (testicular) torsion must be maintained in men who present with a sudden onset of symptoms associated with epididymitis, as this condition is a surgical emergency.

Among sexually active men aged <35 years, acute epididymitis is most frequently caused by *C. trachomatis* or *N. gonorrhoeae*. Acute epididymitis caused by sexually transmitted enteric organisms (e.g., *Escherichia coli*) also occurs among men who are the insertive partner during anal intercourse. Sexually transmitted acute epididymitis usually is accompanied by urethritis, which frequently is asymptomatic. Other nonsexually transmitted infectious causes of acute epididymitis (e.g., Fournier gangrene) are uncommon and should be managed in consultation with a urologist.

In men aged ≥35 years who do not report insertive anal intercourse, sexually transmitted acute epididymitis is less common. In this group, the epididymis usually becomes infected in the setting of bacteriuria secondary to bladder outlet obstruction (e.g., benign prostatic hyperplasia). In older men, nonsexually transmitted acute epididymitis is also associated with prostate biopsy, urinary tract instrumentation or surgery, systemic disease, and/or immunosuppression.

Chronic epididymitis is characterized by a ≥6 week history of symptoms of discomfort and/or pain in the scrotum, testicle, or epididymis. Chronic infectious epididymitis is most frequently seen in conditions associated with a granulomatous reaction; Mycobacterium tuberculosis (TB) is the most common granulomatous disease affecting the epididymis and should be suspected, especially in men with a known history of or recent exposure to TB. The differential diagnosis of chronic non-infectious epididymitis, sometimes termed "orchalgia/epididymalgia" is broad (i.e., trauma, cancer, autoimmune, and idiopathic conditions); men with this diagnosis should be referred to a urologist for clinical management.

Diagnostic Considerations

Men who have acute epididymitis typically have unilateral testicular pain and tenderness, hydrocele, and palpable swelling of the epididymis. Although inflammation and swelling usually begins in the tail of the epididymis, it can spread to involve the rest of the epididymis and testicle. The spermatic cord is usually tender and swollen. Spermatic cord (testicular) torsion, a surgical emergency, should be considered in all cases, but it occurs more frequently among adolescents and in men without evidence of inflammation or infection. In men with severe, unilateral pain with sudden onset, those whose test results do not support a diagnosis of urethritis or urinary-tract infection, or men in whom diagnosis of acute epididymitis is questionable, immediate referral to a urologist for evaluation of testicular torsion is important because testicular viability might be compromised.

Bilateral symptoms should raise suspicion of other causes of testicular pain. Radionuclide scanning of the scrotum is the most accurate method to diagnose epididymitis, but it is not routinely available. Ultrasound should be primarily used for ruling out torsion of the spermatic cord in cases of acute, unilateral, painful scrotum swelling. However, because partial spermatic cord torsion can mimic epididymitis on scrotal ultrasound, when torsion is not ruled out by ultrasound, differentiation between spermatic cord torsion and epididymitis must be made on the basis of clinical evaluation. Although ultrasound can demonstrate epididymal hyperemia and swelling associated with epididymitis, it provides minimal utility for men with a clinical presentation consistent with epididymitis, because a negative ultrasound does not alter clinical management. Ultrasound should be reserved for men with scrotal pain who cannot receive an accurate diagnosis by history, physical examination, and objective laboratory findings or if torsion of the spermatic cord is suspected.

All suspected cases of acute epididymitis should be evaluated for objective evidence of inflammation by one of the following point-of-care tests:

- Gram or methylene blue or gentian violet (MB/GV) stain of urethral secretions demonstrating ≥2 WBC per oil immersion field. These stains are preferred point-of-care diagnostic tests for evaluating urethritis because they are highly sensitive and specific for documenting both urethral inflammation and the presence or absence of gonococcal infection. Gonococcal infection is established by documenting the presence of WBC-containing intracellular Gram-negative or purple diplococci on urethral Gram stain or MB/GV smear, respectively.

- Positive leukocyte esterase test on first-void urine.

- Microscopic examination of sediment from a spun first-void urine demonstrating ≥10 WBC per high power field.

All suspected cases of acute epididymitis should be tested for *C. trachomatis* and for *N. gonorrhoeae* by nucleic acid amplification tests (NAAT). Urine is the preferred specimen for NAAT testing in men. Urine cultures for chlamydia and gonococcal epididymitis are insensitive and are not recommended. Urine bacterial culture might have a higher yield in men with sexually transmitted enteric infections and in older men with acute epididymitis caused by genitourinary bacteruria.

Treatment

To prevent complications and transmission of sexually transmitted infections, presumptive therapy is indicated at the time of the visit before all laboratory test results are available. Selection of presumptive therapy is based on risk for chlamydia and gonorrhea and/or enteric organisms. The goals of treatment of acute epididymitis are:

1. microbiologic cure of infection

2. improvement of signs and symptoms

3. prevention of transmission of chlamydia and gonorrhea to others

4. a decrease in potential chlamydia/gonorrhea epididymitis complications (e.g., infertility and chronic pain)

Although most men with acute epididymitis can be treated on an outpatient basis, referral to a specialist and hospitalization should be considered when severe pain or fever suggests other diagnoses (e.g., torsion, testicular infarction, abscess, and necrotizing fasciitis) or when men are unable to comply with an antimicrobial regimen. Because high fever is uncommon and indicates a complicated infection, hospitalization for further evaluation is recommended.

Therapy including levofloxacin or ofloxacin should be considered if the infection is most likely caused by enteric organisms and gonorrhea has been ruled out by gram, MB, or GV stain. This includes men who have undergone prostate biopsy, vasectomy, and other urinary-tract instrumentation procedures. As an adjunct to therapy, bed rest, scrotal elevation, and nonsteroidal anti-inflammatory drugs are recommended until fever and local inflammation have subsided. Complete resolution of discomfort might not occur until a few weeks after completion of the antibiotic regimen.

Other Management Considerations

Men who have acute epididymitis confirmed or suspected to be caused by *N. gonorrhoeae* or *C. trachomatis* should be advised to abstain from sexual intercourse until they and their partners have been adequately treated and symptoms have resolved. All men with acute epididymitis should be tested for other STDs, including HIV.

Follow-Up

Men should be instructed to return to their healthcare providers if their symptoms fail to improve within 72 hours of the initiation of treatment. Signs and symptoms of epididymitis that do not subside within 3 days require re-evaluation of the diagnosis and therapy. Men who experience swelling and tenderness that persist after completion of antimicrobial therapy should be evaluated for alternative diagnoses, including tumor, abscess, infarction, testicular cancer, tuberculosis, and fungal epididymitis.

Management of Sex Partners

Men who have acute sexually transmitted epididymitis confirmed or suspected to be caused by *N. gonorrhoeae* or *C. trachomatis* should be instructed to refer for evaluation, testing, and presumptive treatment all sex partners with whom they have had sexual contact within the 60 days preceding onset of symptoms. If the last sexual intercourse was >60 days before onset of symptoms or diagnosis, the most recent sex partner should be treated. Arrangements should be made to link female partners to care. Expedited partner therapy (EPT) and enhanced referral are effective strategies for treating female sex partners of men who have chlamydia or gonorrhea for whom linkage to care is anticipated to be delayed. Partners should be instructed to abstain from sexual intercourse until they and their sex partners are adequately treated and symptoms have resolved.

Special Considerations

Allergy, Intolerance, and Adverse Reactions

The cross reactivity between penicillins and cephalosporins is <2.5 percent in persons with a history of penicillin allergy. The risk for penicillin cross-reactivity is highest with first-generation cephalosporins, but is negligible between most second-generation (cefoxitin) and all third-generation (ceftriaxone) cephalosporins. Alternative regimens have not been studied; therefore, clinicians should consult infectious-disease specialists if such regimens are required.

HIV Infection

Men with HIV infection who have uncomplicated acute epididymitis should receive the same treatment regimen as those who are HIV negative. Other etiologic agents have been implicated in acute epididymitis in men with HIV infection, including CMV, salmonella, toxoplasmosis, *Ureaplasma urealyticum*, *Corynebacterium* sp., *Mycoplasma* sp., and *Mima polymorpha*. Fungi and mycobacteria also are more likely to cause acute epididymitis in men with HIV infection than in those who are immunocompetent.

Section 31.2

Hydrocele

"Hydrocele," © 2017 Omnigraphics.
Reviewed August 2016.

A hydrocele is a generally harmless, painless build-up of fluid around one or both testicles that causes swelling in the scrotum.

Hydroceles can be described as primary or secondary. A primary hydrocele, also called an idiopathic hydrocele, often occurs as a result of an imbalance between the secretion and absorption of fluids in the membranes covering the testes. A secondary hydrocele may follow trauma, infection, or neoplasms.

Common in newborns, congenital hydroceles may form a few weeks prior to birth when the testes descend from the abdomen into the scrotum, surrounded by a fluid-filled sac. Normally, this sac closes and the fluid is absorbed. In some newborns, however, the sac fails to close, which causes a route to the abdominal cavity to remain open. This is called a communicating hydrocele, since it allows the passage of fluid between the abdomen and scrotum. A non-communicating hydrocele, on the other hand, develops when the sac closes but traps some fluid in the scrotum. Congenital hydroceles are found in about 10 percent of newborns and may regress spontaneously within the first two years of life.

Hydroceles may also affect adolescents and adults, most often men over 40. In these cases, the hydrocele may be caused by a condition in which the passage from abdomen to scrotum either hasn't closed all the way or has reopened. Other causes of hydroceles in adults include injury to the scrotum or inflammation resulting from an infection.

Symptoms

A hydrocele commonly presents as an enlargement of the scrotum, just below the testes, and is usually painless unless there is infection or some other underlying cause of discomfort. In the case of communicating hydroceles, the size of the swelling may vacillate during the day, typically growing larger with coughing, straining, crying, or any activity that raises intra-abdominal pressure.

Diagnosis

A simple physical examination involving palpation (feeling with the hand) is the first step in diagnosing a hydrocele. The doctor may also use a technique called transillumination, in which. a bright light is focused on the scrotum. The presence of clear fluid allows transmission of light, and the scrotum "lights up," revealing the presence of a hydrocele or other testicular abnormalities. The doctor may also recommend blood and urine tests or a scrotal ultrasound to confirm the initial diagnosis.

Treatment

Hydroceles generally don't require treatment unless they attain a critical size, and the patient experiences discomfort or difficulty moving. However, it is prudent to check with your healthcare provider to rule out other complications, such as infection, testicular tumor, or inguinal hernia. An inguinal hernia, one of the most common risks associated with hydrocele, develops when a loop of the intestine protrudes into the scrotum and may require surgical intervention.

When medical intervention is required, some possible treatments for hydrocele include:

Needle Aspiration

The safest, cheapest, and most non-invasive treatment option involves drainage of fluid from the hydrocele using a syringe. While this procedure is often successful in providing symptomatic relief in large hydroceles, it carries a high likelihood of recurrence and is most often recommended when surgery is not an option.

Sclerotherapy

This form of treatment is often used in conjunction with aspiration to prevent or delay the recurrence of a hydrocele. Sclerotherapy involves the injection of medication after the fluid has been drained.

Hydrocelectomy

A hydrocelectomy is a surgical repair that is used to correct large, painful, recurring hydroceles. If the hydrocele is uncomplicated, the surgery generally takes less than an hour and is typically performed on an outpatient basis under either general or local anesthesia. An incision is made in the scrotum or lower abdomen. The hydrocele sac is drained of its fluid and is partially or totally removed. Related conditions, such as inguinal hernia, may also be corrected during hydrocelectomy. Some surgeons use laparoscopy—a minimally invasive procedure using a camera-tipped instrument called a laparoscope—to repair hydroceles. Hydrocelectomy is generally considered safe, and most patients experience minimal complications and have a successful long-term outcome.

References

1. "Hydrocele—Topic Overview," WebMD, November 14, 2014.

2. Parks, Kelly and Leung, Lawrence. "Recurrent Hydrocoele," National Center for Biotechnology Information (NCBI), U.S. National Library of Medicine (NLM), 2013.

3. "Hydrocele," Mayo Clinic, October 9, 2014.

Section 31.3

Inguinal Hernia

This section includes text excerpted from "Inguinal Hernia," National Institute of Diabetes and Digestive and Kidney Diseases (NIDDK), June 2014.

What Is an Inguinal Hernia?

An inguinal hernia happens when contents of the abdomen—usually fat or part of the small intestine—bulge through a weak area in the lower abdominal wall. The abdomen is the area between the chest and the hips. The area of the lower abdominal wall is also called the inguinal or groin region.

Two types of inguinal hernias are:

1. Indirect inguinal hernias, which are caused by a defect in the abdominal wall that is congenital, or present at birth.

2. Direct inguinal hernias, which usually occur only in male adults and are caused by a weakness in the muscles of the abdominal wall that develops over time.

Inguinal hernias occur at the inguinal canal in the groin region.

What Is the Inguinal Canal?

The inguinal canal is a passage through the lower abdominal wall. People have two inguinal canals—one on each side of the lower abdomen. In males, the spermatic cords pass through the inguinal canals and connect to the testicles in the scrotum—the sac around the testicles. The spermatic cords contain blood vessels, nerves, and a duct, called the spermatic duct, that carries sperm from the testicles to the penis. In females, the round ligaments, which support the uterus, pass through the inguinal canals.

What Causes Inguinal Hernias?

The cause of inguinal hernias depends on the type of inguinal hernia.

Indirect inguinal hernias. A defect in the abdominal wall that is present at birth causes an indirect inguinal hernia.

During the development of the fetus in the womb, the lining of the abdominal cavity forms and extends into the inguinal canal. In males, the spermatic cord and testicles descend out from inside the abdomen and through the abdominal lining to the scrotum through the inguinal canal. Next, the abdominal lining usually closes off the entrance to the inguinal canal a few weeks before or after birth. In females, the ovaries do not descend out from inside the abdomen, and the abdominal lining usually closes a couple of months before birth.

Sometimes the lining of the abdomen does not close as it should, leaving an opening in the abdominal wall at the upper part of the inguinal canal. Fat or part of the small intestine may slide into the

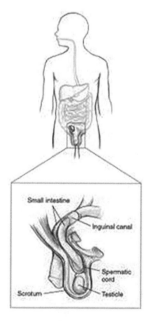

Figure 31.1. *Indirect Inguinal Hernia In a Male*

inguinal canal through this opening, causing a hernia. In females, the ovaries may also slide into the inguinal canal and cause a hernia.

Indirect hernias are the most common type of inguinal hernia. Indirect inguinal hernias may appear in 2 to 3 percent of male children; however, they are much less common in female children, occurring in less than 1 percent.

Direct inguinal hernias. Direct inguinal hernias usually occur only in male adults as aging and stress or strain weaken the abdominal muscles around the inguinal canal. Previous surgery in the lower abdomen can also weaken the abdominal muscles.

Females rarely form this type of inguinal hernia. In females, the broad ligament of the uterus acts as an additional barrier behind the muscle layer of the lower abdominal wall. The broad ligament of the uterus is a sheet of tissue that supports the uterus and other reproductive organs.

Who Is More Likely to Develop an Inguinal Hernia?

Males are much more likely to develop inguinal hernias than females. About 25 percent of males and about 2 percent of females will develop an inguinal hernia in their lifetimes. Some people who have an inguinal hernia on one side will have or will develop a hernia on the other side.

People of any age can develop inguinal hernias. Indirect hernias can appear before age 1 and often appear before age 30; however, they may appear later in life. Premature infants have a higher chance of developing an indirect inguinal hernia. Direct hernias, which usually only occur in male adults, are much more common in men older than age 40 because the muscles of the abdominal wall weaken with age.

People with a family history of inguinal hernias are more likely to develop inguinal hernias. Studies also suggest that people who smoke have an increased risk of inguinal hernias.

What Are the Signs and Symptoms of an Inguinal Hernia?

The first sign of an inguinal hernia is a small bulge on one or, rarely, on both sides of the groin—the area just above the groin crease between the lower abdomen and the thigh. The bulge may increase in size over time and usually disappears when lying down.

Other signs and symptoms can include:

- Discomfort or pain in the groin—especially when straining, lifting, coughing, or exercising—that improves when resting.

- Feelings such as weakness, heaviness, burning, or aching in the groin.

- A swollen or an enlarged scrotum in men or boys.

Indirect and direct inguinal hernias may slide in and out of the abdomen into the inguinal canal. A healthcare provider can often move them back into the abdomen with gentle massage.

What Are the Complications of Inguinal Hernias?

Inguinal hernias can cause the following complications:

- **Incarceration**. An incarcerated hernia happens when part of the fat or small intestine from inside the abdomen becomes stuck in the groin or scrotum and cannot go back into the abdomen. A healthcare provider is unable to massage the hernia back into the abdomen.

- **Strangulation**. When an incarcerated hernia is not treated, the blood supply to the small intestine may become obstructed, causing "strangulation" of the small intestine. This lack of blood supply is an emergency situation and can cause the section of the intestine to die.

Seek Immediate Care

People who have symptoms of an incarcerated or a strangulated hernia should seek emergency medical help immediately. A strangulated hernia is a life-threatening condition. Symptoms of an incarcerated or a strangulated hernia include:

- extreme tenderness or painful redness in the area of the bulge in the groin

- sudden pain that worsens quickly and does not go away

- the inability to have a bowel movement and pass gas

- nausea and vomiting

- fever

How Are Inguinal Hernias Diagnosed?

A healthcare provider diagnoses an inguinal hernia with:

- a medical and family history

- a physical exam

- imaging tests, including X-rays

Medical and family history. Taking a medical and family history may help a healthcare provider diagnose an inguinal hernia. Often the symptoms that the patient describes will be signs of an inguinal hernia.

Physical exam. A physical exam may help diagnose an inguinal hernia. During a physical exam, a healthcare provider usually examines the patient's body. The healthcare provider may ask the patient to stand and cough or strain so the healthcare provider can feel for a bulge caused by the hernia as it moves into the groin or scrotum. The healthcare provider may gently try to massage the hernia back into its proper position in the abdomen.

Imaging tests. A healthcare provider does not usually use imaging tests, including X-rays, to diagnose an inguinal hernia unless he or she:

- Is trying to diagnose a strangulation or an incarceration.

- Cannot feel the inguinal hernia during a physical exam, especially in patients who are overweight.

- Is uncertain if the hernia or another condition is causing the swelling in the groin or other symptoms.

Specially trained technicians perform imaging tests at a healthcare provider's office, an outpatient center, or a hospital.

A radiologist—a doctor who specializes in medical imaging—interprets the images. A patient does not usually need anesthesia.

Tests may include the following:

- **Abdominal X-ray.** An X-ray is a picture recorded on film or on a computer using a small amount of radiation. The patient will lie on a table or stand during the X-ray. The technician positions the X-ray machine over the abdominal area. The patient will hold his or her breath as the technician takes the picture so that the picture will not be blurry. The technician may ask the patient to change position for additional pictures.

- **Computerized tomography (CT) scan.** CT scans use a combination of X-rays and computer technology to create images. For a CT scan, the technician may give the patient a solution to drink and an injection of a special dye, called contrast medium. A healthcare provider injects the contrast medium into a vein, and the injection will make the patient feel warm all over for a minute or two. The contrast medium allows the healthcare provider to see the blood vessels and blood flow on the X-rays. CT scans require the patient to lie on a table that slides into a tunnel-shaped device where the technician takes the X-rays. A healthcare provider may give children a sedative to help them fall asleep for the test.

- **Abdominal ultrasound.** Ultrasound uses a device, called a transducer, that bounces safe, painless sound waves off organs to create an image of their structure.

How Are Inguinal Hernias Treated?

Repair of an inguinal hernia via surgery is the only treatment for inguinal hernias and can prevent incarceration and strangulation. Healthcare providers recommend surgery for most people with inguinal hernias and especially for people with hernias that cause symptoms. Research suggests that men with hernias that cause few or no symptoms may be able to safely delay surgery until their symptoms increase. Men who delay surgery should watch for symptoms and see a healthcare provider regularly. Healthcare providers usually recommend surgery for infants and children to prevent incarceration. Emergent, or immediate, surgery is necessary for incarcerated or strangulated hernias.

A general surgeon—a doctor who specializes in abdominal surgery—performs hernia surgery at a hospital or surgery center, usually on an outpatient basis. Recovery time varies depending on the size of the hernia, the technique used, and the age and health of the person.

Hernia surgery is also called herniorrhaphy. The two main types of surgery for hernias are:

- **Open hernia repair.**During an open hernia repair, a healthcare provider usually gives a patient local anesthesia in the abdomen with sedation; however, some patients may have

  - sedation with a spinal block, in which a healthcare provider injects anesthetics around the nerves in the spine, making the body numb from the waist down

  - general anesthesia

The surgeon makes an incision in the groin, moves the hernia back into the abdomen, and reinforces the abdominal wall with stitches. Usually the surgeon also reinforces the weak area with a synthetic mesh or "screen" to provide additional support.

- **Laparoscopic hernia repair.** A surgeon performs laparoscopic hernia repair with the patient under general anesthesia. The surgeon makes several small, half-inch incisions in the lower abdomen and inserts a laparoscope—a thin tube with a tiny video camera attached. The camera sends a magnified image from inside the body to a video monitor, giving the surgeon a close-up view of the hernia and surrounding tissue. While watching the monitor, the surgeon repairs the hernia using synthetic mesh or "screen."

People who undergo laparoscopic hernia repair generally experience a shorter recovery time than those who have an open hernia repair. However, the surgeon may determine that laparoscopy is not the best option if the hernia is large or if the person has had previous pelvic surgery.

Most adults experience discomfort and require pain medication after either an open hernia repair or a laparoscopic hernia repair. Intense activity and heavy lifting are restricted for several weeks. The surgeon will discuss when a person may safely return to work. Infants and children also experience some discomfort; however, they usually resume normal activities after several days.

Surgery to repair an inguinal hernia is quite safe, and complications are uncommon. People should contact their healthcare provider if any of the following symptoms appear:

- redness around or drainage from the incision

- fever

- bleeding from the incision

- pain that is not relieved by medication or pain that suddenly worsens

Possible long-term complications include:

- long-lasting pain in the groin

- recurrence of the hernia, requiring a second surgery

- damage to nerves near the hernia

How Can Inguinal Hernias Be Prevented?

People cannot prevent the weakness in the abdominal wall that causes indirect inguinal hernias. However, people may be able to prevent direct inguinal hernias by maintaining a healthy weight and not smoking.

People can keep inguinal hernias from getting worse or keep inguinal hernias from recurring after surgery by:

- avoiding heavy lifting
- using the legs, not the back, when lifting objects
- preventing constipation and straining during bowel movements
- maintaining a healthy weight
- not smoking

Eating, Diet, and Nutrition

Researchers have not found that eating, diet, and nutrition play a role in causing inguinal hernias. A person with an inguinal hernia may be able to prevent symptoms by eating high-fiber foods. Fresh fruits, vegetables, and whole grains are high in fiber and may help prevent the constipation and straining that cause some of the painful symptoms of a hernia.

The surgeon will provide instructions on eating, diet, and nutrition after inguinal hernia surgery. Most people drink liquids and eat a light diet the day of the operation and then resume their usual diet the next day.

Section 31.4

Spermatocele

"Spermatocele," © 2017 Omnigraphics.
Reviewed August 2016.

What Is a Spermatocele?

A spermatocele—often called a spermatic cyst—is a benign fluid-filled mass within the scrotum. The cyst is an accumulation of fluid and sperm cells that typically arises from the caput (head) of the epididymis, a tightly coiled tube located above each testicle that collects and transports sperm. Spermatoceles are common and generally do not require treatment. However, discomfort, pain, or a bothersome enlargement may require surgical intervention.

Spermatoceles are found in an estimated 30 percent of adult men. They are usually asymptomatic, do not affect fertility, and are most often discovered during self-examination or in an imaging test carried out for other conditions.

Causes

The exact cause of spermatoceles is unknown, although a number of possible etiologies have been proposed:

- They could be caused by an obstruction in the epididymal ducts.

- Sperm may accumulate in the head of the epididymis and lead to the formation of a cyst.

- Although they usually form spontaneously without any preceding injury, infection, or inflammation, they could result from a previous medical condition.

Symptoms

Symptoms of spermatoceles include the following:

- A lump or mass in the scrotum

- Enlarged scrotum

- Pain, swelling, or redness of the scrotum

- Pressure felt at the base of the penis

Diagnosis

A spermatocele can be felt as a firm, smooth lump by palpating (feeling) the scrotum during a medical examination or self-exam.

Diagnosis can be confirmed by a transillumination exam, in which a doctor shines a light behind each testicle. An ultrasound may be used for further confirmation, and a sonogram can help determine if the lump is a spermatocele or a benign or cancerous tumor. If the lump is painful, a blood count and urinalysis may be required to detect infection or inflammation.

Treatment

Spermatoceles are not dangerous, and if the cyst is small and does not change in size, treatment may not be needed. However, treatment might be required for pain alleviation or, in rare cases, if there is decreased blood supply to the penis.

Oral analgesics are often prescribed for symptomatic pain relief. If the pain and discomfort are caused by underlying epididymitis—inflammation of the epididymis—antibiotics may be prescribed.

If the spermatocele becomes larger and causes considerable discomfort, a procedure to remove it surgically, known as a spermatocelectomy, may be carried out. Needle aspiration, often used to treat other types of cysts, is contraindicated in spermatoceles because it could result in infection due to spillage of sperm within the scrotum.

Spermatocelectomy is generally an outpatient surgical procedure, performed under anesthesia. A post-operative evaluation is done after 2–6 weeks to ensure that the incision is healing properly and that there are no complications. Spermatocelectomy has an excellent outcome and prognosis, with a 94 percent recovery rate.

References

1. Mayo Clinic Staff. "Diseases and Conditions: Spermatocele," Mayo Clinic, December 16, 2014.

2. "Spermatoceles," Urology Care Foundation, n.d.

3. Paris, Vernon M. "Spermatocele Treatment & Management," Medscape, October 15, 2015.

4. Thomson, Gregory E., Wood, Christopher G. "Spermatocele (Epididymal Cyst)," WebMD, November 14, 2014.

Section 31.5

Testicular Torsion

Text in this section is excerpted from "Testicular Torsion,"
© 1995–2016. The Nemours Foundation/KidsHealth®.
Reprinted with permission.

Genital pain is usually nothing more than a mild, brief discomfort. But when it's more painful, it can be caused by a very serious condition called testicular torsion. **Testicular torsion is a medical emergency** that usually requires immediate surgery to save the testicle.

About Testicular Torsion

Testicular torsion (also called testis torsion) happens when the spermatic cord that provides blood flow to the testicle rotates and becomes twisted, usually due to an injury or medical condition. This cuts off the testicle's blood supply and causes sudden, severe pain and swelling.

Testicular torsion requires immediate surgery to fix. If it goes on too long, it can result in severe damage to the testicle and even its removal.

Torsion can happen to males of any age, including newborns and babies, but is most common in 10- to 25-year-olds and teens who've recently gone through puberty.

Causes

The scrotum is the sack of skin beneath the penis. Inside the scrotum are two testes, or testicles. Each testicle is connected to the rest of the body by a blood vessel called the spermatic cord.

Testicular torsion is when a spermatic cord becomes twisted, cutting off the flow of blood to the attached testicle.

Most cases of testicular torsion are in males who have a genetic condition called the bell clapper deformity. Normally, the testicles are attached to the scrotum, but in this condition the testicles aren't attached, and therefore are more likely to turn and twist within the scrotum.

Testicular torsion also can happen after strenuous exercise, while someone is sleeping, or after an injury to the scrotum. Often, though, the exact cause isn't known.

Symptoms

If your son has sudden groin pain, get him to a hospital emergency room as soon as you can. Testicular torsion is a surgical emergency—when it happens, immediate surgery is needed to save the testicle.

Because surgery may be necessary, it's important to not give a boy with testicular pain anything to eat or drink before seeking medical care.

If your son has testicular torsion, he'll feel a sudden, possibly severe pain in his scrotum and one of his testicles. The pain can get worse or ease a bit, but probably won't go away completely.

Other symptoms:

- swelling, especially on one side of the scrotum

- nausea and vomiting

- abdominal pain

- one testicle appears to be higher than the other

Sometimes, the spermatic cord can become twisted and then untwist itself without treatment. This is called **torsion and detorsion**, and it can make testicular torsion more likely to happen again in the future.

If your son's spermatic cord untwists and the pain goes away, it might be easy to dismiss the episode, but you should still call a doctor. Surgery can be done to secure the testicles and make testicular torsion unlikely to happen again.

Diagnosis

When you get to the hospital, a doctor will examine your son's scrotum, testicles, abdomen, and groin and might test his reflexes by rubbing or pinching the inside of his thigh. This normally causes the testicle to contract, which probably won't happen if he has a testicular torsion.

The doctor also might do tests to see if the spermatic cord is twisted, including:

- **Ultrasound**: High-frequency waves are used to make an image of the testicle and check blood flow.

- **Urine tests or blood tests**: These can help determine whether symptoms are being caused by an infection instead of a torsion.

Sometimes, a doctor will have to perform surgery to make a diagnosis of testicular torsion. Other times, when the physical exam clearly points to a torsion, the doctor will perform emergency surgery without any other testing in order to save the testicle.

Saving a testicle becomes more difficult the longer the spermatic cord stays twisted. The degree of twisting (whether it's one entire revolution or several) determines how quickly the testicle will become damaged. As a general rule:

- within about 4-6 hours of the start of the torsion, the testicle can be saved 90 percent of the time

- after 12 hours, this drops to 50%

- after 24 hours, the testicle can be saved only 10 percent of the time

Treatment

Testicular torsion almost always needs surgery to fix. In rare cases, the doctor may be able to untwist the spermatic cord by physically manipulating the scrotum, but surgery usually is still needed to attach one or both testicles to the scrotum to prevent torsion from happening again.

Most torsion surgeries are done on an outpatient basis (with no overnight hospital stay). If your son has a torsion, he'll be given a painkiller and a general anesthetic that will make him unconscious for the procedure.

Surgery consists of making a small cut in the scrotum, untwisting the spermatic cord, and stitching the testicles to the inside of the scrotum to prevent future torsions. Afterward, your son will be taken to a recovery room to rest for an hour or two before he's released.

Following the surgery, your son will need to avoid strenuous activities for a few weeks, and if he's sexually active, he'll need to avoid all sexual activity. Talk to the doctor about when it will be safe for your son to return to his normal activities.

Testicle Removal

If a torsion goes on too long, doctors won't be able to save the affected testicle and it will have to be removed surgically, a procedure known as an **orchiectomy**. Most boys who have a testicle removed but still have a viable testicle can father children later in life. However, many also opt for a prosthetic, or artificial, testicle a few months after surgery. This can help make some boys feel more comfortable about their appearance.

With newborn boys, saving the testicle depends on when the torsion happens. If it's before a boy is born, it may be impossible to save the testicle. In this case, the doctor may recommend a surgery at a later date to remove the affected testicle. If torsion symptoms appear after a boy is born, the doctor may recommend emergency surgery to correct the testicle.

Don't Ignore Symptoms!

Boys need to know that genital pain is serious and shouldn't be ignored. Ignoring pain for too long or simply hoping it goes away can result in severe damage to the testicle and even its removal.

Even if your son has pain in his scrotum that goes away, he still needs to tell you or a doctor and get checked out. A torsion that goes away makes him more likely to have another one in the future. Doctors can greatly reduce the risk of another torsion by performing a simple surgical procedure that secures the testicles to the scrotum.

If your son had a torsion that resulted in the loss of a testicle, it's important to let him know that he can still lead a normal life, just like anyone else. The loss of one testicle won't prevent a man from having normal sexual relations or fathering children.

Section 31.6

Perineal Injury in Males

This section includes text excerpted from "Perineal Injury in Males," National Institute of Diabetes and Digestive and Kidney Diseases (NIDDK), March 2014.

What Is Perineal Injury in Males?

Perineal injury is an injury to the perineum, the part of the body between the anus and the genitals, or sex organs. In males, the perineum is the area between the anus and the scrotum, the external pouch of skin that holds the testicles. Injuries to the perineum can happen suddenly, as in an accident, or gradually, as the result of an activity that persistently puts pressure on the perineum. Sudden damage to the perineum is called an acute injury, while gradual damage is called a chronic injury.

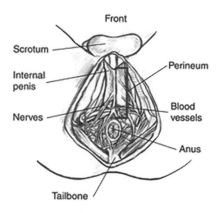

Figure 31.2. *Male Perineum*

Why Is the Perineum Important?

The perineum is important because it contains blood vessels and nerves that supply the urinary tract and genitals with blood and

407

nerve signals. The perineum lies just below a sheet of muscles called the pelvic floor muscles. Pelvic floor muscles support the bladder and bowel.

What Are the Complications of Perineal Injury?

Injury to the blood vessels, nerves, and muscles in the perineum can lead to complications such as:

- bladder control problems
- sexual problems

Bladder control problems. The nerves in the perineum carry signals from the bladder to the spinal cord and brain, telling the brain when the bladder is full. Those same nerves carry signals from the brain to the bladder and pelvic floor muscles, directing those muscles to hold or release urine. Injury to those nerves can block or interfere with the signals, causing the bladder to squeeze at the wrong time or not to squeeze at all. Damage to the pelvic floor muscles can cause bladder and bowel control problems.

Sexual problems. The perineal nerves also carry signals between the genitals and the brain. Injury to those nerves can interfere with the sensations of sexual contact.

Signals from the brain direct the smooth muscles in the genitals to relax, causing greater blood flow into the penis. In men, damaged blood vessels can cause erectile dysfunction (ED), the inability to achieve or maintain an erection firm enough for sexual intercourse. An internal portion of the penis runs through the perineum and contains a section of the urethra. As a result, damage to the perineum may also injure the penis and urethra.

What Are the Most Common Causes of Acute Perineal Injury?

Common causes of acute perineal injury in males include:

- perineal surgery
- straddle injuries
- sexual abuse
- impalement

Perineal Surgery

Acute perineal injury may result from surgical procedures that require an incision in the perineum:

- A **prostatectomy** is the surgical removal of the prostate to treat prostate cancer. The prostate, a walnut-shaped gland in men, surrounds the urethra at the neck of the bladder and supplies fluid that goes into semen. The surgeon chooses the location for the incision based on the patient's physical characteristics, such as size and weight, and the surgeon's experience and preferences. In one approach, called the radical perineal prostatectomy, the surgeon makes an incision between the scrotum and the anus. In a retropubic prostatectomy, the surgeon makes the incision in the lower abdomen, just above the penis. Both approaches can damage blood vessels and nerves affecting sexual function and bladder control.

- **Perineal urethroplasty** is surgery to repair stricture, or narrowing, of the portion of the urethra that runs through the perineum. Without this procedure, some men would not be able to pass urine. However, the procedure does require an incision in the perineum, which can damage blood vessels or nerves.

- **Colorectal or anal cancer surgery** can injure the perineum by cutting through some of the muscle around the anus to remove a tumor. One approach to anal cancer surgery involves making incisions in the abdomen and the perineum.

Surgeons try to avoid procedures that damage a person's blood vessels, perineal nerves, and muscles. However, sometimes a perineal incision may achieve the best angle to remove a life-threatening cancer.

People should discuss the risks of any planned surgery with their healthcare provider so they can make an informed decision and understand what to expect after the operation.

Straddle Injuries

Straddle injuries result from falls onto objects such as metal bars, pipes, or wooden rails, where the person's legs are on either side of the object and the perineum strikes the object forcefully. These injuries include motorcycle and bike riding accidents, saddle horn injuries during horseback riding, falls on playground equipment such as monkey bars, and gymnastic accidents on an apparatus such as the parallel bars or pommel horse.

In rare situations, a blunt injury to the perineum may burst a blood vessel inside the erectile tissue of the penis, causing a persistent partial erection that can last for days to years. This condition is called high-flow priapism. If not treated, ED may result.

Sexual Abuse

Forceful and inappropriate sexual contact can result in perineal injury. When healthcare providers evaluate injuries in the genital area, they should consider the possibility of sexual abuse, even if the person or family members say the injury is the result of an accident such as a straddle injury. The law requires that healthcare providers report cases of sexual abuse that come to their attention. The person and family members should understand the healthcare provider may ask some uncomfortable questions about the circumstances of the injury.

Impalement

Impalement injuries may involve metal fence posts, rods, or weapons that pierce the perineum. Impalement is rare, although it may occur where moving equipment and pointed tools are in use, such as on farms or construction sites. Impalement can also occur as the result of a fall, such as from a tree or playground equipment, onto something sharp. Impalement injuries are most common in combat situations. If an impalement injury pierces the skin and muscles, the injured person needs immediate medical attention to minimize blood loss and repair the injury.

What Are the Most Common Causes of Chronic Perineal Injury?

Chronic perineal injury most often results from a job-or sport-related practice—such as bike, motorcycle, or horseback riding—or a long-term condition such as chronic constipation.

Bike Riding

Sitting on a narrow, saddle-style bike seat—which has a protruding "nose" in the front—places far more pressure on the perineum than sitting in a regular chair. In a regular chair, the flesh and bone of the buttocks partially absorb the pressure of sitting, and the pressure occurs farther toward the back than on a bike seat. The straddling position on a narrow seat pinches the perineal blood vessels and nerves, possibly causing blood vessel and nerve damage over time. Research shows wider, noseless seats reduce perineal pressure.

Occasional bike riding for short periods of time may pose no risk. However, men who ride bikes several hours a week—such as competitive bicyclists, bicycle couriers, and bicycle patrol officers—have a significantly higher risk of developing mild to severe ED. The ED may be caused by repetitive pressure on blood vessels, which constricts them and results in plaque buildup in the vessels.

Other activities that involve riding saddle-style include motorcycle and horseback riding. Researchers have studied bike riding more extensively than these other activities; however, the few studies published regarding motorcycle and horseback riding suggest motorcycle riding increases the risk of ED and urinary symptoms. Horseback riding appears relatively safe in terms of chronic injury, although the action of bouncing up and down, repeatedly striking the perineum, has the potential for causing damage.

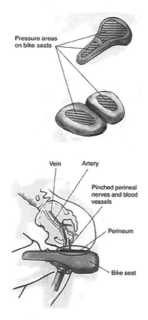

Figure 31.3. *Chronic Perineal Injury due to Bike Riding*

The straddling position on a narrow seat pinches the perineal blood vessels and nerves.

Constipation

Constipation is defined as having a bowel movement fewer than three times per week. People with constipation usually have hard, dry stools that are small in size and difficult to pass. Some people with constipation need to strain to pass stools. This straining creates internal pressure that squeezes the perineum and can damage the perineal blood vessels and nerves.

Who Is Most at Risk for Perineal Injury?

Men who have perineal surgery are most likely to have an acute perineal injury. Straddle injuries are most common among people who ride motorcycles, bikes, or horses and children who use playground equipment. Impalement injuries are most common in military personnel engaged in combat. Impalement injuries can also occur in construction or farm workers.

Chronic perineal injuries are most common in people who ride bikes as part of a job or sport, or in people with constipation.

How Is Perineal Injury Evaluated?

Healthcare providers evaluate perineal injury based on the circumstances and severity of the injury. In general, the evaluation process includes a physical examination and one or more imaging tests.

During a physical examination, the patient lies face up with legs spread and feet in stirrups. The healthcare provider looks for cuts, bruises, or bleeding from the anus. The healthcare provider may insert a gloved, lubricated finger into the rectum to feel for internal injuries.

To look for internal injuries, the healthcare provider may order one or more imaging tests. Imaging is the general term for any technique used to provide pictures of bones and organs inside the body. An X-ray technician performs these procedures in an outpatient center or a hospital, and a radiologist—a doctor who specializes in medical imaging—interprets the images. The person does not need anesthesia. However, people with a fear of confined spaces may receive light sedation before a magnetic resonance imaging (MRI) test.

Computerized tomography (CT) scans use a combination of X-rays and computer technology to create images. For a CT scan, a healthcare provider may give the patient a solution to drink and an injection of a special dye, called contrast medium. CT scans require the patient to lie on a table that slides into a tunnel-shaped device where an X-ray technician takes the X-rays. CT scans can show traumatic injury to the perineum.

MRI is a test that takes pictures of the body's internal organs and soft tissues without using X-rays. An MRI may include the injection of contrast medium. With most MRI machines, the patient will lie on a table that slides into a tunnel-shaped device that may be open ended or closed at one end. During an MRI, the patient, although usually awake, remains perfectly still while the technician takes the images, which usually only takes a few minutes. The technician will take a sequence of images from different angles to create a detailed picture of the perineum. The patient will hear loud mechanical knocking and humming noises. MRI results can show damage to blood vessels and muscles.

Ultrasound uses a device, called a transducer, that bounces safe, painless sound waves off organs to create an image of their structure. Color Doppler is enhanced ultrasound technology that shows blood flowing through arteries and veins. Blood flowing through arteries appears red, while blood flowing through veins appears blue. The color Doppler is useful in showing damage to blood vessels in the perineum.

How Is Perineal Injury Treated?

Treatments for perineal injury vary with the severity and type of injury. Tears or incisions may require stitches. Traumatic or piercing injuries may require surgery to repair damaged pelvic floor muscles, blood vessels, and nerves. Treatment for these acute injuries may also include antibiotics to prevent infection. After a healthcare provider stabilizes an acute injury so blood loss is no longer a concern, a person may still face some long-term effects of the injury, such as bladder control and sexual function problems. A healthcare provider can treat high-flow priapism caused by a blunt injury to the perineum with medication, blockage of the burst blood vessel under X-ray guidance, or surgery.

In people with a chronic perineal injury, a healthcare provider will treat the complications of the condition.

How Can Perineal Injury Be Prevented?

Preventing perineal injury requires being aware of and taking steps to minimize the dangers of activities such as construction work or bike riding:

- People should talk with their healthcare provider about the benefits and risks of perineal surgery well before the operation.

- People who play or work around moving equipment or sharp objects should wear protective gear whenever possible.

- People who ride bikes, motorcycles, or horses should find seats or saddles designed to place the most pressure on the buttocks and minimize pressure on the perineum. Many healthcare providers advise bike riders to use noseless bike seats and to ride in an upright position rather than lean over the handle bars. The National Institute for Occupational Safety and Health, part of the Centers for Disease Control and Prevention, recommends noseless seats for people who ride bikes as part of their job.

- People with constipation should talk with their healthcare provider about whether to take a laxative or stool softener to minimize straining during a bowel movement.

Eating, Diet, and Nutrition

To prevent constipation, a diet with 20 to 35 grams of fiber each day helps the body form soft, bulky stool that is easier to pass. High-fiber foods include beans, whole grains and bran cereals, fresh fruits, and vegetables such as asparagus, brussels sprouts, cabbage, and carrots. For people prone to constipation, limiting foods that have little or no fiber, such as ice cream, cheese, meat, and processed foods, is also important. A healthcare provider can give information about how changes in eating, diet, and nutrition could help with constipation.

Section 31.7

Undescended Testicle

Text in this section is excerpted from "Undescended Testicles,"
© 1995–2016. The Nemours Foundation/KidsHealth®.
Reprinted with permission.

As a baby boy grows inside his mother's womb, his testicles typically form inside his abdomen and move down (descend) into the scrotum shortly before birth. But in some cases, that move or descent doesn't occur, and the baby is born with a condition known as undescended testicles (or cryptorchidism).

Cryptorchidism is the most common genital abnormality in boys, affecting approximately 30 percent of baby boys born prematurely and about 4 percent born at term.

In about half of the babies, the undescended testicles move down or descend on their own by the sixth month of life. If descent doesn't happen by then, it's important to get treatment because testicles that remain undescended may be damaged, which could affect fertility later or lead to other medical problems.

Diagnosis

Doctors usually diagnose cryptorchidism during a physical exam at birth or at a checkup shortly after. In 7 of 10 boys with an undescended testicle (or "testis"), it can be located or "palpated" on examination by the pediatric specialist.

In 3 of 10 boys, the testicle may not be in a location where it can be located or palpated, and may appear to be missing. In some of these cases, the testicle could be inside the abdomen. In some boys with a "non-palpable" testicle, however, the testicle may not be present because it was lost while the baby was inside the womb.

In some boys, the testicles (or "testes") may appear to be outside of the scrotum from time to time, which can raise the concern of an undescended testicle. Some of these boys may have the condition known as retractile testes. This is a normal condition in which the testes reside in the scrotum but on occasion temporarily retract or pull back up into the groin.

There is no need to treat a retractile testicle, since it is a normal condition, but it might require examination by a pediatric specialist to distinguish it from an undescended testicle.

Treatment

If a baby's testicle has not descended on its own within the first 6 months of life, the boy should undergo evaluation by a pediatric specialist and treatment if the condition is confirmed. This usually involves surgically repositioning the testicle into the scrotum.

Treatment is necessary for several reasons:

- The higher temperature of the body may inhibit the normal development of the testicle, which could impair normal production of sperm in the undescended testicle in the future, which could lead to infertility.

- The undescended testicle is at a greater risk to form a tumor than the normally descended testicle.

- The undescended testicle may be more vulnerable to injury or testicular torsion.

- An asymmetrical or empty scrotum may cause a boy worry and embarrassment.

- Sometimes boys with undescended testicles develop inguinal hernias.

If surgery is done, it's likely to be an orchiopexy, in which a small cut is made in the groin and the testicle is brought down into the scrotum where it is fixed (or pexed) in place. Doctors typically do this on an outpatient basis, and most boys recover fully within a week.

Most doctors believe that boys who've had a single undescended testicle will have normal fertility potential and testicular function as adults, while those who've had two undescended testicles might be more likely to have diminished fertility as adults.

It is recommended that all boys who've had undescended testicles undergo follow-up evaluations by a urologist for years after their corrective surgeries.

It is important for all boys—even those whose testicles have properly descended—to learn how to do a testicular self-exam when they are teenagers so that they can detect any lumps or bumps that might be early signs of medical problems.

Section 31.8

Varicocele

Text in this section is excerpted from "Varicocele," © 1995–2016.
The Nemours Foundation/KidsHealth®. Reprinted with permission.

You've heard of varicose veins—those swollen veins that sometimes show up in the legs. Maybe you heard your grandma talking about her varicose veins and never thought twice about them.

But you might never have heard of a varicocele, which is also a swelling of the veins. A varicocele happens just to guys. That's because it's not in the legs but in a place a bit more private and a lot more tender—the scrotum. It's generally harmless and basically the same kind of thing as varicose veins in the legs.

But what exactly is a varicocele and how do you get rid of it?

What Is a Varicocele?

In all guys, a structure called the spermatic cord (which contains arteries, veins, nerves, and tubes) provides a connection and circulates blood to and from the testicles. Veins carry the blood flowing from the body back toward the heart, and a bunch of valves in the veins keep the blood flowing one way and stop it from flowing backward. In other words, the valves regulate your blood flow and make sure everything is flowing in the right direction.

But sometimes these valves can fail. When this happens, some of the blood can flow in reverse. This backed-up blood can collect in pools in the veins, which then causes the veins to stretch and get bigger, or become swollen. This is called a varicocele.

Who Gets Them?

They don't happen to every guy, but varicoceles are fairly common. They appear in about 15 percent of guys between 15-25 years old, mostly during puberty. That's because during puberty, the testicles grow quickly and need more blood delivered to them. If the valves in the veins in the scrotum aren't working quite as well as they should, the veins can't handle carrying this extra blood. So, although most of the blood continues to flow correctly, blood begins to back up, creating a varicocele.

An interesting fact is that varicoceles occur mostly on the left side of the scrotum. This is because a guy's body is organized so that blood flow on that side of the scrotum is greater, so varicoceles happen more often in the left testicle than the right. Although it's less common, they can sometimes happen on both sides.

What Are the Signs and Symptoms?

In most cases, guys have no symptoms at all. A guy might not even be aware that he has a varicocele. However, if there are symptoms, they tend to occur during hot weather, after heavy exercise, or when a guy has been standing or sitting for a long time.

417

Signs include:

- a dull ache in the testicle(s)

- a feeling of heaviness or dragging in the scrotum

- dilated veins in the scrotum that can be felt (described as feeling like worms or spaghetti)

- discomfort in the testicle or on that particular side of the scrotum

- the testicle is smaller on the side where the dilated veins are (due to difference in blood flow)

What Do Doctors Do?

It's a good idea to get a testicular exam regularly, which is normally part of a guy's regular checkup. In addition to visually checking for any unusual lumps or bumps, the doctor generally feels the testicles and the area around them to make sure a guy's equipment is in good shape and there are no problems.

A testicular exam may be done while a guy is standing up so that the scrotum is relaxed. (Some abnormalities like a varicocele can be more easily felt in a standing position.) The doctor checks things like the size, weight, and position of the testicles, and gently rolls each testicle back and forth to feel for lumps or swelling. The doctor also feels for any signs of tenderness along the epididymis, the tube that transports sperm from the testicles.

The spermatic cord is also examined for any sign of swelling. If the doctor thinks there might be a varicocele, he or she might do an ultrasound, which can measure blood flow and identify veins that aren't working correctly.

Do Varicoceles Cause Permanent Damage?

Although there is no way to prevent a varicocele, most need no special treatment. A varicocele is usually harmless and more than likely won't affect a guy's ability to father a child later in life.

Some experts believe, though, that in some cases a varicocele might damage the testicle or decrease sperm production. In those cases, a doctor will probably recommend surgery.

What If the Doctor Finds a Varicocele?

Varicoceles are generally harmless, but if there is any pain and swelling the doctor may prescribe an anti-inflammatory medication to relieve it. If the varicocele causes discomfort or aching, wearing snug underwear (like briefs) or a jock strap for support may bring relief.

If the doctor thinks the testicle is being affected by the varicocele or if there's still pain and support doesn't help, a type of surgery called a varicocelectomy may be recommended. A varicocelectomy is done by a urologist, a doctor who specializes in urinary and genital problems. There are different ways to repair the varicocele, and the urologist will discuss the different ways and recommend the best approach for the patient.

The procedure is usually done on an outpatient basis (meaning there's no need for an overnight hospital stay). The patient usually gets general or local anesthesia. Then, the doctor simply ties off the affected vein to redirect the flow of blood into other normal veins.

In some cases, instead of surgery, doctors can pass a plastic tube into the vein that's causing the varicocele and treat the problem by blocking blood flow to the enlarged vein. Talk with your doctor about whether this form of treatment might be an option for you.

After surgery, the doctor probably will recommend that a guy wear a scrotal support and use a cold pack on the area to bring down any swelling. There may be discomfort in the testicle for a few weeks, but after that, any aches and pains will go away and everything should be back in full working order.

Chapter 32

Noncancerous Prostate Disorders

Chapter Contents

Section 32.1—Benign Prostatic Hyperplasia 422

Section 32.2—Prostatitis 428

Section 32.1

Benign Prostatic Hyperplasia

This section includes text excerpted from "Understanding
Prostate Changes," National Cancer Institute (NCI), August 2011.
Reviewed August 2016.

What Is Benign Prostatic Hyperplasia (Enlarged Prostate)?

BPH stands for benign prostatic hyperplasia.

Benign means "not cancer," and **hyperplasia** means abnormal cell growth. The result is that the prostate becomes enlarged. BPH is not linked to cancer and does not increase your risk of getting
prostate cancer—yet the symptoms for BPH and prostate cancer can be similar.

BPH Symptoms

BPH symptoms usually start after the age of 50. They can include:

- trouble starting a urine stream or making more than a dribble

- passing urine often, especially at night

- feeling that the bladder has not fully emptied

- a strong or sudden urge to pass urine

- weak or slow urine stream

- stopping and starting again several times while passing urine

- pushing or straining to begin passing urine

At its worst, BPH can lead to:

- a weak bladder

- backflow of urine, causing bladder or **kidney** infections

- complete block in the flow of urine

- kidney failure

BPH affects most men as they get older. It can lead to urinary problems like those with prostatitis. BPH rarely causes symptoms before age 40, but more than half of men in their 60s and most men in their 70s and 80s will have signs of BPH.

The prostate gland is about the size of a walnut when a man is in his 20s. By the time he is 40, it may have grown slightly larger, to the size of an apricot. By age 60, it may be the size of a lemon.

The enlarged prostate can press against the bladder and the urethra. This can slow down or block urine flow. Some men might find it hard to start a urine stream, even though they feel the need to go. Once the urine stream has started, it may be hard to stop. Other men may feel like they need to pass urine all the time, or they are awakened during sleep with the sudden need to pass urine.

Early BPH symptoms take many years to turn into bothersome problems. These early symptoms are a cue to see your doctor.

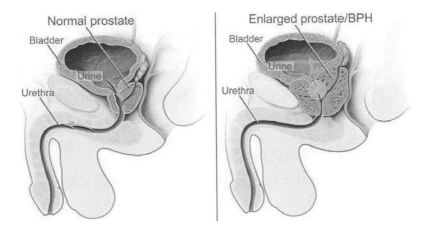

Figure 32.1. *Urine Flow in a Normal (Left) and Enlarged (Right) Prostate*

In diagram on the left, urine flows freely. On the right, urine flow is affected because the enlarged prostate is pressing on the bladder and urethra.

How Is BPH Treated?

Some men with BPH eventually find their symptoms to be bothersome enough to need treatment. BPH cannot be cured, but drugs or **surgery** can often relieve its symptoms.

There are three ways to manage BPH:

- **watchful waiting** (regular follow-up with your doctor)
- drug therapy
- surgery

Talk with your doctor about the best choice for you. Your symptoms may change over time, so be sure to tell your doctor about any new changes.

Watchful Waiting

Men with mild symptoms of BPH who do not find them bothersome often choose this approach.

Watchful waiting means getting annual check-ups. The check-ups can include DREs and other tests.

Treatment is started only when the symptoms become too much of a problem.

If you choose watchful waiting, these simple steps may help lessen your symptoms:

- Limit drinking in the evening, especially drinks with alcohol or caffeine.
- Empty your bladder all the way when you pass urine.
- Use the restroom often. Don't wait for long periods without passing urine.

Some medications can make BPH symptoms worse, so talk with your doctor or pharmacist about any medicines you are taking, such as:

- **over-the-counter** cold and cough medicines (especially **antihistamines**)
- tranquilizers
- **antidepressants**
- **blood pressure** medicine

Your doctor may be able to prescribe other medication that does not increase BPH symptoms.

Drug Therapy

Many American men with mild to moderate BPH symptoms have chosen **prescription** drugs over surgery since the early 1990s. Two main types of drugs are used. One type relaxes muscles near the prostate, and the other type shrinks the prostate gland. Some evidence shows that taking both drugs together may work best to keep BPH symptoms from getting worse.

Alpha-Blockers

These drugs help relax muscles near the prostate to relieve pressure and let urine flow more freely, but they don't shrink the size of the prostate. For many men, these drugs can improve urine flow and reduce the symptoms of BPH within days. Possible side effects include dizziness, headache, and fatigue.

5-Alpha Reductase Inhibitors

These drugs help shrink the prostate. They relieve symptoms by blocking the activity of an enzyme known as 5-alpha reductase. This **enzyme** changes the male hormone **testosterone** into **dihydrotestosterone** (DHT), which stimulates prostate growth. When the action of 5-alpha reductase is blocked, DHT production is lowered and prostate growth slows.

This helps shrink the prostate, reduce blockage, and limit the need for surgery.

Taking these drugs can help increase urine flow and reduce your symptoms. You must continue to take these drugs to prevent symptoms from coming back.

5-alpha reductase inhibitors can cause the following side effects in a small percentage of men:

- decreased interest in sex

- trouble getting or keeping an **erection**

- smaller amount of semen with ejaculation

It's important to note that taking these drugs may lower your PSA test number. There is also evidence that these drugs lower the risk of getting prostate cancer, but whether they can help lower the risk of dying from prostate cancer is still unclear.

Table 32.1. BPH Medications

Category	Activity	Generic Name	Brand Name
Alpha-blockers	Relax muscles near prostate	alfuzosin	Uroxatral
		doxazosin	Cardura
		silodosin	Rapaflo
		tamsulosin	Flomax
		terazosin	Hytrin
5-alpha reductase inhibitors	Slows prostate growth, shrinks prostate	finasteride	Proscar or Propecia
		dutasteride	Avodart

Surgery

The number of prostate surgeries has gone down over the years. But operations for BPH are still among the most common surgeries for American men. Surgery is used when symptoms are severe or drug therapy has not worked well.

Types of surgery for BPH include:

- **TURP (transurethral resection of the prostate).** The most common surgery for BPH, TURP accounts for 90 percent of all BPH surgeries. The doctor passes an instrument through the urethra and trims away extra prostate tissue. A **spinal block (anesthesia)** is used to numb the area. Tissue is sent to the laboratory to check for prostate cancer.

  TURP generally avoids the two main dangers linked to another type of surgery called open prostatectomy (complete removal of the prostate gland through a cut in the lower abdomen):

  - Incontinence (not being able to hold in urine)

  - Impotence (not being able to have an erection)

  However, TURP can have serious side effects, such as bleeding. In addition, men may have to stay in the hospital and need a **catheter** for a few days after surgery.

- **TUIP (transurethral incision of the prostate).** This surgery, which is similar to TURP, is used on slightly enlarged prostate glands. The surgeon places one or two small cuts in the prostate. This relieves pressure without trimming away tissue. It has a low risk of side effects. Like TURP, this treatment helps with urine flow by widening the urethra.

- **TUNA (transurethral needle ablation).** Radio waves are used to burn away excess prostate tissue. TUNA helps with urine flow, relieves symptoms, and may have fewer side effects than TURP. Most men need a catheter to drain urine for a period of time after the procedure.

- **TUMT (transurethral microwave thermotherapy).** Microwaves sent through a catheter are used to destroy excess prostate tissue. This can be an option for men who should not have major surgery because they have other medical problems.

- **TUVP (transurethral electroevaporation of the prostate).** An electrical current is used to vaporize prostate tissue.

- **Laser surgery.** The doctor passes a laser fiber through the urethra into the prostate, using a cystoscope, and then delivers several bursts of laser energy. The laser energy destroys prostate tissue and helps improve urine flow. Like TURP, laser surgery requires anesthesia. One advantage of laser surgery over TURP is that laser surgery causes little blood loss. The recovery period for laser surgery may be shorter too. However, laser surgery may not be effective on larger prostates.

- **Open prostatectomy.** This may be the only option in rare cases, such as when the **obstruction** is severe, the prostate is very large, or other procedures can't be done. **General anesthesia** or a spinal block is used, and a catheter remains for 3 to 7 days after the surgery. This surgery carries the highest risk of **complications**. Tissue is sent to the laboratory to check for prostate cancer.

Be sure to discuss options with your doctor and ask about the potential short- and long-term benefits and risks with each procedure.

Section 32.2

Prostatitis

This section includes text excerpted from "Prostatitis:
Inflammation of the Prostate," National Institute Diabetes and
Digestive and Kidney Diseases (NIDDK), July 2014.

What Is Prostatitis?

Prostatitis is a frequently painful condition that involves inflammation of the prostate and sometimes the areas around the prostate. Scientists have identified four types of prostatitis:

- chronic prostatitis/chronic pelvic pain syndrome

- acute bacterial prostatitis

- chronic bacterial prostatitis

- asymptomatic inflammatory prostatitis

Men with asymptomatic inflammatory prostatitis do not have symptoms. A healthcare provider may diagnose asymptomatic inflammatory prostatitis when testing for other urinary tract or reproductive tract disorders. This type of prostatitis does not cause complications and does not need treatment.

What Is the Prostate?

The prostate is a walnut-shaped gland that is part of the male reproductive system. The main function of the prostate is to make a fluid that goes into semen. Prostate fluid is essential for a man's fertility. The gland surrounds the urethra at the neck of the bladder. The bladder neck is the area where the urethra joins the bladder. The bladder and urethra are parts of the lower urinary tract. The prostate has two or more lobes, or sections, enclosed by an outer layer of tissue, and it is in front of the rectum, just below the bladder. The urethra is the tube that carries urine from the bladder to the outside of the body. In men, the urethra also carries semen out through the penis.

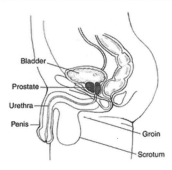

Figure 32.2. *Prostate*

The prostate is a walnut-shaped gland that is part of the male reproductive system.

What Causes Prostatitis?

The causes of prostatitis differ depending on the type.

Chronic prostatitis/chronic pelvic pain syndrome. The exact cause of chronic prostatitis/chronic pelvic pain syndrome is unknown. Researchers believe a microorganism, though not a bacterial infection, may cause the condition. This type of prostatitis may relate to chemicals in the urine, the immune system's response to a previous urinary tract infection (UTI), or nerve damage in the pelvic area.

Acute and chronic bacterial prostatitis. A bacterial infection of the prostate causes bacterial prostatitis. The acute type happens suddenly and lasts a short time, while the chronic type develops slowly and lasts a long time, often years. The infection may occur when bacteria travel from the urethra into the prostate.

How Common Is Prostatitis?

Prostatitis is the most common urinary tract problem for men younger than age 50 and the third most common urinary tract problem for men older than age 50. Prostatitis accounts for about two million visits to healthcare providers in the United States each year.

Chronic prostatitis/chronic pelvic pain syndrome is the most common and least understood form of prostatitis. Chronic prostatitis/chronic pelvic pain syndrome can occur in men of any age group and affects 10 to 15 percent of the U.S. male population.

Who Is More Likely to Develop Prostatitis?

The factors that affect a man's chances of developing prostatitis differ depending on the type.

Chronic prostatitis/chronic pelvic pain syndrome. Men with nerve damage in the lower urinary tract due to surgery or trauma may be more likely to develop chronic prostatitis/chronic pelvic pain syndrome. Psychological stress may also increase a man's chances of developing the condition.

Acute and chronic bacterial prostatitis. Men with lower UTIs may be more likely to develop bacterial prostatitis. UTIs that recur or are difficult to treat may lead to chronic bacterial prostatitis.

What Are the Symptoms of Prostatitis?

Each type of prostatitis has a range of symptoms that vary depending on the cause and may not be the same for every man. Many symptoms are similar to those of other conditions.

Chronic prostatitis/chronic pelvic pain syndrome. The main symptoms of chronic prostatitis/chronic pelvic pain syndrome can include pain or discomfort lasting 3 or more months in one or more of the following areas:

- between the scrotum and anus
- the central lower abdomen
- the penis
- the scrotum
- the lower back

Pain during or after ejaculation is another common symptom. A man with chronic prostatitis/chronic pelvic pain syndrome may have pain spread out around the pelvic area or may have pain in one or more areas at the same time. The pain may come and go and appear suddenly or gradually. Other symptoms may include

- pain in the urethra during or after urination.
- pain in the penis during or after urination.
- urinary frequency—urination eight or more times a day. The bladder begins to contract even when it contains small amounts of urine, causing more frequent urination.
- urinary urgency—the inability to delay urination.
- a weak or an interrupted urine stream.

Acute bacterial prostatitis. The symptoms of acute bacterial prostatitis come on suddenly and are severe. Men should seek immediate medical care. Symptoms of acute bacterial prostatitis may include

- urinary frequency
- urinary urgency
- fever
- chills
- a burning feeling or pain during urination
- pain in the genital area, groin, lower abdomen, or lower back
- noctur
- ia—frequent urination during periods of sleep
- nausea and vomiting
- body aches
- urinary retention—the inability to empty the bladder completely
- trouble starting a urine stream
- a weak or an interrupted urine stream
- urinary blockage—the complete inability to urinate
- a UTI—as shown by bacteria and infection-fighting cells in the urine

Chronic bacterial prostatitis. The symptoms of chronic bacterial prostatitis are similar to those of acute bacterial prostatitis, though not as severe. This type of prostatitis often develops slowly and can last 3 or more months. The symptoms may come and go, or they may be mild all the time. Chronic bacterial prostatitis may occur after previous treatment of acute bacterial prostatitis or a UTI. The symptoms of chronic bacterial prostatitis may include

- urinary frequency
- urinary urgency
- a burning feeling or pain during urination
- pain in the genital area, groin, lower abdomen, or lower back
- noctu
- ria

- painful ejaculation
- urinary retention
- trouble starting a urine stream
- a weak or an interrupted urine stream
- urinary blockage
- a UTI

What Are the Complications of Prostatitis?

The complications of prostatitis may include

- bacterial infection in the bloodstream
- prostatic abscess—a pus-filled cavity in the prostate
- sexual dysfunction
- inflammation of reproductive organs near the prostate

When to Seek Medical Care

A person may have urinary symptoms unrelated to prostatitis that are caused by bladder problems, UTIs, or benign prostatic hyperplasia. Symptoms of prostatitis also can signal more serious conditions, including prostate cancer.

Men with symptoms of prostatitis should see a healthcare provider.

Men with the following symptoms should seek immediate medical care:

- complete inability to urinate
- painful, frequent, and urgent need to urinate, with fever and chills
- blood in the urine
- great discomfort or pain in the lower abdomen and urinary tract

How Is Prostatitis Diagnosed?

A healthcare provider diagnoses prostatitis based on

- a personal and family medical history
- a physical exam
- medical tests

A healthcare provider may have to rule out other conditions that cause similar signs and symptoms before diagnosing prostatitis.

Personal and Family Medical History

Taking a personal and family medical history is one of the first things a healthcare provider may do to help diagnose prostatitis.

Physical Exam

A physical exam may help diagnose prostatitis. During a physical exam, a healthcare provider usually

- examines a patient's body, which can include checking for

  - discharge from the urethra

  - enlarged or tender lymph nodes in the groin

  - a swollen or tender scrotum

- performs a digital rectal exam

A digital rectal exam, or rectal exam, is a physical exam of the prostate. To perform the exam, the healthcare provider asks the man to bend over a table or lie on his side while holding his knees close to his chest. The healthcare provider slides a gloved, lubricated finger into the rectum and feels the part of the prostate that lies next to the rectum. The man may feel slight, brief discomfort during the rectal exam. A healthcare provider usually performs a rectal exam during an office visit, and the man does not need anesthesia. The exam helps the healthcare provider see if the prostate is enlarged or tender or has any abnormalities that require more testing.

Many healthcare providers perform a rectal exam as part of a routine physical exam for men age 40 or older, whether or not they have urinary problems.

Medical Tests

A healthcare provider may refer men to a urologist—a doctor who specializes in the urinary tract and male reproductive system. A urologist uses medical tests to help diagnose lower urinary tract problems related to prostatitis and recommend treatment. Medical tests may include

- urinalysis

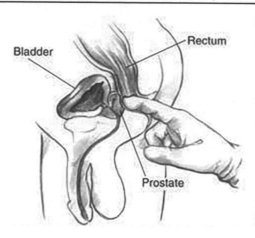

Figure 32.3. *Digital Rectal Exam*

- blood tests
- urodynamic tests
- cystoscopy
- transre
- ctal ultrasound
- biopsy
- semen analysis

Urinalysis. Urinalysis involves testing a urine sample. The patient collects a urine sample in a special container in a healthcare provider's office or a commercial facility. A healthcare provider tests the sample during an office visit or sends it to a lab for analysis. For the test, a nurse or technician places a strip of chemically treated paper, called a dipstick, into the urine. Patches on the dipstick change color to indicate signs of infection in urine.

The healthcare provider can diagnose the bacterial forms of prostatitis by examining the urine sample with a microscope. The healthcare provider may also send the sample to a lab to perform a culture. In a urine culture, a lab technician places some of the urine sample in a tube or dish with a substance that encourages any bacteria present to grow; once the bacteria have multiplied, a technician can identify them.

Blood tests. Blood tests involve a healthcare provider drawing blood during an office visit or in a commercial facility and sending the sample to a lab for analysis. Blood tests can show signs of infection and other prostate problems, such as prostate cancer.

Urodynamic tests. Urodynamic tests include a variety of procedures that look at how well the bladder and urethra store and release urine. A healthcare provider performs urodynamic tests during an office visit or in an outpatient center or a hospital. Some urodynamic tests do not require anesthesia; others may require local anesthesia. Most urodynamic tests focus on the bladder's ability to hold urine and empty steadily and completely and may include the following:

- uroflowmetry, which measures how rapidly the bladder releases urine

- postvoid residual measurement, which evaluates how much urine remains in the bladder after urination

Cystoscopy. Cystoscopy is a procedure that uses a tubelike instrument, called a cystoscope, to look inside the urethra and bladder. A urologist inserts the cystoscope through the opening at the tip of the penis and into the lower urinary tract. He or she performs cystoscopy during an office visit or in an outpatient center or a hospital. He or she will give the patient local anesthesia. In some cases, the patient may require sedation and regional or general anesthesia. A urologist may use cystoscopy to look for narrowing, blockage, or stones in the urinary tract.

Transrectal ultrasound. Transrectal ultrasound uses a device, called a transducer, that bounces safe, painless sound waves off organs to create an image of their structure. The healthcare provider can move the transducer to different angles to make it possible to examine different organs. A specially trained technician performs the procedure in a healthcare provider's office, an outpatient center, or a hospital, and a radiologist—a doctor who specializes in medical imaging—interprets the images; the patient does not require anesthesia. Urologists most often use transrectal ultrasound to examine the prostate. In a transrectal ultrasound, the technician inserts a transducer slightly larger than a pen into the man's rectum next to the prostate. The ultrasound image shows the size of the prostate and any abnormalities, such as tumors. Transrectal ultrasound cannot reliably diagnose prostate cancer.

Biopsy. Biopsy is a procedure that involves taking a small piece of prostate tissue for examination with a microscope. A urologist performs the biopsy in an outpatient center or a hospital. He or she will give the patient light sedation and local anesthetic; however, in some cases, the patient will require general anesthesia. The urologist uses imaging techniques such as ultrasound, a computerized tomography scan, or magnetic resonance imaging to guide the biopsy needle into the prostate. A pathologist—a doctor who specializes in examining tissues to diagnose diseases—examines the prostate tissue in a lab. The test can show whether prostate cancer is present.

Semen analysis. Semen analysis is a test to measure the amount and quality of a man's semen and sperm. The man collects a semen sample in a special container at home, a healthcare provider's office, or a commercial facility. A healthcare provider analyzes the sample during an office visit or sends it to a lab for analysis. A semen sample can show blood and signs of infection.

How Is Prostatitis Treated?

Treatment depends on the type of prostatitis.

Chronic prostatitis/chronic pelvic pain syndrome. Treatment for chronic prostatitis/chronic pelvic pain syndrome aims to decrease pain, discomfort, and inflammation. A wide range of symptoms exists and no single treatment works for every man. Although antibiotics will not help treat nonbacterial prostatitis, a urologist may prescribe them, at least initially, until the urologist can rule out a bacterial infection. A urologist may prescribe other medications:

- silodo
- sin (Rapaflo)
- 5-alpha reductase inhibitors such as finasteride (Proscar) and dutasteride (Avodart)
- nonsteroidal anti-inflammatory drugs—also called NSAIDs—such as aspirin, ibuprofen, and naproxen sodium
- glycosaminogly
- cans such as chondroitin sulfate
- muscle relaxants such as cyclobenzaprine (Amrix, Flexeril) and clonazepam (Klonopin)
- neuromodulators such as amitriptyline, nortriptyline (Aventyl, Pamelor), and pregabalin (Lyrica)

Alternative treatments may include

- warm baths, called sitz baths

- local heat therapy with hot water bottles or heating pads

- physical therapy, such as

  - Kegel exercises—tightening and relaxing the muscles that hold urine in the bladder and hold the bladder in its proper position. Also called pelvic muscle exercises.

  - myofascial release—pressing and stretching, sometimes with cooling and warming, of the muscles and soft tissues in the lower back, pelvic region, and upper legs. Also known as myofascial trigger point release.

- relaxation exercises

- biofeedback

- phytotherapy with plant extracts such as quercetin, bee pollen, and saw palmetto

- acupuncture

To help ensure coordinated and safe care, people should discuss their use of complementary and alternative medical practices, including their use of dietary supplements, with their healthcare provider.

For men whose chronic prostatitis/chronic pelvic pain syndrome symptoms are affected by psychological stress, appropriate psychiatric treatment and stress reduction may reduce the recurrence of symptoms.

To help measure the effectiveness of treatment, a urologist may ask a series of questions from a standard questionnaire called the National Institutes of Health (NIH) Chronic Prostatitis Symptom Index. The questionnaire helps a urologist assess the severity of symptoms and how they affect the man's quality of life. A urologist may ask questions several times, such as before, during, and after treatment.

Acute bacterial prostatitis. A urologist treats acute bacterial prostatitis with antibiotics. The antibiotic prescribed may depend on the type of bacteria causing the infection. Urologists usually prescribe oral antibiotics for at least 2 weeks. The infection may come back; therefore, some urologists recommend taking oral antibiotics for 6 to 8 weeks. Severe cases of acute prostatitis may require a short hospital stay so men can receive fluids and antibiotics through an intravenous

(IV) tube. After the IV treatment, the man will need to take oral antibiotics for 2 to 4 weeks. Most cases of acute bacterial prostatitis clear up completely with medication and slight changes to diet. The urologist may recommend

- Avoiding or reducing intake of substances that irritate the bladder, such as alcohol, caffeinated beverages, and acidic and spicy foods.

- Increasing intake of liquids—64 to 128 ounces per day—to urinate often and help flush bacteria from the bladder.

Chronic bacterial prostatitis. A urologist treats chronic bacterial prostatitis with antibiotics; however, treatment requires a longer course of therapy. The urologist may prescribe a low dose of antibiotics for up to 6 months to prevent recurrent infection. The urologist may also prescribe a different antibiotic or use a combination of antibiotics if the infection keeps coming back. The urologist may recommend increasing intake of liquids and avoiding or reducing intake of substances that irritate the bladder.

A urologist may use alpha blockers that treat chronic prostatitis/chronic pelvic pain syndrome to treat urinary retention caused by chronic bacterial prostatitis. These medications help relax the bladder muscles near the prostate and lessen symptoms such as painful urination. Men may require surgery to treat urinary retention caused by chronic bacterial prostatitis. Surgically removing scar tissue in the urethra often improves urine flow and reduces urinary retention.

How Can Prostatitis Be Prevented?

Men cannot prevent prostatitis. Researchers are currently seeking to better understand what causes prostatitis and develop prevention strategies.

Eating, Diet, and Nutrition

Researchers have not found that eating, diet, and nutrition play a role in causing or preventing prostatitis. During treatment of bacterial prostatitis, urologists may recommend increasing intake of liquids and avoiding or reducing intake of substances that irritate the bladder. Men should talk with a healthcare provider or dietitian about what diet is right for them.

Chapter 33

Sexual Dysfunction

Sexual dysfunction can refer to any physical or psychological problem that disrupts the sexual response cycle and prevents an individual or couple from achieving satisfaction. More than 30% of men report experiencing some sort of sexual dysfunction during their lives. The most common types of male sexual dysfunction include erectile dysfunction (ED) and premature ejaculation (PE). Less common conditions that may result in male sexual dysfunction include priapism and retrograde ejaculation. A variety of treatment options are available to help men overcome sexual dysfunction and enjoy satisfying intimate relations.

Erectile Dysfunction

Erectile dysfunction (formerly known as impotence) is a condition in which a man has trouble achieving an erection or sustaining it long enough for sexual intercourse. Researchers believe that ED affects 30 million men in the United States, including about 30% of men over age 70. ED can be caused by a variety of diseases and conditions that affect the nerves and arteries, as well as by some medications commonly prescribed to treat such conditions. Lifestyle choices can also contribute to ED, as can psychological or emotional issues. Some of the conditions that are often related to ED include:

- high blood pressure
- diabetes

"Sexual Dysfunction," © 2017 Omnigraphics. Reviewed August 2016.

- cardiovascular disease

- atherosclerosis (formation of plaque in the arteries)

- kidney disease

- multiple sclerosis

- Peyronie disease (formation of scar tissue in the penis)

- injury to the penis, prostate, pelvis, or spinal cord

- prostate cancer and related treatments

- lifestyle choices such as smoking, excessive alcohol consumption, illegal drug use, poor diet, lack of exercise, and being overweight

- psychological issues such as anxiety, depression, stress, guilt, low self-esteem, or fear of sexual failure

- medications such as antihistamines, antidepressants, appetite suppressants, blood pressure medications, and ulcer medications

Although some men may feel reluctant to acknowledge or discuss erectile dysfunction, it is important to seek medical attention if the problem persists for more than a few weeks or months. ED can be a sign of other health conditions, such as diabetes or heart disease, that may be developing or worsening. In addition, ED can cause both health and relationship complications if left untreated.

Diagnosis of ED

To diagnose erectile dysfunction, a urologist or other healthcare provider will typically begin by discussing the patient's medical and sexual history. The doctor will ask about health conditions, medications, and lifestyle decisions that may contribute to ED. They will also inquire about the patient's ability to get an erection, maintain an erection hard enough for penetration and intercourse, and reach climax and ejaculate. The doctor may also use a questionnaire or other tools to assess psychological or emotional factors that may contribute to ED.

The next step in diagnosing ED typically involves a physical examination. The doctor may check for high blood pressure, circulatory problems, or hormonal changes that may contribute to ED. Blood tests may be ordered to check for signs of underlying health conditions such as diabetes, cardiovascular disease, or kidney disease. The doctor may also examine the penis for unusual characteristics or lack of sensitivity.

There are three main diagnostic tests that are used to help determine the underlying cause of ED:

- Injection test

  This test involves injecting medication into the urethra or into the base of the penis to cause an erection. It allows the doctor to evaluate the hardness of the penis and the duration of the erection.

- Doppler ultrasound

  This imaging exam, which is often conducted in combination with an injection test, enables the doctor to measure the speed and direction of blood flow through the penis.

- Nocturnal erection test

  Most men have between three and five erections each night while asleep. This test is used to determine whether a patient is physically capable of having an erection, which may indicate that the cause of ED is psychological in nature. It may be performed in a sleep laboratory using electronic monitoring equipment to record the number of erections, their firmness, and how long they last. A simpler version may be done at home by placing a plastic ring around the penis that will break if the patient has a nocturnal erection.

Treatment of ED

Erectile dysfunction can be treated in a variety of ways, depending on the extent of the problem and the underlying cause. Some of the treatment options include:

- Lifestyle changes, such as eating a healthy diet, exercising regularly, losing weight, and not smoking or consuming excessive alcohol

- Treatment of underlying health conditions, such as diabetes or cardiovascular disease

- Psychological counseling to address self-esteem issues or performance anxiety

- Oral medications designed to increase blood flow to the penis, such as sildenafil (Viagra), vardenafil (Levitra), or tadalafil (Cialis)

- Medications such asalprostadil (Caverject, Edex) that are administered directly to the penis, either via injection or a suppository that is inserted into the urethra

- Use of a vacuum device to pump blood into the penis manually, coupled with an elastic ring at the base of the penis to help maintain the erection

- Surgery to reconstruct arteries that supply blood to the penis

- Surgery to implant an inflatable or malleable prosthetic device in the penis

Some forms of treatment involve risks or side effects, so men with ED should research their options carefully and choose the one that works best for them and their partners.

Premature Ejaculation

Premature ejaculation (PE) is a common form of sexual dysfunction in which a man consistently reaches orgasm and ejaculates sooner than he or his partner would like during sexual activity. Ejaculation occurs when muscles at the base of the penis contract, forcing semen from the prostate gland to be released from the erect penis. It usually takes place at the same time as orgasm or sexual climax, and the erection typically dissipates afterward. Premature ejaculation usually occurs with very little stimulation, or within one to two minutes of penetration.

Surveys suggest that one-third of men experience PE at least occasionally, although doctors believe that only about 2% suffer from primary or lifelong PE, meaning that they climax too early during nearly every sexual encounter. PE can lead to negative personal consequences for men, including frustration, embarrassment, worry, anxiety, and avoidance of sexual intimacy. In many cases, however, the man who experiences PE is much more concerned about it than is his sexual partner.

Causes of PE

Some cases of PE are related to underlying medical conditions, such as diabetes, high blood pressure, multiple sclerosis, prostate disease, thyroid problems, or nerve damage due to injury or surgery. Lifestyle choices such as illegal drug use or alcohol abuse can also increase the likelihood of PE. In addition, some studies suggest that low levels of serotonin in the brain may act to shorten the time to ejaculation.

In most cases, however, the primary causes of PE are not biological but psychological in nature. Some of the common factors that can lead to PE include:

- sexual inexperience

- overexcitement or overstimulation

- unrealistic expectations about sexual performance

- lack of confidence or self-esteem

- relationship problems

- intimacy issues

- guilt, anxiety, stress, or depression

- early sexual trauma or history of sexual repression

- conditioning oneself to ejaculate quickly while masturbating

Diagnosis and Treatment of PE

To diagnose PE, a urologist or other healthcare provider will usually take a medical and sexual history and conduct a physical examination. They will typically ask a series of questions to assess the patient's symptoms and help determine the cause of the problem, such as how often PE occurs, whether it happens in every sexual encounter or only under certain circumstances, how long the patient is able to delay ejaculation, and the extent to which PE has affected the patient's sexual activity and quality of life.

Most treatments for PE involve therapy to address the psychological issues that contribute to the problem as well as exercises and medications to help the patient delay ejaculation. Up to 95% of patients with PE show improvement through some combination of the following treatments:

- Psychological therapy to help patients uncover the source of negative feelings that may interfere with sexual performance

- Couples counseling or sex therapy to improve communication, intimacy, and sexual satisfaction

- Relaxation techniques to reduce performance anxiety and increase confidence

- Exercises to help the patient learn to control and delay ejaculation, such as the squeeze method (squeezing the penis firmly just before the point of climax) or the start-stop method (stimulating the penis to the point of climax and then stopping until the patient regains control)

- Condom use to reduce sensation in the penis

- Topical anesthetic creams or sprays, such as lidocaine or prilocaine, applied 30 minutes before intercourse to numb the penis

- Antidepressant medications such as fluoxetine, paroxetine, sertraline, and clomipramine that affect serotonin levels in the brain and delay orgasm in some patients.

Priapism

Priapism is a rare but serious medical condition in which an erection lasts more than four hours. This persistent erection is not caused by sexual stimulation, and it does not dissipate after ejaculation. Instead, it occurs when blood becomes trapped in the penis due to problems with nerves or blood vessels. Left untreated, priapism can cause permanent damage to the penis and result in sexual dysfunction. There are three main types of priapism:

- Low blood flow or ischemic priapism

    The most common form of priapism, it occurs due to blockage of a blood vessel that prevents blood from flowing normally through the penis. The blockage prevents oxygen- and nutrient-rich blood from reaching the penile tissue, which can cause permanent damage if not treated promptly.

- High blood flow priapism

    This rare condition occurs when a blood vessel ruptures, causing excessive blood to flow into the penile tissue. It usually results from an injury to the genital area.

- Stuttering or episodic priapism

    This condition involves recurring, painful erections that last between two and three hours. They may occur during sleep or before or after sexual stimulation, and their frequency may increase over time. The causes and risk factors are usually similar to low blood flow priapism.

Causes of Priapism

Priapism can have a number of underlying causes, including the following:

- Prescription medications that are commonly used to treat high blood pressure, attention deficit hyperactivity disorder, depression, schizophrenia, and hormone imbalances

- Injectable medications that are used to treat erectile dysfunction

- Illegal drugs such as marijuana, ecstasy, cocaine, or methamphetamine (crystal meth)

- Sickle cell disease (an inherited condition in which the body produces abnormally shaped red blood cells that can interfere with the function of blood vessels)

- Blood cancers, such as leukemia and multiple myeloma

- Injuries or medical conditions that affect the nervous system, brain, or spinal cord

- Tumors of the prostate, bladder, or kidney

- Infections in the genital area

Diagnosis and Treatment of Priapism

In addition to taking a medical history and performing a physical examination, a urologist or other practitioner will likely order blood tests and diagnostic tests to determine the type of priapism. These tests may include blood-gas analysis of blood taken from the penile tissue, color duplex ultrasound to measure blood flow in the penis, or magnetic resonance imaging (MRI) to detect possible tumors or blood clots.

To relieve the immediate symptoms of priapism and restore normal blood flow, applying ice packs to the penis and perineum or exercising vigorously may be helpful. In other cases, a doctor may need to drain the trapped blood manually by inserting a needle into the penis. A vasoconstrictor medication may also be injected to help reduce the size of blood vessels and improve blood flow.

The recommended treatment for priapism depends on the underlying cause. If priapism occurs as a side effect of medication, the doctor may recommend stopping the medication and trying an alternative prescription. For stuttering priapism, a medication called phenylephrine may be prescribed to help control blood flow to the penis and prevent further episodes. For priapism resulting from a blood clot, surgery may be needed to remove the clot. High blood flow priapism resolves itself without treatment in about two-thirds of men, while the remaining cases require surgery to repair the ruptured blood vessels.

If priapism causes tissue damage, resulting in sexual dysfunction, the patient may require surgery to implant a penile prosthesis.

Retrograde Ejaculation

Retrograde ejaculation (also known as dry climax) is a rare condition in which semen flows backwards and enters the bladder during ejaculation, rather than flowing out of the body through the penis. Under normal circumstances, the bladder sphincter muscle contracts just before ejaculation, which prevents semen from entering the bladder and forces it out through the urethra. In retrograde ejaculation, the sphincter malfunctions and remains open. The condition is not harmful—and the semen is soon eliminated in the form of urine—but it can decrease fertility.

Symptoms and Causes of Retrograde Ejaculation

Men with retrograde ejaculation will notice that little to no fluid is released from the penis when they ejaculate. In addition, their urine may appear cloudy following orgasms, and urinalysis results will show the presence of sperm.

The most common causes of retrograde ejaculation include uncontrolled diabetes and side effects of medications used to treat high blood pressure, depression, and anxiety. Surgery for prostate or urethra disorders can also cause retrograde ejaculation. Nerve damage from multiple sclerosis or a spinal cord injury can also affect the function of the bladder sphincter muscle.

Treatment of Retrograde Ejaculation

Since retrograde ejaculation is not harmful, no treatment is needed unless the condition interferes with fertility. In that case, a urologist or other healthcare provider may recommend that the patient reduce the dosage or stop taking any medications that may contribute to the condition. For retrograde ejaculation caused by diabetes, the condition may improve if the patient maintains good control over blood sugar. Medications such as pseudoephedrine or imipramine have also shown positive results in improving muscle tone in the bladder sphincter so that it closes during ejaculation. Collagen injections into the bladder neck or surgical reconstruction of the sphincter muscles are other possible treatments to improve contraction.

If retrograde ejaculation persists following treatment, assisted reproductive technologies can be used to improve the chances of conception. One approach involves harvesting sperm from the bladder or gathering them from a urine sample for use in artificial insemination procedures. Of course, the success of such infertility procedures depends not only on the viability of the man's sperm, but also on his partner's fertility.

References

1. "Erectile Dysfunction." National Institute of Diabetes and Digestive and Kidney Diseases, November 2015.

2. MacGill, Markus. "Premature Ejaculation: Causes and Treatments." Medical News Today, July 5, 2016.

3. "Priapism." MyDr, June 25, 2016.

4. "Retrograde Ejaculation." Norman Regional Health Center, 2012.

5. "Retrograde Ejaculation Treatments." Urologists.org, n.d.

6. "What Is Premature Ejaculation?" Urology Care Foundation, 2016.

Chapter 34

Male Infertility

What Are the Causes of Male Infertility?

Men can also contribute to infertility in a couple. In fact, men are found to be the only cause or a contributing cause of infertility problems in couples in 30% to 40% of cases.

To conceive a child, a male's sperm must combine with a female's egg. The testicles make and store sperm, which are ejaculated by the penis to deliver sperm to the female reproductive tract during sexual intercourse.

The most common issues that lead to infertility in men are problems that affect how the testicles work.

Other problems are hormone imbalances or blockages in the male reproductive organs. In about 50% of cases, the cause of male infertility cannot be determined.

A complete lack of sperm is the cause of infertility in about 10% to 15% of men who are infertile. When a man does not produce sperm, it is called azoospermia. A hormone imbalance or a blockage of sperm movement can cause azoospermia.

This chapter contains text excerpted from the following sources: Text beginning with the heading "What Are the Causes of Male Infertility?" is excerpted from "What Are the Causes of Male Infertility?" *Eunice Kennedy Shriver* National Institute of Child Health and Human Development (NICHD), July 2, 2013. Reviewed August 2016; Text under the heading "What Treatment Options Are Available for Male Infertility?" is excerpted from "What Treatment Options Are Available for Male Infertility?" *Eunice Kennedy Shriver* National Institute of Child Health and Human Development (NICHD), November 30, 2012. Reviewed August 2016.

In some cases of infertility, a man produces less sperm than normal. This condition is called oligospermia. The most common cause of oligospermia is varicocele, an enlarged vein in the testicle.

Conditions That Affect Sperm Formation

Many different issues can affect the formation of sperm in the testicles. These conditions can lead to sperm that is abnormally shaped or malformed or to low amounts of sperm. Some of the more common issues include:

- chromosome defects

- diabetes

- hyperprolactinemia, which is overproduction of a hormone called prolactin made by the pituitary gland

- injury to the testicle

- insensitivity to hormones called androgens, which include testosterone

- radiation

- reactions to medications

- swelling of the testicles from infections such as mumps, gonorrhea, or chlamydia

- chromosome disorder called Klinefelter syndrome

- thyroid problems

- cryptorchidism, which occurs when one or both testicles are not descended

- Varicocele, which is the enlargement of veins in the scrotum; enlarged veins disrupt the blood flow in the testicle and cause an increase in temperature, which negatively affects sperm production. This condition is present in about 40% of men with fertility problems.

- chemotherapy and radiation

Conditions That Affect Transport of Sperm

Even if the male's body produces enough viable sperm, sometimes factors and conditions that affect how or if the sperm moves can also contribute to infertility. Sperm may move too slowly or not at all, so that they die before they can reach the egg. Sometimes the seminal fluid, which contains the sperm, is too thick for the sperm to move around properly.

An inability to transport sperm from the testicles to the penis causes about 10% to 20% of the cases of male infertility. The inability can be caused by natural obstructions in the tubes that transport sperm from the testicles to the penis or from vasectomy, a surgical procedure that cuts and seals the ends of the tubes.

Many men with cystic fibrosis lack the tubes that carry the sperm out of the testicles, making them infertile (but not sterile, because they produce sperm).

Some men have problems getting an erection, called erectile dysfunction, which makes having sex difficult.

A condition called retrograde ejaculation can also cause infertility. This condition causes sperm to move into the bladder instead of out of the penis.

What Treatment Options Are Available for Male Infertility?

Other than the inability to conceive within a stated period of time or the inability to deliver a live-born infant, in most cases, infertility has no other outward symptoms.

The evaluation of a man's fertility includes looking for signs of hormone deficiency, such as increased body fat, decreased muscle mass, and decreased facial and body hair. The evaluation also includes questions about the man's health history, including past injury to the testicles or penis, recent high fevers, and childhood diseases such as mumps. A physical examination allows for the identification of problems such as infection, hernia, or varicocele. A healthcare provider may also ask a man to provide a semen sample to assess the health and quality of his sperm. Other tests may include measurement of hormones in the blood, a biopsy of the testicle, or genetic screening.

Treatments for male infertility may be based on the underlying cause of the problem, or in the case of no identified problem, evidence-based treatments that improve fertility may be recommended. Treatments include surgery to correct or repair anatomic abnormalities or damage to reproductive organs, use of medical procedures to deliver sperm to the woman, fertilization of the egg in a laboratory, and using a third party for donating sperm or eggs and/or carrying a pregnancy. Medication can treat some issues that affect male fertility, including hormone imbalances and erectile dysfunction. Surgery can be effective for repairing blockages in the tubes that transport sperm. Surgery can also be used for repair of varicocele. Assistive reproductive technologies, such as in vitro fertilization, can be effective if other treatments do not restore fertility.

Chapter 35

Vasectomy and Vasectomy Reversal

A vasectomy is a surgical procedure performed as a method of birth control. It involves cutting the vas deferens in order to close off the tubes that carry sperm from the testicles (there is one vas deferens per testicle). If a man has a successful vasectomy, he can no longer get a woman pregnant.

Sperm are made in the two testicles, which are inside the scrotum. Sperm is stored in a tube attached to each testicle called the epididymis. When a man ejaculates, the sperm travel from the epididymis, through the vas deferens, and then mix with seminal fluid to form semen. The semen then travels through the urethra and out the penis.

Before a vasectomy, semen contains sperm and seminal fluid. After a vasectomy, sperm are no longer in the semen. The man's testicles will make less sperm over time, and his body will harmlessly absorb any sperm that are made.

How Is a Vasectomy Done?

A vasectomy is usually performed in the office of urologist, a doctor who specializes in the male urinary tract and reproductive system. In

This chapter includes text excerpted from "Vasectomy: Condition Information," *Eunice Kennedy Shriver* National Institute of Child Health and Human Development (NICHD), June 3, 2013. Reviewed August 2016.

some cases, the urologist may decide to do a vasectomy in an outpatient surgery center or a hospital. This could be because of patient anxiety or because other procedures will be done at the same time.

There are two ways to perform a vasectomy. In either case, the patient is awake during the procedure, but the urologist uses a local anesthetic to numb the scrotum.

With the conventional method, the doctor makes one or two small cuts in the scrotum to access the vas deferens. A small section of the vas deferens is cut out and then removed. The urologist may cauterize (seal with heat) the ends and then tie the ends with stitches. The doctor will then perform the same procedure on the other testicle, either through the same opening or through a second scrotal incision. For both testicles, when the vas deferens has been tied off, the doctor will use a few stitches or skin "glue" to close the opening(s) in the scrotum.

With the "no-scalpel" method, a small puncture hole is made on one side of the scrotum. The healthcare provider will find the vas deferens under the skin and pull it through the hole. The vas deferens is then cut and a small section is removed. The ends are either cauterized or tied off and then put back in place. The procedure is then performed on the other testicle. No stitches are needed with this method because the puncture holes are so small.

After a vasectomy, most men go home the same day and fully recover in less than a week.

How Effective Is Vasectomy?

Vasectomy is one of the most effective forms of birth control. In the first year after vasectomy, only 15 to 20 of every 10,000 couples will experience a pregnancy. In comparison, 1,400 of every 10,000 couples have a pregnancy each year using condoms, and 500 of every 10,000 couples experience a pregnancy each year using oral contraceptive pills.

However, a vasectomy is not effective right away. Men still need to use other birth control until the remaining sperm are cleared out of the semen. This takes 15 to 20 ejaculations, or about 3 months. Even then, 1 of every 5 men will still have sperm in his semen and will need to wait longer for the sperm to clear.

A healthcare provider will check a man's semen for sperm at least once after the surgery. Once the sperm count has dropped to zero, it is safe to assume that the vasectomy is now an effective form of birth control. Until that time, men need to use another form of birth control to make sure their partner does not become pregnant.

What Are the Risks of Vasectomy?

Although vasectomy is safe and highly effective, men should be aware of problems that could occur after surgery and over time.

Surgical Risks

After surgery, most men have discomfort, bruising, and some swelling, all of which usually go away within 2 weeks. Problems that can occur after surgery and need to be checked by a healthcare provider include:

- Hematoma. Bleeding under the skin that can lead to painful swelling.

- Infection. Fever and scrotal redness and tenderness are signs of infection.

Other Risks

The risk of other problems is small, but they do occur. These include:

- A lump in the scrotum, called a granuloma. This is formed from sperm that leak out of the vas deferens into the tissue.

- Pain in the testicles that doesn't go away. This is called postvasectomy pain syndrome and occurs in about 10% of men.

- Vasectomy failure. There is a small risk that the vasectomy will fail. This can lead to unintended pregnancy. Among 1,000 vasectomies, 11 will likely fail over 2 years; and half of these failures will occur within the first 3 months after surgery. The risk of failure depends on a number of factors. For example, some surgical techniques are more likely to fail than others. Additionally, there is a very small risk that the two ends of the vas deferens will grow back together. If this happens, sperm may be able to enter the semen and make pregnancy possible.

- Risk of regret. Vasectomy may be a good choice for men and/ or couples who are certain that they do not want more or any children. Most men who have vasectomy, as well as spouses of men who have vasectomy, do not regret the decision. Men who have vasectomy before age 30 are the group most likely to want a vasectomy reversal in the future.

Will Vasectomy Affect My Sex Life?

Vasectomy will not affect your sex life. It does not decrease your sex drive because it does not affect the production of the male hormone testosterone. It also does not affect your ability to get an erection or ejaculate semen. Because the sperm make up a very small amount of the semen, you will not notice a difference in the amount of semen you ejaculate.

Can Vasectomy Be Reversed?

Almost all vasectomies can be reversed. In a reversal, the cut ends of the vas deferens are surgically reattached. Or, one end of the vas deferens is surgically connected to the part of the testicle where mature sperm are stored.

Vasectomy reversal is usually done in an outpatient surgery center or the outpatient area of a hospital. The surgeon may use general anesthesia.

To reverse a vasectomy, the surgeon makes a small cut in the side of the scrotum and finds the closed ends of the vas deferens. Then a fluid sample is taken from the end closest to the testicle to test for the presence of sperm. If sperm is found in the fluid, the two closed ends of the vas deferens can be reattached.

Many doctors perform the reversal using a microsurgical approach. Here, a high-powered microscope is used to magnify the ends of the vas deferens. It allows the surgeon to use smaller stitches—as small as an eyelash—which reduces scarring. Microsurgery returns sperm to the semen in 75% to 99% of reversals.

If no sperm is found in the fluid, there is a blockage in the epididymis or vas deferens. The surgeon gets around this by attaching the upper part of the vas deferens to the epididymis in a place that bypasses the blockage. This procedure is more involved but has nearly as high a success rate as a standard reversal.

Recovery from a reversal usually takes 1 to 3 weeks. As with vasectomy, complications from surgery are possible. Most men who undergo vasectomy reversal report the same or less discomfort during recovery than they had after vasectomy.

Sperm start appearing in the semen about 3 months after the surgery. However, if the surgeon has to work around a blockage, it can take as long as 15 months for sperm to reappear.

On average, it takes 1 year to achieve a pregnancy after a vasectomy reversal. However, a successful reversal (sperm is returned to the semen) does not guarantee pregnancy. The chance of restored fertility and pregnancy is highest when the reversal is performed not long after the vasectomy. The likelihood of restored fertility and pregnancy decreases as more time elapses between the vasectomy and the vasectomy reversal.

Chapter 36

Nonsurgical Contraception

Chapter Contents

Section 36.1—Birth Control Methods: How Well Do
    They Work?... 460

Section 36.2—Condoms 462

Section 36.3—Withdrawal... 464

Section 36.1

Birth Control Methods: How Well Do They Work?

This section includes text excerpted from "Birth Control Methods
Fact Sheet," Office on Women's Health (OWH), U.S. Department of
Health and Human Services (HHS), July 16, 2012.
Reviewed August 2016.

What Is the Best Method of Birth Control (or Contraception)?

There is no "best" method of birth control. Each method has its
pros and cons.

All women and men can have control over when, and if, they
become parents. Making choices about birth control, or contraception, isn't easy. There are many things to think about. To get started,
learn about birth control methods you or your partner can use to
prevent pregnancy. You can also talk with your doctor about the
choices.

Before choosing a birth control method, think about:

- Your overall health

- How often you have sex

- The number of sex partners you have

- If you want to have children someday

- How well each method works to prevent pregnancy

- Possible side effects

- Your comfort level with using the method

Keep in mind, even the most effective birth control methods can
fail. But your chances of getting pregnant are lowest if the method you
choose always is used correctly and every time you have sex.

How Well Do Different Kinds of Birth Control Work? Do They Have Side Effects?

All birth control methods work the best if used correctly and every time you have sex. Be sure you know the right way to use them. Sometimes doctors don't explain how to use a method because they assume you already know. Talk with your doctor if you have questions. They are used to talking about birth control. So don't feel embarrassed about talking to him or her.

Some birth control methods can take time and practice to learn. For example, some people don't know you can put on a male condom "inside out." Also, not everyone knows you need to leave a little space at the tip of the condom for the sperm and fluid when a man ejaculates, or has an orgasm.

Here is a list of some birth control methods with their failure rates.

Table 36.1. Birth Control Methods, Failure Rates

Method	Failure rate (the number of pregnancies expected per 100 women)
Sterilization surgery for women	Less than 1 pregnancy
Sterilization implant for women (Essure)	Less than 1 pregnancy
Sterilization surgery for men	Less than 1 pregnancy
Implantable rod (Implanon)	Less than 1 pregnancy
Intrauterine device (ParaGard, Mirena)	Less than 1 pregnancy
Shot/injection (Depo-Provera)	Less than 1 pregnancy
Oral contraceptives (combination pill, or "the pill")	5 pregnancies
Oral contraceptives (continuous/ extended use, or "no-period pill")	5 pregnancies
Oral contraceptives (progestin-only pill, or "mini-pill")	5 pregnancies
Skin patch (Ortho Evra)	5 pregnancies
Vaginal ring (NuvaRing)	5 pregnancies
Male condom	11–16 pregnancies

Table 36.1. Continued

Method	Failure rate (the number of pregnancies expected per 100 women)
Diaphragm with spermicide	15 pregnancies
Cervical cap with spermicide	17–23 pregnancies
Female condom	20 pregnancies
Natural family planning (rhythm method)	25 pregnancies
Spermicide alone	30 pregnancies
Emergency contraception ("morning-after pill," "Plan B One-Step," "Next Choice")	1 pregnancy

Section 36.2

Condoms

This section includes text excerpted from documents published by two public domain sources. Text under headings marked 1 are excerpted from "Male Condom Fact Sheet," Office of Population Affairs (OPA), U.S. Department of Health and Human Services (HHS), November 4, 2014; Text under headings marked 2 are excerpted from "Using Condoms," AIDS.gov, U.S. Department of Health and Human Services (HHS), September 29, 2014.

What Is the Male Condom?[1]

A male condom is a thin film sheath that's placed over the penis. Condoms prevent pregnancy by keeping sperm from entering a woman's body.

Condoms—sometimes called "rubbers"—made from latex rubber are the most common type. For people who get skin irritation from latex, polyurethane condoms are a good choice

Condoms come either lubricated or non-lubricated. You can also add water-based lubricant, such as KY jelly, to a condom to make sex more comfortable. Avoid oil-based lubricants (e.g., petroleum jelly, massage oil, body lotion) as these weaken condoms and may cause them to break.

Used correctly each time you have sex, latex and polyurethane condoms do a good job of preventing pregnancy and many sexually transmitted infections (STIs). Condoms made from natural or lamb-skin materials also protect against pregnancy, but they won't protect against some STIs.

How to Use a Condom Consistently and Correctly[2]

Male and female condoms can be used to protect you from HIV or other STDs. But don't use them both at the same time. If used together, they won't stay in place, and they can tear or become damaged. Read the instructions on the condom package and practice before using them for the first time. Also, follow these guidelines:

- Keep male condoms in a cool, dry place. Don't keep them in your wallet or in your car. This can cause them to break or tear.

- Check the wrapper for tears and for the expiration date, to make sure the condom is not too old to use. Carefully open the wrapper. Don't use your teeth or fingernails. Make sure the condom looks okay to use. Don't use a condom that is gummy, brittle, discolored, or has even a tiny hole.

- Put on the condom as soon as the penis is erect, but before it touches the vagina, mouth, or anus.

- If the condom does not have a reservoir tip, pinch the tip enough to leave a half-inch space for semen to collect. Holding the tip, unroll the condom all the way to the base of the erect penis.

- Be sure to use adequate lubrication during vaginal and anal sex. Only use water-based or silicone-based lubricants. Don't use oil-based lubricants (e.g., petroleum jelly, shortening, mineral oil, massage oils, body lotions, and cooking oil) with latex condoms because they can weaken latex and cause breakage. Put the lubricant on the outside of the condom.

- After ejaculation and before the penis gets soft, grip the rim of the condom and carefully withdraw. Then gently pull the condom off the penis, making sure that semen doesn't spill out.

- Wrap the condom in a tissue and throw it in the trash where others won't handle it.

463

- If you feel the condom break at any point during sexual activity, stop immediately, withdraw, remove the broken condom, and put on a new condom.

- Use a new condom if you want to have sex again or in a different way.

How Effective Are Male Condoms?[1]

Of 100 couples each year whose partners use male condoms, about 18 women may get pregnant. Condoms are more effective at preventing pregnancy when they are used correctly and when you use them every time you have sex.

Advantages of the Male Condom[1]

- You don't need a prescription.

- Anyone can buy them.

- Male condoms are safe and easy to use.

- They can be used for vaginal, anal, and oral sex. Ask for flavored condoms to improve the experience when using them for protection against STIs with oral sex.

- Latex and polyurethane condoms offer protection against STIs, including HIV, as well as pregnancy.

Section 36.3

Withdrawal

"Withdrawal," © 2016 Omnigraphics, Inc.
Reviewed November 2015.

What Is Withdrawal All About?

Withdrawal, or the pull-out method, has been practiced for centuries, to avoid the risk of unwanted pregnancy during sexual intercourse.

Scientifically known as *Coitus interruptus* (Latin for interrupted intercourse), withdrawal happens when a man removes his penis from the vagina before ejaculating (the moment when semen spurts out of the penis).

What Is the Logic behind Withdrawal?

Withdrawal prevents sperm from entering the woman's vagina, thereby preventing contact between the sperm and the egg.

Why Use Withdrawal?

Withdrawal continues to be a popular birth control method among younger couples. There are a number of factors that make this an attractive option including:

- it can be used when no other method is available
- is free
- has none of the side effects that can be associated with other birth control methods.

Is Withdrawal Fail Proof?

No. For a number of reasons withdrawal is an unreliable form of birth control.

The practice of withdrawal requires a lot of trust, self-control and experience. It requires the male partner to know the sexual responses of his own body so as to know when to pull out. It is generally not recommended for teens and sexually inexperienced men. If done incorrectly and a man is unable to predict, and unable to control the exact moment of his ejaculation this method could be very ineffective.

What Are the Risks?

Even if the guy pulls out in time, there is still a risk of pregnancy from pre-ejaculate, or precum sperm that is still in the urinary tract from a previous ejaculation. It is advisable for a guy to urinate, to get rid of all the pre-cum from the urethra before intercourse and clean properly to get rid of any fluid, before having intercourse again.

While withdrawal may prevent unwanted pregnancy if practiced correctly, it does not protect the couple engaged in intercourse from the risk of sexually transmitted diseases (STDs) and human immunodeficiency virus (HIV). It is always wiser to protect yourself from the risk of pregnancy, STDs and the transmission of HIV by correctly and consistently using male latex condoms and/or other contraceptive methods.

For women who do not want to risk pregnancy due to medical or personal reasons, it is always better to rely on other forms of birth control such as diaphragms, caps, or a female condom.

References

1. "Withdrawal method (*Coitus interruptus*)." Mayo Clinic Staff, March 5, 2015.

2. Dr. David Delvin. "*Coitus interruptus* (Withdrawal method)." NetDoctor, December 22, 2014.

Chapter 37

Safer Sex Guidelines

Practice Safer Sex

Safer Sex

Taking simple steps to prevent getting or spreading HIV will pay off both for you and for those you love. The only 100 percent effective way to prevent the spread of HIV through sex is to abstain—to not have sex of any kind. If you do have sex, practice safer sex methods. These are the steps you can take to help prevent HIV infection from sex:

- **Abstain from sex.** Not having vaginal, anal, or oral sex is the surest way to avoid HIV. If you do decide to have sex, you can reduce your risk of HIV by practicing safer sex.

- **Get tested.** Be sure you know yours and your partner's HIV status before ever having sex.

- **Use condoms.** Use them correctly and every time you have sex. Using a male condom for all types of sex can greatly lower your risk of getting HIV during sex. If you or your partner is allergic to latex, use polyurethane condoms. If your partner won't use a male condom, you can use a female condom. It may protect against HIV, but we don't have much evidence that it does, so it is better to use a male condom, which we know has a high rate

This chapter includes text excerpted from "HIV/AIDS," Office on Women's Health (OWH), U.S. Department of Health and Human Services (HHS), July 1, 2011. Reviewed August 2016.

of preventing HIV infection. Do not use a male and female condom at the same time. They do not work together and can break. **"Natural" or "lambskin" condoms don't protect against HIV.** Condoms are easy to find, and some places give them out for free. Contact your local health department or a health clinic for information about places in your area that may give away free condoms. For instance, the New York State Health Department offers a cellphone app that can help youth find free condoms in their area.

- **Talk with your partner.** It's up to you to make sure you are protected. Remember, it's *your body*!

- **Practice monogamy (be faithful to one partner).** Being in a sexual relationship with only one partner who is also faithful to you can help protect you.

- **Limit your number of sexual partners.** Your risk of getting HIV goes up with the number of partners you have. Condoms should be used for any sexual activity with a partner who has HIV. They should also be used with any partner outside of a long-term, faithful sexual relationship.

- **Use protection for all kinds of sexual contact.** Remember that you don't only get HIV from penile-vaginal sex. Use a condom during oral sex and during anal sex. Dental dams also can be used to help lower your risk as well as your partner's risk of getting HIV during oral-vaginal or oral-anal sex.

- **Know that other types of birth control will not protect you from HIV.** Other methods of birth control, like birth control pills, shots, implants, or diaphragms, will not protect you from HIV. If you use one of these, be sure to also use a male condom or dental dam correctly every time you have sex.

- **Don't use nonoxynol-9 (N-9).** Some contraceptives, like condoms, suppositories, foams, and gels contain the spermicide N-9. You shouldn't be using gels, foams, or suppositories to prevent against HIV—these methods only lower chances of pregnancy, not of HIV and other sexually transmitted infections (STIs). N-9 actually makes your risk of HIV infection higher, because it can irritate the vagina, which might make it easier for HIV to get into your body.

- **Get screened for STIs.** Having an STI, particularly genital herpes, increases your chances of becoming infected with HIV during sex. If your partner has an STI in addition to HIV, that also increases your risk of HIV infection. If you have an STI, you should also get tested for HIV.

- **Don't douche.** Douching removes some of the normal bacteria in the vagina that protects you from infection. This can increase your risk of getting HIV.

- **Don't abuse alcohol or drugs, which are linked to sexual risk-taking.** Drinking too much alcohol or using drugs also puts you at risk of sexual assault and possible exposure to HIV.

Take Time to Talk before Having Sex

Talking about sex is hard for some people. So, they don't bring up safe sex or STIs with their partners. But keep in mind that it's your body, and it's up to you to protect yourself. Before having sex, talk with your partner about his or her past and present sexual behavior and HIV status, and talk about using condoms and dental dams. Ask if he or she has been tested for HIV or other STIs. Having the talk ahead of time can help you avoid misunderstandings during a moment of passion. Let your partner know that you will not have any type of sex at any time without using a condom or dental dam. If your partner gives an excuse, be ready with a response.

Chapter 38

Sexually Transmitted Diseases

Chapter Contents

Section 38.1—What Are Sexually Transmitted
    Diseases?.. 472

Section 38.2—Chlamydia 475

Section 38.3—Genital Herpes 480

Section 38.4—Gonorrhea 485

Section 38.5—Hepatitis B... 488

Section 38.6—Human Papillomavirus..................................... 490

Section 38.7—Pubic Lice (Crabs) 494

Section 38.8—Scabies 498

Section 38.9—Syphilis 501

Section 38.10—Trichomoniasis 507

Section 38.1

What Are Sexually Transmitted Diseases?

This section includes text excerpted from "Sexually
Transmitted Diseases," Centers for Disease Control and
Prevention (CDC), May 22, 2014.

What Are Sexually Transmitted Diseases (STDs)?

STDs are diseases that are passed from one person to another
through sexual contact. These include chlamydia, gonorrhea, genital
herpes, human papillomavirus (HPV), syphilis, and HIV. Many of
these STDs do not show symptoms for a long time, but they can still
be harmful and passed on during sex.

How Are STDs Spread?

You can get an STD by having sex (vaginal, anal or oral) with
someone who has an STD. Anyone who is sexually active can get an
STD. You don't even have to "go all the way" (have anal or vaginal sex)
to get an STD, since some STDs, like herpes and HPV, are spread by
skin-to-skin contact.

How Common Are STDs?

STDs are common, especially among young people. There are about
20 million new cases of STDs each year in the United States, and about
half of these are in people between the ages of 15 and 24. Young people
are at greater risk of getting an STD for several reasons:

- Young women's bodies are biologically more susceptible to STDs.

- Some young people do not get the recommended STD tests.

- Many young people are hesitant to talk openly and honestly
  with a doctor or nurse about their sex lives.

- Not having insurance or transportation can make it more difficult for young people to access STD testing.

- Some young people have more than one sex partner.

What Can I Do to Protect Myself?

- The surest way to protect yourself against STDs is to not have sex. That means not having any vaginal, anal, or oral sex ("abstinence"). There are many things to consider before having sex, and it's okay to say "no" if you don't want to have sex.

- If you do decide to have sex, you and your partner should get tested beforehand and make sure that you and your partner use a condom—every time you have oral, anal, or vaginal sex, from start to finish. Know where to get condoms and how to use them correctly. It is not safe to stop using condoms unless you've both been tested, know your status, and are in a mutually monogamous relationship.

- Mutual monogamy means that you and your partner both agree to only have sexual contact with each other. This can help protect against STDs, as long as you've both been tested and know you're STD-free.

- Before you have sex, talk with your partner about how you will prevent STDs and pregnancy. If you think you're ready to have sex, you need to be ready to protect your body and your future. You should also talk to your partner ahead of time about what you will and will not do sexually. Your partner should always respect your right to say no to anything that doesn't feel right.

- Make sure you get the healthcare you need. Ask a doctor or nurse about STD testing and about vaccines against HPV and hepatitis B.

- Avoid using alcohol and drugs. If you use alcohol and drugs, you are more likely to take risks, like not using a condom or having sex with someone you normally wouldn't have sex with.

If I Get an STD, How Will I Know?

Many STDs don't cause any symptoms that you would notice, so the only way to know for sure if you have an STD is to get tested. You can get an STD from having sex with someone who has no symptoms. Just like you, that person might not even know he or she has an STD.

Where Can I Get Tested?

There are places that offer teen-friendly, confidential, and free STD tests. This means that no one has to find out you've been tested.

Can STDs Be Treated?

Your doctor can prescribe medicines to cure some STDs, like chlamydia and gonorrhea. Other STDs, like herpes, can't be cured, but you can take medicine to help with the symptoms.

If you are ever treated for an STD, be sure to finish all of your medicine, even if you feel better before you finish it all. Ask the doctor or nurse about testing and treatment for your partner, too. You and your partner should avoid having sex until you've both been treated. Otherwise, you may continue to pass the STD back and forth. It is possible to get an STD again (after you've been treated), if you have sex with someone who has an STD.

What Happens If I Don't Treat an STD?

Some curable STDs can be dangerous if they aren't treated. For example, if left untreated, chlamydia and gonorrhea can make it difficult—or even impossible—for a woman to get pregnant. You also increase your chances of getting HIV if you have an untreated STD. Some STDs, like HIV, can be fatal if left untreated.

What If My Partner or I Have an Incurable STD?

Some STDs—like herpes and HIV—aren't curable, but a doctor can prescribe medicine to treat the symptoms.

If you are living with an STD, it's important to tell your partner before you have sex. Although it may be uncomfortable to talk about your STD, open and honest conversation can help your partner make informed decisions to protect his or her health.

If I Have Questions, Who Can Answer Them?

If you have questions, talk to a parent or other trusted adult. Don't be afraid to be open and honest with them about your concerns. If you're ever confused or need advice, they're the first place to start. Remember, they were young once, too.

Talking about sex with a parent or another adult doesn't need to be a one-time conversation. It's best to leave the door open for conversations in the future.

It's also important to talk honestly with a doctor or nurse. Ask which STD tests and vaccines they recommend for you.

Section 38.2

Chlamydia

This section includes text excerpted from "Chlamydia—CDC
Fact Sheet (Detailed)," Centers for Disease Control and
Prevention (CDC), September 24, 2015.

Chlamydia is a common sexually transmitted disease (STD) caused
by infection with *Chlamydia trachomatis*. It can cause cervicitis in
women and urethritis and proctitis in both men and women. Lympho-
granuloma venereum (LGV), another type of STD caused by different
serovars of the same bacterium, occurs commonly in the developing
world, and has more recently emerged as a cause of outbreaks of proctitis among men who have sex with men (MSM) worldwide.

How Common Is Chlamydia?

Chlamydia is the most frequently reported bacterial sexually transmitted infection in the United States. In 2014, 1,441,789 cases of chlamydia were reported to Centers for Disease Control and Prevention
(CDC) from 50 states and the District of Columbia, but an estimated
2.86 million infections occur annually. A large number of cases are not
reported because most people with chlamydia are asymptomatic and
do not seek testing. Chlamydia is most common among young people.
Almost two-thirds of new chlamydia infections occur among youth aged
15–24 years. It is estimated that 1 in 20 sexually active young women
aged 14–24 years has chlamydia.

Substantial racial/ethnic disparities in chlamydial infection exist,
with prevalence among non-Hispanic blacks 6.7 times the prevalence
among non-Hispanic whites. Chlamydia is also common among men
who have sex with men (MSM). Among MSM screened for rectal chlamydial infection, positivity has ranged from 3.0% to 10.5%. Among
MSM screened for pharyngeal chlamydial infection, positivity has
ranged from 0.5% to 2.3%.

How Do People Get Chlamydia?

Chlamydia is transmitted through sexual contact with the penis,
vagina, mouth, or anus of an infected partner. Ejaculation does not

have to occur for chlamydia to be transmitted or acquired. Chlamydia can also be spread perinatally from an untreated mother to her baby during childbirth, resulting in ophthalmia neonatorum (conjunctivitis) or pneumonia in some exposed infants. In published prospective studies, chlamydial conjunctivitis has been identified in 18–44% and chlamydial pneumonia in 3–16% of infants born to women with untreated chlamydial cervical infection at the time of delivery. While rectal or genital chlamydial infection has been shown to persist one year or longer in infants infected at birth, the possibility of sexual abuse should be considered in prepubertal children beyond the neonatal period with vaginal, urethral, or rectal chlamydial infection.

People who have had chlamydia and have been treated may get infected again if they have sexual contact with a person infected with chlamydia.

Who Is at Risk for Chlamydia?

Any sexually active person can be infected with chlamydia. It is a very common STD, especially among young people. It is estimated that 1 in 20 sexually active young women aged 14–19 years has chlamydia.

Sexually active young people are at high risk of acquiring chlamydia for a combination of behavioral, biological, and cultural reasons. Some young people don't use condoms consistently. Some adolescents may move from one monogamous relationship to the next more rapidly than the likely infectivity period of chlamydia, thus increasing risk of transmission. The higher prevalence of chlamydia among young people also may reflect multiple barriers to accessing STD prevention services, such as lack of transportation, cost, and perceived stigma.

Men who have sex with men (MSM) are also at risk for chlamydial infection since chlamydia can be transmitted by oral or anal sex. Among MSM screened for rectal chlamydial infection, positivity has ranged from 3.0% to 10.5%.Among MSM screened for pharyngeal chlamydial infection, positivity has ranged from 0.5% to 2.3%.

What Are the Symptoms of Chlamydia?

Chlamydia is known as a 'silent' infection because most infected people are asymptomatic and lack abnormal physical examination findings. Estimates of the proportion of chlamydia-infected people who develop symptoms vary by setting and study methodology; two published studies that incorporated modeling techniques to address limitations of point prevalence surveys estimated that only about 10%

of men and 5–30% of women with laboratory-confirmed chlamydial infection develop symptoms. The incubation period of chlamydia is poorly defined. However, given the relatively slow replication cycle of the organism, symptoms may not appear until several weeks after exposure in those persons who develop symptoms.

Men who are symptomatic typically have urethritis, with a mucoid or watery urethral discharge and dysuria. A minority of infected men develop epididymitis (with or without symptomatic urethritis), presenting with unilateral testicular pain, tenderness, and swelling.

Chlamydia can infect the rectum in men and women, either directly (through receptive anal sex), or possibly via spread from the cervix and vagina in a woman with cervical chlamydial infection. While these infections are often asymptomatic, they can cause symptoms of proctitis (e.g., rectal pain, discharge, and/or bleeding).

Sexually acquired chlamydial conjunctivitis can occur in both men and women through contact with infected genital secretions.

While chlamydia can also be found in the throats of women and men having oral sex with an infected partner, it is typically asymptomatic and not thought to be an important cause of pharyngitis.

What Complications Can Result from Chlamydia Infection?

The initial damage that chlamydia causes often goes unnoticed. However, chlamydial infections can lead to serious health problems with both short- and long-term consequences.

Some patients with chlamydial PID develop perihepatitis, or "Fritz-Hugh-Curtis Syndrome", an inflammation of the liver capsule and surrounding peritoneum, which is associated with right upper quadrant pain.

Reactive arthritis can occur in men and women following symptomatic or asymptomatic chlamydial infection, sometimes as part of a triad of symptoms (with urethritis and conjunctivitis) formerly referred to as Reiter Syndrome.

What about Chlamydia and HIV?

Untreated chlamydia may increase a person's chances of acquiring or transmitting HIV–the virus that causes AIDS.

Who Should Be Tested for Chlamydia?

Any sexually active person can be infected with chlamydia. Anyone with genital symptoms such as discharge, burning during urination, unusual sores, or rash should refrain from having sex until they are able to see a healthcare provider about their symptoms.

Also, anyone with an oral, anal, or vaginal sex partner who has been recently diagnosed with an STD should see a healthcare provider for evaluation.

Routine screening is not recommended for men. However, the screening of sexually active young men should be considered in clinical settings with a high prevalence of chlamydia (e.g., adolescent clinics, correctional facilities, and STD clinics) when resources permit and do not hinder screening efforts in women.

Sexually active men who have sex with men (MSM) who had insertive intercourse should be screened for urethral chlamydial infection and MSM who had receptive anal intercourse should be screened for rectal infection at least annually; screening for pharyngeal infection is not recommended.. More frequent chlamydia screening at 3-month intervals is indicated for MSM, including those with HIV infection, if risk behaviors persist or if they or their sexual partners have multiple partners.

At the initial HIV care visit, providers should test all sexually active persons with HIV infection for chlamydia and perform testing at least annually during the course of HIV care. A patient's healthcare provider might determine more frequent screening is necessary, based on the patient's risk factors.

How Is Chlamydia Diagnosed?

There are a number of diagnostic tests for chlamydia, including nucleic acid amplification tests (NAATs), cell culture, and others. NAATs are the most sensitive tests, and can be performed on easily obtainable specimens such as vaginal swabs (either clinician- or patient-collected) or urine.

Vaginal swabs, either patient- or clinician-collected, are the optimal specimen to screen for genital chlamydia using NAATs in women; urine is the specimen of choice for men, and is an effective alternative specimen type for women. Patients may prefer self-collected vaginal swabs or urine-based screening to the more invasive endocervical or urethral swab specimens.

Chlamydial culture can be used for rectal or pharyngeal specimens, but is not widely available. NAATs have demonstrated improved sensitivity and specificity compared with culture for the detection of *C. trachomatis* at non-genital sites. Most tests, including NAATs, are not FDA-cleared for use with rectal or pharyngeal swab specimens; however, NAATS have demonstrated improved sensitivity and specificity compared with culture for the detection of *C. trachomatis* at rectal sites and however, some laboratories have met regulatory requirements and have validated NAAT testing on rectal and pharyngeal swab specimens.

What Is the Treatment for Chlamydia?

Chlamydia can be easily cured with antibiotics. HIV-positive persons with chlamydia should receive the same treatment as those who are HIV-negative.

Persons with chlamydia should abstain from sexual activity for 7 days after single dose antibiotics or until completion of a 7-day course of antibiotics, to prevent spreading the infection to partners. It is important to take all of the medication prescribed to cure chlamydia. Medication for chlamydia should not be shared with anyone. Although medication will cure the infection, it will not repair any permanent damage done by the disease. If a person's symptoms continue for more than a few days after receiving treatment, he or she should return to a healthcare provider to be reevaluated.

Repeat infection with chlamydia is common. Women and men with chlamydia should be retested about three months after treatment of an initial infection, regardless of whether they believe that their sex partners were successfully treated.

Infants infected with chlamydia may develop ophthalmia neonatorum (conjunctivitis) and/or pneumonia. Chlamydial infection in infants can be treated with antibiotics.

What about Partners?

If a person has been diagnosed and treated for chlamydia, he or she should tell all recent anal, vaginal, or oral sex partners (all sex partners within 60 days before the onset of symptoms or diagnosis) so they can see a healthcare provider and be treated. This will reduce the risk that the sex partners will develop serious complications from chlamydia and will also reduce the person's risk of becoming re-infected. A person with chlamydia and all of his or her sex partners must avoid having sex until they have completed their treatment for chlamydia (i.e., seven days after single dose antibiotics or until completion of a seven-day course of antibiotics) and until they no longer have symptoms.

To help get partners treated quickly, healthcare providers in some states may give infected individuals extra medicine or prescriptions to give to their sex partners. This is called expedited partner therapy or

EPT. In published clinical trials comparing EPT to traditional patient referral (i.e., asking the patient to refer their partners in for treatment), EPT was associated with fewer persistent or recurrent chlamydial infections in the index patient, and a larger reported number of partners treated. For providers, EPT represents an additional strategy for partner management of persons with chlamydial infection; partners should still be encouraged to seek medical evaluation, regardless of whether they receive EPT. To obtain further information regarding EPT, including the legal status of EPT in a specific area, see the Legal Status of Expedited Partner Therapy.

How Can Chlamydia Be Prevented?

Latex male condoms, when used consistently and correctly, can reduce the risk of getting or giving chlamydia. The surest way to avoid chlamydia is to abstain from vaginal, anal, and oral sex, or to be in a long-term mutually monogamous relationship with a partner who has been tested and is known to be uninfected.

Section 38.3

Genital Herpes

This section includes text excerpted from "Genital Herpes—
CDC Fact Sheet (Detailed)," Centers for Disease Control and
Prevention (CDC), September 24, 2015.

What Is Genital Herpes?

Genital herpes is a sexually transmitted disease (STD) caused by the herpes simplex viruses type 1 (HSV-1) or type 2 (HSV-2).

How Common Is Genital Herpes?

Genital herpes infection is common in the United States. CDC estimates that, annually, 776,000 people in the United States get new herpes infections. Nationwide, 15.5 % of persons aged 14 to 49 years have HSV-2 infection. The overall prevalence of genital herpes is likely higher than 15.5% because an increasing number of genital herpes infections are caused by HSV-1. HSV-1 is typically acquired in childhood; as the prevalence of HSV-1 infection has declined in recent decades, people may have become more susceptible to genital herpes from HSV-1.

HSV-2 infection is more common among women than among men (20.3% versus 10.6% in 14 to 49 year olds). Infection is more easily transmitted from men to women than from women to men. HSV-2 infection is more common among non-Hispanic blacks (41.8%) than among non-Hispanic whites (11.3%). This disparity remains even among persons with similar numbers of lifetime sexual partners. For example, among persons with 2–4 lifetime sexual partners, HSV-2 is still more prevalent among non-Hispanic blacks (34.3%) than among non-Hispanic whites (9.1%) or Mexican Americans (13%). Most infected persons are unaware of their infection. In the United States, an estimated 87.4% of 14–49 year olds infected with HSV-2 have never received a clinical diagnosis.

The percentage of persons in the United States who are infected with HSV-2 decreased from 21.2% in 1988–1994 to 15.5% in 2007–2010.

How Do People Get Genital Herpes?

Infections are transmitted through contact with lesions, mucosal surfaces, genital secretions, or oral secretions. HSV-1 and HSV-2 can also be shed from skin that looks normal. Generally, a person can only get HSV-2 infection during sexual contact with someone who has a genital HSV-2 infection. Transmission most commonly occurs from an infected partner who does not have visible sores and who may not know that he or she is infected. In persons with asymptomatic HSV-2 infections, genital HSV shedding occurs on 10% of days, and on most of those days the person has no signs or symptoms.

What Are the Symptoms of Genital Herpes?

Most individuals infected with HSV-1 or HSV-2 are asymptomatic or have very mild symptoms that go unnoticed or are mistaken for another skin condition. As a result, 87.4% of infected individuals remain unaware of their infection. When symptoms do occur, they typically appear as one or more vesicles on or around the genitals, rectum or mouth. The average incubation period after exposure is 4 days (range, 2 to 12). The vesicles break and leave painful ulcers that may take two to four weeks to heal. Experiencing these symptoms is referred to as having an "outbreak" or episode.

Clinical manifestations of genital herpes differ between the first and recurrent outbreaks of HSV. The first outbreak of herpes is often associated with a longer duration of herpetic lesions, increased viral shedding (making HSV transmission more likely) and systemic symptoms including fever, body aches, swollen lymph nodes, or headache. Recurrent outbreaks of genital herpes are common, in particular during the first year of infection. Approximately half of patients who recognize recurrences have prodromal symptoms, such as mild tingling or shooting pains in the legs, hips or buttocks, which occur hours to days before the eruption of herpetic lesions. Symptoms of recurrent outbreaks are typically shorter in duration and less severe than the first outbreak of genital herpes. Although the infection can stay in the body indefinitely, the number of outbreaks tends to decrease over time. Recurrences and subclinical shedding are much less frequent for genital HSV-1 infection than for genital HSV-2 infection.

What Are the Complications of Genital Herpes?

Genital herpes may cause painful genital ulcers that can be severe and persistent in persons with suppressed immune systems, such as HIV-infected persons. Both HSV-1 and HSV-2 can also cause rare but serious complications such as blindness, encephalitis (inflammation of the brain), and aseptic meningitis (inflammation of the linings of the brain). Development of extragenital lesions in the buttocks, groin, thigh, finger, or eye may occur during the course of infection.

Some persons who contract genital herpes have concerns about how it will impact their overall health, sex life, and relationships. There can be can be considerable embarrassment, shame, and stigma associated with a herpes diagnosis that can substantially interfere with a patient's relationships. Clinicians can address these concerns by encouraging patients to recognize that while herpes is not curable, it is a manageable condition. Three important steps that providers can take for their newly-diagnosed patients are: giving information, providing support resources, and helping define options. Since a diagnosis of genital herpes may affect perceptions about existing or future sexual relationships, it is important for patients to understand how to talk to sexual partners about STDs.

What Is the Link between Genital Herpes and HIV?

Genital ulcerative disease caused by herpes make it easier to transmit and acquire HIV infection sexually. There is an estimated 2- to

4-fold increased risk of acquiring HIV, if exposed to HIV when genital herpes is present. Ulcers or breaks in the skin or mucous membranes (lining of the mouth, vagina, and rectum) from a herpes infection may compromise the protection normally provided by the skin and mucous membranes against infections, including HIV. Herpetic genital ulcers can bleed easily, and when they come into contact with the mouth, vagina, or rectum during sex, they may increase the risk of HIV transmission.

How Is Genital Herpes Diagnosed?

The preferred HSV tests for patients with active genital ulcers include viral culture or detection of HSV DNA by polymerase chain reaction (PCR). HSV culture requires collection of a sample from the sore and, once viral growth is seen, specific cell staining to differentiate between HSV-1 and HSV-2. However, culture sensitivity is low, especially for recurrent lesions, and declines as lesions heal. PCR is more sensitive, allows for more rapid and accurate results, and is increasingly being used. Because viral shedding is intermittent, failure to detect HSV by culture or PCR does not indicate and absence of HSV infection. Tzanck preparations are insensitive and nonspecific and should not be used.

Serologic tests are blood tests that detect antibodies to the herpes virus. Several ELISA-based serologic tests are FDA approved and available commercially. Older assays that do not accurately distinguish HSV-1 from HSV-2 antibody remain on the market, so providers should specifically request serologic type-specific assays when blood tests are performed for their patients. The sensitivities of type-specific serologic tests for HSV-2 vary from 80–98%; false-negative results might be more frequent at early stages of infection. Additionally, false positive results may occur at low index values and should be confirmed with another test such as Biokit or the Western Blot. Negative HSV-1 results should be interpreted with caution because some ELISA-based serologic tests are insensitive for detection of HSV-1 antibody.

For the symptomatic patient, testing with both virologic and serologic assays can determine whether it is a new infection or a newly-recognized old infection. A primary infection would be supported by a positive virologic test and a negative serologic test, while the diagnosis of recurrent disease would be supported by positive virologic and serologic test results.

CDC does not recommend screening for HSV-1 or HSV-2 in the general population. Several scenarios where type-specific serologic HSV tests may be useful include

- patients with recurrent genital symptoms or atypical symptoms and negative HSV PCR or culture

- patients with a clinical diagnosis of genital herpes but no laboratory confirmation

- patients who report having a partner with genital herpes

- patients presenting for an STD evaluation (especially those with multiple sex partners)

- persons with HIV infection and

- MSM at increased risk for HIV acquisition

Is There a Cure or Treatment for Herpes?

There is no cure for herpes. Antiviral medications can, however, prevent or shorten outbreaks during the period of time the person takes the medication. In addition, daily suppressive therapy (i.e., daily use of antiviral medication) for herpes can reduce the likelihood of transmission to partners.

Several clinical trials have tested vaccines against genital herpes infection, but there is currently no commercially available vaccine that is protective against genital herpes infection. One vaccine trial showed efficacy among women whose partners were HSV-2 infected, but only among women who were not infected with HSV-1. No efficacy was observed among men whose partners were HSV-2 infected. A subsequent trial testing the same vaccine showed some protection from genital HSV-1 infection, but no protection from HSV-2 infection.

How Can Herpes Be Prevented?

Correct and consistent use of latex condoms can reduce the risk of genital herpes. However, outbreaks can occur in areas that are not covered by a condom.

The surest way to avoid transmission of sexually transmitted diseases, including genital herpes, is to abstain from sexual contact, or to be in a long-term mutually monogamous relationship with a partner who has been tested and is known to be uninfected.

Persons with herpes should abstain from sexual activity with partners when sores or other symptoms of herpes are present. It is important to know that even if a person does not have any symptoms, he or she can still infect sex partners. Sex partners of infected persons should be advised that they may become infected and they should use condoms to reduce the risk. Sex partners can seek testing to determine if they are infected with HSV.

Section 38.4

Gonorrhea

This section includes text excerpted from "Gonorrhea—CDC Fact Sheet (Detailed Version)," Centers for Disease Control and Prevention (CDC), August 27, 2015.

What Is Gonorrhea?

Gonorrhea is a sexually transmitted disease (STD) caused by infection with the *Neisseria gonorrhoeae* bacterium. *N. gonorrhoeae* infects the mucous membranes of the reproductive tract, including the cervix, uterus, and fallopian tubes in women, and the urethra in women and men. *N. gonorrhoeae* can also infect the mucous membranes of the mouth, throat, eyes, and rectum.

How Common Is Gonorrhea?

Gonorrhea is a very common infectious disease. Centers for Disease Control and Prevention (CDC) estimates that approximately 820,000 new gonorrheal infections occur in the United States each year, and that less than half of these infections are detected and reported to CDC. CDC estimates that 570,000 of them were among young people 15–24 years of age. In 2014, 350,062 cases of gonorrhea were reported to CDC.

How Do People Get Gonorrhea?

Gonorrhea is transmitted through sexual contact with the penis, vagina, mouth, or anus of an infected partner. Ejaculation does not have to occur for gonorrhea to be transmitted or acquired. Gonorrhea can also be spread perinatally from mother to baby during childbirth.

People who have had gonorrhea and received treatment may be reinfected if they have sexual contact with a person infected with gonorrhea.

Who Is at Risk for Gonorrhea?

Any sexually active person can be infected with gonorrhea. In the United States, the highest reported rates of infection are among sexually active teenagers, young adults, and African Americans.

What Are the Signs and Symptoms of Gonorrhea?

Many men with gonorrhea are asymptomatic. When present, signs and symptoms of urethral infection in men include dysuria or a white, yellow, or green urethral discharge that usually appears one to fourteen days after infection. In cases where urethral infection is complicated by epididymitis, men with gonorrhea may also complain of testicular or scrotal pain.

Symptoms of rectal infection in both men and women may include discharge, anal itching, soreness, bleeding, or painful bowel movements. Rectal infection also may be asymptomatic. Pharyngeal infection may cause a sore throat, but usually is asymptomatic.

What Are the Complications of Gonorrhea?

Untreated gonorrhea can cause serious and permanent health problems in both women and men.

In men, gonorrhea may be complicated by epididymitis. In rare cases, this may lead to infertility.

If left untreated, gonorrhea can also spread to the blood and cause disseminated gonococcal infection (DGI). DGI is usually characterized by arthritis, tenosynovitis, and/or dermatitis. This condition can be life threatening.

What about Gonorrhea and HIV?

Untreated gonorrhea can increase a person's risk of acquiring or transmitting HIV, the virus that causes AIDS.

Who Should Be Tested for Gonorrhea?

Any sexually active person can be infected with gonorrhea. Anyone with genital symptoms such as discharge, burning during urination, unusual sores, or rash should stop having sex and see a healthcare provider immediately.

Also, anyone with an oral, anal, or vaginal sex partner who has been recently diagnosed with an STD should see a healthcare provider for evaluation.

Some people should be tested (screened) for gonorrhea even if they do not have symptoms or know of a sex partner who has gonorrhea. Anyone who is sexually active should discuss his or her risk factors with a healthcare provider and ask whether he or she should be tested for gonorrhea or other STDs.

People who have gonorrhea should also be tested for other STDs.

How Is Gonorrhea Diagnosed?

Urogenital gonorrhea can be diagnosed by testing urine, urethral (for men), or endocervical or vaginal (for women) specimens using nucleic acid amplification testing (NAAT). It can also be diagnosed using gonorrhea culture, which requires endocervical or urethral swab specimens.

If a person has had oral and/or anal sex, pharyngeal and/or rectal swab specimens should be collected either for culture or for NAAT (if the local laboratory has validated the use of NAAT for extra-genital specimens).

What Is the Treatment for Gonorrhea?

Gonorrhea can be cured with the right treatment. CDC now recommends dual therapy (i.e., using two drugs) for the treatment of gonorrhea. It is important to take all of the medication prescribed to cure gonorrhea. Medication for gonorrhea should not be shared with anyone. Although medication will stop the infection, it will not repair any permanent damage done by the disease. Antimicrobial resistance in gonorrhea is of increasing concern, and successful treatment of gonorrhea is becoming more difficult. If a person's symptoms continue for more than a few days after receiving treatment, he or she should return to a healthcare provider to be reevaluated.

What about Partners?

If a person has been diagnosed and treated for gonorrhea, he or she should tell all recent anal, vaginal, or oral sex partners (all sex partners within 60 days before the onset of symptoms or diagnosis) so they can see a health provider and be treated. This will reduce the risk that the sex partners will develop serious complications from gonorrhea and will also reduce the person's risk of becoming reinfected. A person with gonorrhea and all of his or her sex partners must avoid having sex until they have completed their treatment for gonorrhea and until they no longer have symptoms.

How Can Gonorrhea Be Prevented?

Latex condoms, when used consistently and correctly, can reduce the risk of transmission of gonorrhea. The surest way to avoid transmission of gonorrhea or other STDs is to abstain from vaginal, anal, and oral sex, or to be in a long-term mutually monogamous relationship with a partner who has been tested and is known to be uninfected.

Section 38.5

Hepatitis B

This section includes text excerpted from "Hepatitis B," Centers for Disease Control and Prevention (CDC), March 9, 2016.

What Is Hepatitis B?

Hepatitis B is a contagious virus that is transmitted through blood, blood products, and other body fluids (such as semen). Travelers can become infected through unprotected sex with an infected person, injection drug use, and transfusions with unscreened blood.

Symptoms include a sudden fever, tiredness, loss of appetite, nausea, vomiting, stomach pain, dark urine, joint pain, and yellowing of the skin and eyes (jaundice). Symptoms may last from several weeks to several months. Some people who get hepatitis B develop lifelong (chronic) hepatitis B. This can cause people to die early from liver disease and liver cancer.

Who Is at Risk?

Hepatitis B is most common in some countries in Asia, Africa, South America and the Caribbean. However, it occurs in nearly every part of the world. The risk to most travelers is low, but travelers could become infected if they have sex with an infected person, receive a transfusion of unscreened blood, have medical or dental procedures, get tattoos or piercings or receive acupuncture with needles that are not sterile.

What Can Travelers Do to Prevent Disease?

Get Hepatitis B Vaccine

- Ask your doctor or nurse about hepatitis B vaccine. The vaccine is recommended for extended stay travelers, people with chronic conditions, older people, healthcare workers, and people who participate in high-risk activities (such as injection drug use and unprotected sex). Other travelers may consider the vaccine, especially since some countries may not screen their blood supply, and travelers could become infected by a blood transfusion.

- This vaccine is a 3 dose vaccine. The second vaccine is given 1 month after the first dose and the third dose is given 6 months after the first dose.

  - Talk to your doctor about accelerated dosing and the combination vaccine with hepatitis A.

- Routine booster doses are not routinely recommended for any age group.

- The vaccine is over 90% effective, and has been considered a routine childhood vaccine since 1995.

Protect Yourself

- Use latex condoms correctly.

- Do not inject drugs.

- Limit alcohol consumption. People take more risks when intoxicated.

- Do not share needles or any devices that can break the skin. That includes needles for tattoos, piercings, and acupuncture.

  - If you do get tattoos or piercings, make sure equipment is sterile.

- If you receive medical or dental care, make sure the equipment is disinfected or sanitized.

Consider Medical Evacuation Insurance

- An injury or illness that requires invasive medical or dental treatment (e.g., injection, IV drip, transfusion, stitching) could result in hepatitis B infection if the blood supply is not properly screened.

- Medical evacuation insurance may cover the cost to transfer you to the nearest destination where you can get complete care. Some policies may cover your eventual return to your home country.

If You Feel Sick and Think You May Have Hepatitis B

- Talk to your doctor or nurse if you feel seriously ill, especially if you have a fever.

  - Tell them about your travel.

- Take medicine to control your fever and reduce your pain. Take medicine that contains aspirin, ibuprofen (Advil), or naproxen (Aleve). Do NOT take acetaminophen (Tylenol).

- Avoid contact with other people while you are sick.

Section 38.6

Human Papillomavirus

This section includes text excerpted from "HPV and Men—Fact Sheet," Centers for Disease Control and Prevention (CDC), February 16, 2015.

What Is HPV?

HPV is the most common sexually transmitted infection. HPV is a viral infection that can be spread from one person to another person through anal, vaginal, or oral sex, or through other close skin-to-skin touching during sexual activity. If you are sexually active you can get HPV, and nearly all sexually active people get infected with HPV at some point in their lives. It is important to understand that getting HPV is not the same thing as getting HIV or HSV (herpes).

How Do Men Get HPV?

You can get HPV by having sex with someone who is infected with HPV. This disease is spread easily during anal or vaginal sex, and it can also be spread through oral sex or other close skin-to-skin touching during sex. HPV can be spread even when an infected person has no visible signs or symptoms.

Will HPV Cause Health Problems for Me?

Most of the time HPV infections completely go away and don't cause any health problems. However, if an infection does not go away on its own, it is possible to develop HPV symptoms months or years after getting infected. This makes it hard to know exactly when you became infected. Lasting HPV infection can cause genital warts or certain kinds of cancer. It is not known why some people develop health problems from HPV and others do not.

What Are the Symptoms of HPV?

Most men who get HPV never develop symptoms and the infection usually goes away completely by itself. However, if HPV does not go away, it can cause genital warts or certain kinds of cancer.

See your healthcare provider if you have questions about anything new or unusual such as warts, or unusual growths, lumps, or sores on your penis, scrotum, anus, mouth, or throat.

What Are the Symptoms of Genital Warts?

Genital warts usually appear as a small bump or group of bumps in the genital area around the penis or the anus. These warts might be small or large, raised or flat, or shaped like a cauliflower. The warts may go away, or stay the same, or grow in size or number. Usually, a healthcare provider can diagnose genital warts simply by looking at them. Genital warts can come back, even after treatment. The types of HPV that cause warts do not cause cancer.

Can HPV Cause Cancer?

Yes. HPV infection isn't cancer but can cause changes in the body that lead to cancer. HPV infections usually go away by themselves but having an HPV infection can cause certain kinds of cancer to develop. These include cervical cancer in women, penile cancer in men, and anal cancer in both women and men. HPV can also cause cancer in the back of the throat, including the base of the tongue and tonsils (called oropharyngeal cancer). All of these cancers are caused by HPV infections that did not go away. Cancer develops very slowly and may not be diagnosed until years, or even decades, after a person initially gets infected with HPV. Currently, there is no way to know who will have only a temporary HPV infection, and who will develop cancer after getting HPV.

How Common Are HPV-Related Cancers in Men?

Although HPV is the most common sexually transmitted infection, HPV-related cancers are not common in men.

Certain men are more likely to develop HPV-related cancers:

- Men with weak immune systems (including those with HIV) who get infected with HPV are more likely to develop HPV-related health problems.

- Men who receive anal sex are more likely to get anal HPV and develop anal cancer.

Can I Get Tested for HPV?

No, there is currently no approved test for HPV in men.

Routine testing (also called 'screening') to check for HPV or HPV-related disease before there are signs or symptom, is not recommended by the CDC for anal, penile, or throat cancers in men in the United States. However, some healthcare providers do offer anal Pap tests to men who may be at increased risk for anal cancer, including men with HIV or men who receive anal sex. If you have symptoms and are concerned about cancer, please see a healthcare provider.

Can I Get Treated for HPV or Health Problems Caused by HPV?

There is no specific treatment for HPV, but there are treatments for health problems caused by HPV. Genital warts can be treated by your healthcare provider, or with prescription medication. HPV-related cancers are more treatable when diagnosed and treated promptly.

How Can I Lower My Chance of Getting HPV?

There are two steps you can take to lower your chances of getting HPV and HPV-related diseases:

- *Get vaccinated.* HPV vaccines are safe and effective. They can protect men against warts and certain cancers caused by HPV. Ideally, you should get vaccinated before ever having sex. HPV vaccines are given in a series of three shots over a period of about six months.

- *Use condoms the correct way every time you have sex.* This can lower your chances of getting all STIs, including HPV. However, HPV can infect areas that are not covered by a condom, so condoms may not give full protection against getting HPV.

Can I Get an HPV Vaccine?

In the United States, HPV vaccines are recommended for the following men:

- All boys at age 11 or 12 years (or as young as 9 years)

- Older boys through age 21 years, if they did not get vaccinated when they were younger

- Gay, bisexual, and other men who have sex with men through age 26 years, if they did not get vaccinated when they were younger

- Men with HIV or weakened immune systems through age 26 years, if they did not get vaccinated when they were younger

What Does Having HPV Mean for Me or My Sex Partner's Health?

See a healthcare provider if you have questions about anything new or unusual (such as warts, growths, lumps, or sores) on your own or your partner's penis, scrotum, anus, mouth or throat. Even if you are healthy, you and your sex partner(s) may also want to get checked by a healthcare provider for other STIs.

If you or your partner have genital warts, you should avoid having sex until the warts are gone or removed. However, it is not known how long a person is able to spread HPV after warts are gone.

What Does HPV Mean for My Relationship?

HPV infections are usually temporary. A person may have had HPV for many years before it causes health problems. If you or your partner are diagnosed with an HPV-related disease, there is no way to know how long you have had HPV, whether your partner gave you HPV, or whether you gave HPV to your partner. HPV is not necessarily a sign that one of you is having sex outside of your relationship. It is important that sex partners discuss their sexual health, and risk for all STIs, with each other.

Section 38.7

Pubic Lice (Crabs)

This section includes text excerpted from "Pubic "Crab" Lice," Centers for Disease Control and Prevention (CDC), September 24, 2013. Reviewed August 2016.

What Are Pubic Lice?

Also called crab lice or "crabs," pubic lice are parasitic insects found primarily in the pubic or genital area of humans. Pubic lice infestation is found worldwide and occurs in all races, ethnic groups, and levels of society.

What Do Pubic Lice Look Like?

Pubic lice have three forms: the egg (also called a nit), the nymph, and the adult.

Nit: Nits are lice eggs. They can be hard to see and are found firmly attached to the hair shaft. They are oval and usually yellow to white. Pubic lice nits take about 6–10 days to hatch.

Nymph: The nymph is an immature louse that hatches from the nit (egg). A nymph looks like an adult pubic louse but it is smaller. Pubic lice nymphs take about 2–3 weeks after hatching to mature into adults capable of reproducing. To live, a nymph must feed on blood.

Adult: The adult pubic louse resembles a miniature crab when viewed through a strong magnifying glass. Pubic lice have six legs; their two front legs are very large and look like the pincher claws of a crab. This is how they got the nickname "crabs." Pubic lice are tan to grayish-white in color. Females lay nits and are usually larger than males. To live, lice must feed on blood. If the louse falls off a person, it dies within 1–2 days.

Where Are Pubic Lice Found?

Pubic lice usually are found in the genital area on pubic hair; but they may occasionally be found on other coarse body hair, such as hair on the legs, armpits, mustache, beard, eyebrows, or eyelashes. Pubic lice on the eyebrows or eyelashes of children may be a sign of sexual exposure or abuse. Lice found on the head generally are head lice, not pubic lice.

Animals do not get or spread pubic lice.

What Are the Signs and Symptoms of Pubic Lice?

Signs and symptoms of pubic lice include

- Itching in the genital area
- Visible nits (lice eggs) or crawling lice

How Did I Get Pubic Lice?

Pubic lice usually are spread through sexual contact and are most common in adults. Pubic lice found on children may be a sign of sexual exposure or abuse. Occasionally, pubic lice may be spread by close personal contact or contact with articles such as clothing, bed linens, or towels that have been used by an infested person. A common misconception is that pubic lice are spread easily by sitting on a toilet seat. This would be extremely rare because lice cannot live long away from a warm human body and they do not have feet designed to hold onto or walk on smooth surfaces such as toilet seats.

Persons infested with pubic lice should be examined for the presence of other sexually transmitted diseases.

How Is a Pubic Lice Infestation Diagnosed?

A pubic lice infestation is diagnosed by finding a "crab" louse or egg (nit) on hair in the pubic region or, less commonly, elsewhere on the body (eyebrows, eyelashes, beard, mustache, armpit, perianal area, groin, trunk, scalp). Pubic lice may be difficult to find because there may be only a few. Pubic lice often attach themselves to more than one hair and generally do not crawl as quickly as head and body lice. If crawling lice are not seen, finding nits in the pubic area strongly suggests that a person is infested and should be treated. If you are unsure about infestation or if treatment is not successful, see a healthcare provider for a diagnosis. Persons infested with pubic lice should be investigated for the presence of other sexually transmitted diseases.

Although pubic lice and nits can be large enough to be seen with the naked eye, a magnifying lens may be necessary to find lice or eggs.

How Is a Pubic Lice Infestation Treated?

A lice-killing lotion containing 1% permethrin or a mousse containing pyrethrins and piperonyl butoxide can be used to treat pubic ("crab") lice. These products are available over-the-counter without a prescription at a local drug store or pharmacy. These medications are safe and effective when used exactly according to the instructions in the package or on the label.

Lindane shampoo is a prescription medication that can kill lice and lice eggs. However, lindane is not recommended as a first-line therapy. Lindane can be toxic to the brain and other parts of the nervous system; its use should be restricted to patients who have failed treatment with or cannot tolerate other medications that pose less risk. Lindane should not be used to treat premature infants, persons with a seizure disorder, persons who have very irritated skin or sores where the lindane will be applied, infants, children, the elderly, and persons who weigh less than 110 pounds.

Malathion* lotion 0.5% (Ovide*) is a prescription medication that can kill lice and some lice eggs; however, malathion lotion (Ovide*) currently has not been approved by the U.S. Food and Drug Administration (FDA) for treatment of pubic ("crab") lice.

Both topical and oral ivermectin have been used successfully to treat lice; however, only topical ivermectin lotion currently is approved by the U.S. Food and Drug Administration (FDA) for treatment of lice. Oral ivermectin is not FDA-approved for treatment of lice.

How to treat pubic lice infestations: (Warning: See special instructions for treatment of lice and nits on eyebrows or eyelashes. The lice medications described in this section should not be used near the eyes.)

1. Wash the infested area; towel dry.

2. Carefully follow the instructions in the package or on the label. Thoroughly saturate the pubic hair and other infested areas with lice medication. Leave medication on hair for the time recommended in the instructions. After waiting the recommended time, remove the medication by following carefully the instructions on the label or in the box.

3. Following treatment, most nits will still be attached to hair shafts. Nits may be removed with fingernails or by using a fine-toothed comb.

4. Put on clean underwear and clothing after treatment.

5. To kill any lice or nits remaining on clothing, towels, or bedding, machine-wash and machine-dry those items that the infested person used during the 2–3 days before treatment. Use hot water (at least 130°F) and the hot dryer cycle.

6. Items that cannot be laundered can be dry-cleaned or stored in a sealed plastic bag for 2 weeks.

7. All sex partners from within the previous month should be informed that they are at risk for infestation and should be treated.

8. Persons should avoid sexual contact with their sex partner(s) until both they and their partners have been successfully treated and reevaluated to rule out persistent infestation.

9. Repeat treatment in 9–10 days if live lice are still found.

10. Persons with pubic lice should be evaluated for other sexually transmitted diseases (STDs).

Special instructions for treatment of lice and nits found on eyebrows or eyelashes:

- If only a few live lice and nits are present, it may be possible to remove these with fingernails or a nit comb.

- If additional treatment is needed for lice or nits on the eyelashes, careful application of ophthalmic-grade petrolatum

497

ointment (only available by prescription) to the eyelid margins 2–4 times a day for 10 days is effective. Regular petrolatum (e.g., Vaseline)* should not be used because it can irritate the eyes if applied.

Section 38.8

Scabies

This section includes text excerpted from "Sexually Transmitted Diseases Treatment Guidelines," Centers for Disease Control and Prevention (CDC), June 5, 2015.

What Is Scabies?

The predominant symptom of scabies is pruritus. Sensitization to Sarcoptes scabiei occurs before pruritus begins. The first time a person is infested with S. *scabiei*, sensitization takes up to several weeks to develop. However, pruritus might occur within 24 hours after a subsequent reinfestation. Scabies in adults frequently is sexually acquired, although scabies in children usually is not.

Treatment

Permethrin is effective, safe, and less expensive than ivermectin. One study demonstrated increased mortality among elderly, debilitated persons who received ivermectin, but this observation has not been confirmed in subsequent reports. Ivermectin has limited ovicidal activity and may not prevent recurrences of eggs at the time of treatment; therefore, a second dose of ivermectin should be administered 14 days after the first dose. Ivermectin should be taken with food because bioavailability is increased, thereby increasing penetration of the drug into the epidermis. Adjustments to ivermectin dosing are not required in patients with renal impairment, but the safety of multiple doses in patients with severe liver disease is not known.

Lindane is an alternative regimen because it can cause toxicity; it should only be used if the patient cannot tolerate the recommended therapies or if these therapies have failed. Lindane should not be used immediately after a bath or shower, and it should not be used by persons who have extensive dermatitis or children aged <10 years. Seizures have occurred when lindane was applied after a bath or used by patients who had extensive dermatitis. Aplastic anemia after lindane use also has been reported. Lindane resistance has been reported in some areas of the world, including parts of the United States.

Other Management Considerations

Bedding and clothing should be decontaminated (i.e., either machine-washed, machine-dried using the hot cycle, or dry cleaned) or removed from body contact for at least 72 hours.

Fumigation of living areas is unnecessary. Persons with scabies should be advised to keep fingernails closely trimmed to reduce injury from excessive scratching.

Crusted Scabies

Crusted scabies (i.e., Norwegian scabies) is an aggressive infestation that usually occurs in immunodeficient, debilitated, or malnourished persons, including persons receiving systemic or potent topical glucocorticoids, organ transplant recipients, persons with HIV infection or human T-lymphotrophic virus-1-infection, and persons with hematologic malignancies.

Crusted scabies is transmitted more easily than scabies. No controlled therapeutic studies for crusted scabies have been conducted, and the appropriate treatment remains unclear. Substantial treatment failure might occur with a single-dose topical scabicide or with oral ivermectin treatment. Combination treatment is recommended with a topical scabicide, either 25 percent topical benzyl benzoate or 5 percent topical permethrin cream (full-body application to be repeated daily for 7 days then 2x weekly until discharge or cure), and treatment with oral ivermectin 200 ug/kg on days 1,2,8,9, and 15. Additional ivermectin treatment on days 22 and 29 might be required for severe cases. Lindane should be avoided because of the risks for neurotoxicity with heavy applications or denuded skin.

Follow-Up

The rash and pruritus of scabies might persist for up to 2 weeks after treatment. Symptoms or signs persisting for >2 weeks can be attributed to several factors. Treatment failure can occur as a result of resistance to medication or faulty application of topical scabicides. These medications do not easily penetrate into thick, scaly skin of persons with crusted scabies, perpetuating the harboring of mites in these difficultto-penetrate layers. In the absence of appropriate contact treatment and decontamination of bedding and clothing, persisting symptoms can be attributed to reinfection by family members or fomites. Finally, other household mites can cause symptoms to persist as a result of cross reactivity between antigens. Even when treatment is successful, reinfection is avoided, and cross reactivity does not occur, symptoms can persist or worsen as a result of allergic dermatitis. Retreatment 2 weeks after the initial treatment regimen can be considered for those persons who are still symptomatic or when live mites are observed. Use of an alternative regimen is recommended for those persons who do not respond initially to the recommended treatment.

Management of Sex Partners and Household Contacts

Persons who have had sexual, close personal, or household contact with the patient within the month preceding scabies infestation should be examined. Those found to be infested should be provided treatment.

Management of Outbreaks in Communities, Nursing Homes, and Other Institutional Settings

Scabies epidemics frequently occur in nursing homes, hospitals, residential facilities, and other communities. Control of an epidemic can only be achieved by treating the entire population at risk. Ivermectin can be considered in these settings, especially if treatment with topical scabicides fails. Epidemics should be managed in consultation with a specialist.

Section 38.9

Syphilis

This section includes text excerpted from "Syphilis-CDC
Fact Sheet (Detailed)," Centers for Disease Control and
Prevention (CDC), September 24, 2015.

What Is Syphilis?

Syphilis is a sexually transmitted disease (STD) caused by the
bacterium Treponema pallidum. Syphilis can cause long-term complications if not adequately treated.

How Common Is Syphilis?

During 2014, there were 63,450 reported new cases of syphilis, compared to 47,352 estimated new diagnoses of HIV infection in 2013 and
350,062 cases of gonorrhea in 2014. Of syphilis cases, 19.999 were of
primary and secondary (P&S) syphilis, the earliest and most transmis-
sible stages of syphilis. During the 1990s, syphilis primarily occurred
among heterosexual men and women of racial and ethnic minority
groups; during the 2000s, however, cases increased among men who
have sex with men (MSM). In 2014, MSM accounted for 83% of all P&S
syphilis cases among males in which sex of sex partner was known.

How Do People Get Syphilis?

Syphilis is transmitted from person to person by direct contact with
a syphilitic sore, known as a chancre. Chancres occur mainly on the
external genitals, vagina, anus, or in the rectum. Chancres also can
occur on the lips and in the mouth. Transmission of syphilis occurs
during vaginal, anal, or oral sex.

How Quickly Do Symptoms Appear after Infection?

The average time between infection with syphilis and the start of
the first symptom is 21 days, but can range from 10 to 90 days.

What Are the Signs and Symptoms in Adults?

Syphilis has been called "The Great Pretender", as its symptoms can look like many other diseases. However, syphilis typically follows a progression of stages that can last for weeks, months, or even years:

Primary Stage

The appearance of a single chancre marks the primary (first) stage of syphilis symptoms, but there may be multiple sores. The chancre is usually firm, round, and painless. It appears at the location where syphilis entered the body. These painless chancres can occur in locations that make them difficult to find (e.g., the vagina or anus). The chancre lasts 3 to 6 weeks and heals regardless of whether a person is treated or not. However, if the infected person does not receive adequate treatment, the infection progresses to the secondary stage.

Secondary Stage

Skin rashes and/or mucous membrane lesions (sores in the mouth, vagina, or anus) mark the second stage of symptoms. This stage typically starts with the development of a rash on one or more areas of the body. Rashes associated with secondary syphilis can appear when the primary chancre is healing or several weeks after the chancre has healed. The rash usually does not cause itching. The characteristic rash of secondary syphilis may appear as rough, red, or reddish brown spots both on the palms of the hands and the bottoms of the feet. However, rashes with a different appearance may occur on other parts of the body, sometimes resembling rashes caused by other diseases. Sometimes rashes associated with secondary syphilis are so faint that they are not noticed. Large, raised, gray or white lesions, known as condyloma lata, may develop in warm, moist areas such as the mouth, underarm or groin region. In addition to rashes, symptoms of secondary syphilis may include fever, swollen lymph glands, sore throat, patchy hair loss, headaches, weight loss, muscle aches, and fatigue. The symptoms of secondary syphilis will go away with or without treatment, but without treatment, the infection will progress to the latent and possibly late stages of disease.

Latent and Late Stages

The latent (hidden) stage of syphilis begins when primary and secondary symptoms disappear. Without treatment, the infected person will continue to have syphilis infection in their body even though there are no signs or symptoms. Early latent syphilis is latent syphilis where infection occurred within the past 12 months. Late latent syphilis is latent syphilis where infection occurred more than 12 months ago. Latent syphilis can last for years.

The late stages of syphilis can develop in about 15% of people who have not been treated for syphilis, and can appear 10–20 years after infection was first acquired. In the late stages of syphilis, the disease may damage the internal organs, including the brain, nerves, eyes, heart, blood vessels, liver, bones, and joints. Symptoms of the late stage of syphilis include difficulty coordinating muscle movements, paralysis, numbness, gradual blindness, and dementia. This damage may be serious enough to cause death.

Neurosyphilis

Syphilis can invade the nervous system at any stage of infection, and causes a wide range of symptoms varying from no symptoms at all, to headache, altered behavior, and movement problems that look like other neurologic diseases, such as Parkinson or Huntington disease. This invasion of the nervous system is called "neurosyphilis."

Ocular syphilis, a clinical manifestation of neurosyphilis, can involve almost any eye structure, but posterior uveitis and panuveitis are the most common. Ocular syphilis may lead to decreased visual acuity including permanent blindness. Clinicians should be aware of ocular syphilis and screen for visual complaints in any patient at risk for syphilis (e.g., MSM, HIV-infected persons, others with risk factors and persons with multiple or anonymous partners). A 2015 Clinical Advisory and a MMWR: Notes from the Field discuss recent reported cases and provide information for clinicians on the diagnosis and management of ocular syphilis.

HIV Infection and Syphilis Symptoms

Individuals who are HIV-positive can develop symptoms very different from the symptoms described above, including hypopigmented skin rashes. HIV can also increase the chances of developing syphilis with neurological involvement.

How Is Syphilis Diagnosed?

The definitive method for diagnosing syphilis is visualizing the spirochete via darkfield microscopy. This technique is rarely performed today because it is a technologically difficult method. Diagnoses are thus more commonly made using blood tests. There are two types of blood tests available for syphilis: 1) nontreponemal tests and 2) treponemal tests.

Nontreponemal tests (e.g., Venereal Disease Reference Laboratory test (VDRL) and Rapid Plasma Reagin test (RPR)) are simple, inexpensive, and are often used for screening. However, they are not specific for syphilis, can produce false-positive results, and, by themselves, are insufficient for diagnosis. VDRL and RPR should each have their antibody titer results reported quantitatively. Persons with a reactive nontreponemal test should receive a treponemal test to confirm a syphilis diagnosis. This sequence of testing (nontreponemal, then treponemal test) is considered the "classical" testing algorithm.

Treponemal tests (e.g., FTA-ABS, TP-PA, various EIAs, chemiluminescence immunoassays, immunoblots, and rapid treponemal assays) detect antibodies that are specific for syphilis. Treponemal antibodies appear earlier than nontreponemal antibodies and usually remain detectable for life, even after successful treatment. If a treponemal test is used for screening and the results are positive, a nontreponemal test with titer should be performed to confirm diagnosis and guide patient management decisions. Based on the results, further treponemal testing may be indicated. For further guidance, please refer to the 2015 STD Treatment Guidelines. This sequence of testing (treponemal, then nontreponemal, test) is considered the "reverse" sequence testing algorithm. Reverse sequence testing can be more convenient for laboratories, but its clinical interpretation is problematic, as this testing sequence can identify individuals not previously described (e.g., treponemal test positive, nontreponemal test negative), making optimal management choices difficult.

What Is the Link between Syphilis and HIV?

Genital sores caused by syphilis make it easier to transmit and acquire HIV infection sexually. There is an estimated 2- to 5-fold increased risk of acquiring HIV if exposed to that infection when syphilis is present.

Ulcerative STDs that cause sores, ulcers, or breaks in the skin or mucous membranes, such as syphilis, disrupt barriers that provide protection against infections. The genital ulcers caused by syphilis can bleed easily, and when they come into contact with oral and rectal mucosa during sex, increase the infectiousness of and susceptibility to HIV. Studies have observed that infection with syphilis was associated with subsequent HIV infection among MSM.

Having other STDs can also indicate increased risk for becoming HIV infected.

What Is the Treatment for Syphilis?

There are no home remedies or over-the-counter drugs that will cure syphilis, but syphilis is easy to cure in its early stages. A single intramuscular injection of long acting Benzathine penicillin G (2.4 million units administered intramuscularly) will cure a person who has primary, secondary or early latent syphilis. Three doses of long acting Benzathine penicillin G (2.4 million units administered intramuscularly) at weekly intervals is recommended for individuals with late latent syphilis or latent syphilis of unknown duration. Treatment will kill the syphilis bacterium and prevent further damage, but it will not repair damage already done.

Selection of the appropriate penicillin preparation is important to properly treat and cure syphilis. Combinations of some penicillin preparations (e.g., Bicillin C-R, a combination of benzathine penicillin and procaine penicillin) are not appropriate treatments for syphilis, as these combinations provide inadequate doses of penicillin.

Although data to support the use of alternatives to penicillin is limited, options for non-pregnant patients who are allergic to penicillin may include doxycycline, tetracycline, and for neurosyphilis, potentially ceftriaxone. These therapies should be used only in conjunction with close clinical and laboratory follow-up to ensure appropriate serological response and cure.

Persons who receive syphilis treatment must abstain from sexual contact with new partners until the syphilis sores are completely healed. Persons with syphilis must notify their sex partners so that they also can be tested and receive treatment if necessary.

Who Should Be Tested for Syphilis?

Any person with signs or symptoms of primary infection, secondary infection, neurologic infection, or tertiary infection should be tested for syphilis.

Providers should routinely test persons who

- are members of an at-risk subpopulation (i.e., persons in correctional facilities and MSM)
- have HIV infection
- are taking PrEP for HIV prevention
- have partner(s) who have tested positive for syphilis
- are sexually active and live in areas with high syphilis morbidity

Will Syphilis Recur?

Syphilis does not recur. However, having syphilis once does not protect a person from becoming infected again. Even following successful treatment, people can be reinfected. Patients with signs or symptoms that persist or recur or who have a sustained fourfold increase in nontreponemal test titer probably failed treatment or were reinfected. These patients should be retreated.

Because chancres can be hidden in the vagina, rectum, or mouth, it may not be obvious that a sex partner has syphilis. Unless a person knows that their sex partners have been tested and treated, they may be at risk of being reinfected by an untreated partner. For further details on the management of sex partners, refer to the 2015 STD Treatment Guidelines.

How Can Syphilis Be Prevented?

Correct and consistent use of latex condoms can reduce the risk of syphilis only when the infected area or site of potential exposure is protected. However, a syphilis sore outside of the area covered by a latex condom can still allow transmission, so caution should be exercised even when using a condom.

The surest way to avoid transmission of sexually transmitted diseases, including syphilis, is to abstain from sexual contact or to be in a long-term mutually monogamous relationship with a partner who has been tested and is known to be uninfected.

Partner-based interventions include partner notification—a critical component in preventing the spread of syphilis. Sexual partners of infected patients should be considered at risk and provided treatment per the 2015 STD Treatment Guidelines.

Transmission of an STD, including syphilis, cannot be prevented by washing the genitals, urinating, and/or douching after sex. Any unusual discharge, sore, or rash, particularly in the groin area, should be a signal to refrain from having sex and to see a doctor immediately.

Section 38.10

Trichomoniasis

This section includes text excerpted from "Neglected Parasitic Infections in the United States," Centers for Disease Control and Prevention (CDC), November 14, 2013. Reviewed August 2016.

Trichomoniasis

Trichomoniasis is the most common curable sexually transmitted disease (STD) in the United States. Trichomoniasis is caused by infection with a parasite (*Trichomonas vaginalis*). Women and men who have trichomoniasis are at higher risk for getting or spreading other STDs, including HIV. About 3.7 million people in the United States are infected with this parasite, and most do not have any signs or symptoms. Trichomoniasis is treated with prescription antimicrobial medication (one dose of metronidazole or tinidazole) but it is possible to become infected again. Trichomoniasis is considered a Neglected Parasitic Infection, one of a group of diseases that can result in serious illness among those who are infected, yet the burden and impact remain poorly understood.

How People get Trichomoniasis

Trichomoniasis is a sexually transmitted disease (STD); the parasite is passed from an infected person to an uninfected person during sex. Women and men with trichomoniasis may notice redness, soreness, or itching of the genitals, burning with urination, or discharge. Without treatment, infection can last for months or even years. Some people develop symptoms within 5 to 28 days after being infected, but others do not develop symptoms until much later or not at all. About 70% of infected people never have any signs or symptoms. Even without any symptoms, infected people can pass the infection to others.

Risk Factors for Acquiring Trichomoniasis

- Both men and women can get infected.

507

- People with more sexual partners are more likely to become infected.

- Other risk factors for infection may include limited education and low socioeconomic status.

Prevention of Trichomoniasis

Trichomoniasis is a preventable STD. People can reduce their risk by:

- Using latex condoms consistently and correctly

- Consulting a healthcare provider if any signs or symptoms develop

- Notifying any recent sex partners so they can be treated too

Why be Concerned about Trichomoniasis Infection in the United States?

- An estimated 3.7 million people are infected with *T. vaginalis* in the United States. Most infected people do not have any signs or symptoms of trichomoniasis and never know that they are infected.

- Having trichomoniasis increases the risk of getting or spreading other STDs, including HIV.

- Other health consequences of asymptomatic *T. vaginalis* infection are not well defined.

- A recent study found that 4.3% of *T. vaginalis* infections were resistant to the only class of antimicrobial medication available to treat this infection, and this number may be increasing.

What is CDC Doing to Address Trichomoniasis?

- CDC tracks the number of new and existing cases of trichomoniasis, including antimicrobial-resistant *T. vaginalis* infections, in the United States. Creates and publishes informational materials to educate the public about the infection.

- Offers national STD treatment guidelines, with evidence-based clinical recommendations to healthcare providers for screening and treating patients for trichomoniasis, including antimicrobial-resistant *T. vaginalis* infections.

- Provides continuing medical education (CME) courses and training for healthcare providers.

- Conducts laboratory testing to detect antimicrobial-resistant trichomoniasis.

- Works with key stakeholders at the local, state, national, and international levels to address trichomoniasis.

What More is Needed?

- Better estimate of the burden of disease, including accounting for asymptomatic cases

- Improved strategies for reducing age, race, and other health disparities seen with trichomoniasis

- Further investigation of the role *T. vaginalis* infections play in HIV transmission

- Ongoing education for the public regarding steps individuals can take to keep themselves and their sex partners free of infection

- Development of new treatment options, especially for people who have antimicrobial-resistant infections or who are allergic to antimicrobial medications that are available for treatment

- Continued epidemiologic and laboratory support for efforts by key stakeholders including state and local health departments to prevent the spread of trichomoniasis

Part Four

Other Medical Issues of Concern to Men

Chapter 39

Male-Linked Genetic Disorders

Chapter Contents

Section 39.1—Color Vision Deficiency 514

Section 39.2—Fragile X Syndrome 521

Section 39.3—Hemophilia 526

Section 39.4—Klinefelter Syndrome 535

Section 39.5—Muscular Dystrophy.. 543

Section 39.1

Color Vision Deficiency

This section includes text excerpted from "Facts about Color Blindness," National Eye Institute (NEI), February 2015.

What Is Color Blindness?

Most of us share a common color vision sensory experience. Some people, however, have a color vision deficiency, which means their perception of colors is different from what most of us see. The most severe forms of these deficiencies are referred to as color blindness. People with color blindness aren't aware of differences among colors that are obvious to the rest of us. People who don't have the more severe types of color blindness may not even be aware of their condition unless they're tested in a clinic or laboratory.

Inherited color blindness is caused by abnormal photopigments. These color-detecting molecules are located in cone-shaped cells within the retina, called cone cells. In humans, several genes are needed for the body to make photopigments, and defects in these genes can lead to color blindness.

There are three main kinds of color blindness, based on photopigment defects in the three different kinds of cones that respond to blue, green, and red light. Red-green color blindness is the most common, followed by blue-yellow color blindness. A complete absence of color vision—total color blindness—is rare.

Sometimes color blindness can be caused by physical or chemical damage to the eye, the optic nerve, or parts of the brain that process color information. Color vision can also decline with age, most often because of cataract—a clouding and yellowing of the eye's lens.

Who Gets Color Blindness?

As many as 8 percent of men and 0.5 percent of women with Northern European ancestry have the common form of red-green color blindness.

Men are much more likely to be colorblind than women because the genes responsible for the most common, inherited color blindness are on the X chromosome. Males only have one X chromosome, while females have two X chromosomes. In females, a functional gene on only one of the X chromosomes is enough to compensate for the loss on the other. This kind of inheritance pattern is called X-linked, and primarily affects males. Inherited color blindness can be present at birth, begin in childhood, or not appear until the adult years.

How Genes Are Inherited

Genes are bundled together on structures called chromosomes. One copy of each chromosome is passed by a parent at conception through egg and sperm cells. The X and Y chromosomes, known as sex chromosomes, determine whether a person is born female (XX) or male (XY) and also carry other traits not related to gender.

In X-linked inheritance, the mother carries the mutated gene on one of her X chromosomes and will pass on the mutated gene to 50 percent of her children. Because females have two X chromosomes, the effect of a mutation on one X chromosome is offset by the normal gene on the other X chromosome. In this case the mother will not have the disease, but she can pass on the mutated gene and so is called a carrier. If a mother is a carrier of an X-linked disease (and the father is not affected), there is a:

- 1 in 2 chance that a son will have the disease

- 1 in 2 chance that a daughter will be a carrier of the disease

- No chance that a daughter will have the disease

In autosomal recessive inheritance, it takes two copies of the mutant gene to give rise to the disease. An individual who has one copy of a recessive gene mutation is known as a carrier. When two carriers have a child, there is a:

- 1 in 4 chance of having a child with the disease

- 1 in 2 chance of having a child who is a carrier

- 1 in 4 chance of having a child who neither has the disease nor is a carrier

In autosomal dominant inheritance, it takes just one copy of the mutant gene to bring about the disease. When an affected parent with one dominant gene mutation has a child, there is a 1 in 2 chance that a child will inherit the disease.

How Do We See Color?

What color is a strawberry? Most of us would say red, but do we all see the same red? Color vision depends on our eyes and brain working together to perceive different properties of light.

We see the natural and artificial light that illuminates our world as white, although it is actually a mixture of colors that, perceived on their own, would span the visual spectrum from deep blue to deep red. You can see this when rain separates sunlight into a rainbow or a glass prism separates white light into a multi-color band. The color of light is determined by its *wavelength*. Longer wavelength corresponds to red light and shorter wavelength corresponds to blue light.

Strawberries and other objects reflect some wavelengths of light and absorb others. The reflected light we perceive as color. So, a strawberry is red because its surface is only reflecting the long wavelengths we see as red and absorbing the others. An object appears white when it reflects all wavelengths and black when it absorbs all wavelengths.

Vision begins when light enters the eye and the cornea and lens focus it onto the retina, a thin layer of tissue at the back of the eye that contains millions of light-sensitive cells called photoreceptors. Some photoreceptors are shaped like rods and some are shaped like cones. In each eye there are many more rods than cones—approximately 120 million rods compared to only 6 million cones. Rods and cones both contain photopigment molecules that undergo a chemical change when they absorb light. This chemical change acts like an on-switch, triggering electrical signals that are then passed from the retina to the visual parts of the brain.

Rods and cones are different in how they respond to light. Rods are more responsive to dim light, which makes them useful for night vision. Cones are more responsive to bright light, such as in the day-time when light is plentiful.

Another important difference is that all rods contain only one photopigment, while cones contain one of three different photopigments. This makes cones sensitive to long (red), medium (green), or short (blue) wavelengths of light. The presence of three types of photopigments, each sensitive to a different part of the visual spectrum, is what gives us our rich color vision.

Humans are unusual among mammals for our trichromatic vision—named for the three different types of photopigments we have. Most mammals, including dogs, have just two photopigment types. Other creatures, such as butterflies, have more than three. They may be able to see colors we can only imagine.

Most of us have a full set of the three different cone photopigments and so we share a very similar color vision experience, but because the human eye and brain together translate light into color, each of us sees colors differently. The differences may be slight. Your blue may be more blue than someone else's, or in the case of color blindness, your red and green may be someone else's brown.

What Are the Different Types of Color Blindness?

The most common types of color blindness are inherited. They are the result of defects in the genes that contain the instructions for making the photopigments found in cones. Some defects alter the photopigment's sensitivity to color, for example, it might be slightly more sensitive to deeper red and less sensitive to green. Other defects can result in the total loss of a photopigment. Depending on the type of defect and the cone that is affected problems can arise with red, green, or blue color vision.

Red-Green Color Blindness

The most common types of hereditary color blindness are due to the loss or limited function of red cone (known as protan) or green cone (deutran) photopigments. This kind of color blindness is commonly referred to as red-green color blindness.

- **Protanomaly:** In males with protanomaly, the red cone photopigment is abnormal. Red, orange, and yellow appear greener and colors are not as bright. This condition is mild and doesn't usually interfere with daily living. Protanomaly is an X-linked disorder estimated to affect 1 percent of males.

- **Protanopia:** In males with protanopia, there are no working red cone cells. Red appears as black. Certain shades of orange, yellow, and green all appear as yellow. Protanopia is an X-linked disorder that is estimated to affect 1 percent of males.

- **Deuteranomaly:** In males with deuteranomaly, the green cone photopigment is abnormal. Yellow and green appear redder and it is difficult to tell violet from blue. This condition is mild and doesn't interfere with daily living. Deuteranomaly is the most common form of color blindness and is an X-linked disorder affecting 5 percent of males.

- **Deuteranopia:** In males with deuteranopia, there are no working green cone cells. They tend to see reds as brownish-yellow and greens as beige. Deuteranopia is an X-linked disorder that affects about 1 percent of males.

Blue-Yellow Color Blindness

Blue-yellow color blindness is rarer than red-green color blindness. Blue-cone (tritan) photopigments are either missing or have limited function.

- **Tritanomaly:** People with tritanomaly have functionally limited blue cone cells. Blue appears greener and it can be difficult to tell yellow and red from pink. Tritanomaly is extremely rare. It is an autosomal dominant disorder affecting males and females equally.

- **Tritanopia:** People with tritanopia, also known as blue-yellow color blindness, lack blue cone cells. Blue appears green and yellow appears violet or light grey. Tritanopia is an extremely rare autosomal recessive disorder affecting males and females equally.

Complete Color Blindness

People with complete color blindness (monochromacy) don't experience color at all and the clearness of their vision (visual acuity) may also be affected.

There are two types of monochromacy:

1. **Cone monochromacy:** This rare form of color blindness results from a failure of two of the three cone cell photopigments to work. There is red cone monochromacy, green cone monochromacy, and blue cone monochromacy. People with cone monochromacy have trouble distinguishing colors because the brain needs to compare the signals from different types of cones in order to see color. When only one type of cone works, this comparison isn't possible. People with blue cone monochromacy, may also have reduced visual acuity, near-sightedness, and uncontrollable eye movements, a condition known as nystagmus. Cone monochromacy is an autosomal recessive disorder.

2. **Rod monochromacy or achromatopsia:** This type of monochromacy is rare and is the most severe form of color blindness. It is present at birth. None of the cone cells have functional photopigments. Lacking all cone vision, people with rod

monochromacy see the world in black, white, and gray. And since rods respond to dim light, people with rod monochromacy tend to be photophobic—very uncomfortable in bright environments. They also experience nystagmus. Rod monochromacy is an autosomal recessive disorder.

How Is Color Blindness Diagnosed?

Eye care professionals use a variety of tests to diagnose color blindness. These tests can quickly diagnose specific types of color blindness.

The Ishihara Color Test is the most common test for red-green color blindness. The test consists of a series of colored circles, called Ishihara plates, each of which contains a collection of dots in different colors and sizes. Within the circle are dots that form a shape clearly visible to those with normal color vision, but invisible or difficult to see for those with red-green color blindness.

The newer Cambridge Color Test uses a visual array similar to the Ishihara plates, except displayed on a computer monitor. The goal is to identify a C shape that is different in color from the background. The "C" is presented randomly in one of four orientations. When test-takers see the "C," they are asked to press one of four keys that correspond to the orientation.

The anomaloscope uses a test in which two different light sources have to be matched in color. Looking through the eyepiece, the viewer sees a circle. The upper half is a yellow light that can be adjusted in brightness. The lower half is a combination of red and green lights that can be mixed in variable proportions. The viewer uses one knob to adjust the brightness of the top half, and another to adjust the color of the lower half. The goal is to make the upper and lower halves the same brightness and color.

The HRR Pseudoisochromatic Color Test is another red-green color blindness test that uses color plates to test for color blindness.

The Farnsworth-Munsell 100 Hue Test uses a set of blocks or pegs that are roughly the same color but in different hues (shades of the color). The goal is to arrange them in a line in order of hue. This test measures the ability to discriminate subtle color changes. It is used by industries that depend on the accurate color perception of its employees, such as graphic design, photography, and food quality inspection.

The Farnsworth Lantern Test is used by the U.S. military to determine the severity of color blindness. Those with mild forms pass the test and are allowed to serve in the armed forces.

Are There Treatments for Color Blindness?

There is no cure for color blindness. However, people with red-green color blindness may be able to use a special set of lenses to help them perceive colors more accurately. These lenses can only be used outdoors under bright lighting conditions. Visual aids have also been developed to help people cope with color blindness. There are iPhone and iPad apps, for example, that help people with color blindness discriminate among colors. Some of these apps allow users to snap a photo and tap it anywhere on the image to see the color of that area. More sophisticated apps allow users to find out both color and shades of color. These kinds of apps can be helpful in selecting ripe fruits such as bananas, or finding complementary colors when picking out clothing.

How Does Color Blindness Affect Daily Life?

Color blindness can make it difficult to read color-coded information such as bar graphs and pie charts. This can be particularly troubling for children who aren't yet diagnosed with color blindness, since educational materials are often color-coded. Children with red-green color blindness may also have difficulty reading a green chalkboard when yellow chalk is used. Art classes, which require selecting appropriate colors of paint or crayons, may be challenging.

Color blindness can go undetected for some time since children will often try to hide their disorder. It's important to have children tested, particularly boys, if there is a family history of color blindness. Many school systems offer vision screening tests that include color blindness testing. Once a child is diagnosed, he or she can learn to ask for help with tasks that require color recognition.

Simple everyday tasks like cooking meat to the desired color or selecting ripe produce can be a challenge for adults. Children might find food without bright color as less appetizing. Traffic lights pose challenges, since they have to be read by the position of the light. Since most lights are vertical, with green on bottom and red on top, if a light is positioned horizontally, a color blind person has to do a quick mental rotation to read it. Reading maps or buying clothes that match colors can also be difficult. However, these are relatively minor inconveniences and most people with color blindness learn to adapt.

Section 39.2

Fragile X Syndrome

This section includes text excerpted from "Fragile X Syndrome,"
Eunice Kennedy Shriver National Institute of Child Health and
Human Development (NICHD), October 29, 2013.
Reviewed August 2016.

Fragile X Syndrome (FXS): Overview

The genetic disorder FXS, which results from mutations in a gene on the X chromosome, is the most commonly inherited form of developmental and intellectual disability.

Common Name

Fragile X syndrome or Fragile X

Medical or Scientific Names

Martin-Bell syndrome

What Is Fragile X Syndrome?

FXS is a genetic disorder that affects a person's development, especially that person's behavior and ability to learn. In addition, FXS can affect:

- communication skills

- physical appearance

- sensitivity to noise, light, or other sensory information

FXS is the most common form of inherited intellectual and developmental disability (IDD)

People with FXS may not have noticeable symptoms, or they can have more serious symptoms that range from learning disabilities to cognitive and behavior problems.

How Is a Change in the FMR1 Gene Related to Fragile X Syndrome and Associated Disorders?

FXS and its associated conditions are caused by changes (mutations) in the *Fragile X Mental Retardation 1 (FMR1)* gene found on the X chromosome. This mutation affects how the body makes the Fragile X Mental Retardation Protein, or FMRP. The mutation causes the body to make only a little bit or none of the protein, which can cause the symptoms of FXS.

In a gene, the information for making a protein has two parts: the introduction, and the instructions for making the protein itself. Researchers call the introduction the **promoter** because of how it helps to start the process of building the protein.

The promoter part of the *FMR1* gene includes many **repeats**— repeated instances of a specific DNA sequence called the CGG sequence. A normal *FMR1* gene has between 6 and 40 repeats in the promoter; the average is 30 repeats.

People with between 55 and 200 repeats have a premutation of the gene.

The **premutation** may cause the gene to not work properly, but it does not cause intellectual and developmental disability (IDD). The premutation is linked to the disorders FXPOI and FXTAS. However, not all people with the premutation show symptoms of FXPOI or FXTAS.

People with 200 or more repeats in the promoter part of the gene have a full mutation, meaning the gene might not work at all. People with a **full mutation** often have FXS.

The number of repeats, also called the "size of the mutation," affects the type of symptoms and how serious the symptoms of FXS will be.

Inheriting Fragile X Syndrome

FXS is inherited, which means it is passed down from parents to children. Anyone with the *FMR1* gene mutation can pass it to their children. However, a person who inherits the gene mutation may not develop FXS. Males will pass it down to all of their daughters and not their sons. Females have a 50/50 chance to pass it along to both their sons and daughters. In some cases, an *FMR1* premutation can change to a full mutation when it is passed from parent to child.

What Causes Fragile X Syndrome?

FXS results from a change or mutation in the *FMR1* gene, which is found on the X chromosome. The gene normally makes a protein called Fragile X Mental Retardation Protein, or FMRP. This protein is important for creating and maintaining connections between cells in the brain and nervous system. The mutation causes the body to make only a little bit or none of the protein, which often causes the symptoms of FXS.

Not everyone with the mutated *FMR1* gene has symptoms of FXS, because the body may still be able to make FMRP. A few things affect how much FMRP the body can make:

- **The size of the mutation.** Some people have a smaller mutation (a lower number of repeats) in their *FMR1* gene, while others have big mutations (a large number of repeats) in the gene. If the mutation is small, the body may be able to make some of the protein. Having the protein available makes the symptoms milder.

- **The number of cells that have the mutation.** Because not every cell in the body is exactly the same, some cells might have the *FMR1* mutation while others do not. This situation is called mosaicism. If the mutation is in most of the body's cells, the person will probably have symptoms of FXS. If the mutation is in only some of the cells, the person might not have any symptoms at all or only mild symptoms.

- **Being female.** Females have two X chromosomes (XX), while males have only one. In females, if the *FMR1* gene on one X chromosome has the mutation, the *FMR1* gene on the other X chromosome might not have the mutation. Even if one of the female's genes has a very large mutation, the body can usually make at least some FMRP, leading to milder symptoms.

How Many People Are Affected by Fragile X Syndrome?

About 1 in 4,000 males and 1 in 8,000 females have FXS.

How Many People Have the Fragile X Premutation?

Although FXS is relatively rare, premutations in the *FMR1* gene are relatively common: A recent study of 6,747 people found that 1 in 151 women and 1 in 468 men had the premutation. People with the premutation might not have any symptoms of FXS. However, the premutation can sometimes expand in the next generation, which can cause FXS.

What Are the Symptoms of Fragile X Syndrome?

People with FXS do not all have the same signs and symptoms, but they do have some things in common. Symptoms are often milder in females than in males.

- **Intelligence and learning.** Many people with FXS have problems with intellectual functioning.

    - These problems can range from the mild, such as learning disorders or problems with mathematics, to the severe, such as an intellectual or developmental disability.

    - The syndrome may affect the ability to think, reason, and learn.

    - Because many people with FXS also have attention disorders, hyperactivity, anxiety, and language-processing problems, a person with FXS may have more capabilities than his or her IQ (intelligence quotient) score suggests.

- **Physical.** Most infants and younger children with FXS don't have any specific physical features of this syndrome. When these children start to go through puberty, however, many will begin to develop certain features that are typical of those with FXS.

    - These features include a narrow face, large head, large ears, flexible joints, flat feet, and a prominent forehead.

    - These physical signs become more obvious with age.

- **Behavioral, social, and emotional.** Most children with FXS have some behavioral challenges.

    - They may be afraid or anxious in new situations.

    - They may have trouble making eye contact with other people.

    - Boys, especially, may have trouble paying attention or be aggressive.

- **Speech and language.** Most boys with FXS have some problems with speech and language.

    - They may have trouble speaking clearly, may stutter, or may leave out parts of words. They may also have problems understanding other people's social cues, such as tone of voice or specific types of body language.

- Some children with FXS begin talking later than typically developing children. Most will talk eventually, but a few might stay nonverbal throughout their lives.

- **Sensory.** Many children with FXS are bothered by certain sensations, such as bright light, loud noises, or the way certain clothing feels on their bodies.

  - These sensory issues might cause them to act out or display behavior problems.

How Do Healthcare Providers Diagnose Fragile X Syndrome?

Healthcare providers often use a blood sample to diagnose FXS. The healthcare provider will take a sample of blood and will send it to a laboratory, which will determine what form of the *FMR1* gene is present.

Diagnosis of Children

Many parents first notice symptoms of delayed development in their infants or toddlers. These symptoms may include delays in speech and language skills, social and emotional difficulties, and being sensitive to certain sensations. Children may also be delayed in or have problems with motor skills such as learning to walk.

A healthcare provider can perform developmental screening to determine the nature of delays in a child. If a healthcare provider suspects the child has FXS, he/she can refer parents to a clinical geneticist, who can perform a genetic test for FXS.

What Are the Treatments for Fragile X Syndrome?

There is no single treatment for FXS, but there are treatments that help minimize the symptoms of the condition. Individuals with FXS who receive appropriate education, therapy services, and medications have the best chance of using all of their individual capabilities and skills. Even those with an intellectual or developmental disability can learn to master many self-help skills.

Early intervention is important. Because a young child's brain is still forming, early intervention gives children the best start possible and the greatest chance of developing a full range of skills. The sooner a child with FXS gets treatment, the more opportunity there is for learning.

Section 39.3

Hemophilia

This section includes text excerpted from "Hemophilia," National Heart, Lung, and Blood Institute (NHLBI), July 13, 2013. Reviewed August 2016.

What Is Hemophilia?

Hemophilia is a rare bleeding disorder in which the blood doesn't clot normally.

If you have hemophilia, you may bleed for a longer time than others after an injury. You also may bleed inside your body (internally), especially in your knees, ankles, and elbows. This bleeding can damage your organs and tissues and may be life threatening.

Other Names for Hemophilia

Hemophilia A

- Classic hemophilia

- Factor VIII deficiency

Hemophilia B

- Christmas disease

- Factor IX deficiency

What Causes Hemophilia?

A defect in one of the genes that determines how the body makes blood clotting factor VIII or IX causes hemophilia. These genes are located on the X chromosomes.

Chromosomes come in pairs. Females have two X chromosomes, while males have one X and one Y chromosome. Only the X chromosome carries the genes related to clotting factors.

A male who has a hemophilia gene on his X chromosome will have hemophilia. When a female has a hemophilia gene on only one of her X chromosomes, she is a "hemophilia carrier" and can pass the gene to her children. Sometimes carriers have low levels of clotting factor and have symptoms of hemophilia, including bleeding. Clotting factors are proteins in the blood that work together with platelets to stop or control bleeding.

Below are two examples of how the hemophilia gene is inherited.

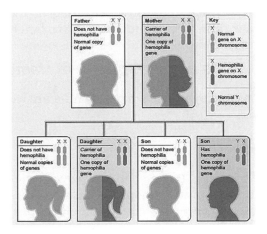

Figure 39.1. *Inheritance Pattern for Hemophilia—Example 1*

In this example, the father doesn't have hemophilia (that is, he has two normal chromosomes—X and Y). The mother is a carrier of hemophilia (that is, she has one hemophilia gene on one X chromosome and one normal X chromosome).

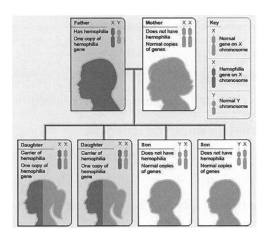

Figure 39.2. *Inheritance Pattern for Hemophilia—Example 2*

In this example, the father has hemophilia (that is, he has the hemophilia gene on the X chromosome). The mother isn't a hemophilia carrier (that is, she has two normal X chromosomes).

- Each daughter has a 50 percent chance of inheriting the hemo-philia gene from her mother and being a carrier. Each son has a 50 percent chance of inheriting the hemophilia gene from his mother and having hemophilia.

- Each daughter will inherit the hemophilia gene from her father and be a carrier. None of the sons will inherit the hemophilia gene from their father; thus, none will have hemophilia.

What Are the Signs and Symptoms of Hemophilia?

The major signs and symptoms of hemophilia are excessive bleeding and easy bruising.

Excessive Bleeding

The extent of bleeding depends on how severe the hemophilia is.

Children who have mild hemophilia may not have signs unless they have excessive bleeding from a dental procedure, an accident, or surgery. Males who have severe hemophilia may bleed heavily after circumcision.

Bleeding can occur on the body's surface (external bleeding) or inside the body (internal bleeding).

Signs of external bleeding may include:

- bleeding in the mouth from a cut or bite or from cutting or losing a tooth

- nosebleeds for no obvious reason

- heavy bleeding from a minor cut

- bleeding from a cut that resumes after stopping for a short time

Signs of internal bleeding may include:

- blood in the urine (from bleeding in the kidneys or bladder)

- blood in the stool (from bleeding in the intestines or stomach)

- large bruises (from bleeding into the large muscles of the body)

Bleeding in the Joints

Bleeding in the knees, elbows, or other joints is another common form of internal bleeding in people who have hemophilia. This bleeding can occur without obvious injury.

At first, the bleeding causes tightness in the joint with no real pain or any visible signs of bleeding. The joint then becomes swollen, hot to touch, and painful to bend.

Swelling continues as bleeding continues. Eventually, movement in the joint is temporarily lost. Pain can be severe. Joint bleeding that isn't treated quickly can damage the joint.

Bleeding in the Brain

Internal bleeding in the brain is a very serious complication of hemophilia. It can happen after a simple bump on the head or a more serious injury. The signs and symptoms of bleeding in the brain include:

- long-lasting, painful headaches or neck pain or stiffness

- repeated vomiting

- sleepiness or changes in behavior

- sudden weakness or clumsiness of the arms or legs or problems walking

- double vision

- convulsions or seizures

How Is Hemophilia Diagnosed?

If you or your child appears to have a bleeding problem, your doctor will ask about your personal and family medical histories. This will reveal whether you or your family members, including women and girls, have bleeding problems. However, some people who have hemophilia have no recent family history of the disease.

You or your child also will likely have a physical exam and blood tests to diagnose hemophilia. Blood tests are used to find out:

- How long it takes for your blood to clot

- Whether your blood has low levels of any clotting factors

- Whether any clotting factors are completely missing from your blood

The test results will show whether you have hemophilia, what type of hemophilia you have, and how severe it is.

Hemophilia A and B are classified as mild, moderate, or severe, depending on the amount of clotting factor VIII or IX in the blood.

Table 39.1. Hemophilia and Clotting Factor

Mild hemophilia	5–40 percent of normal clotting factor
Moderate hemophilia	1–5 percent of normal clotting factor
Severe hemophilia	Less than 1 percent of normal clotting factor

The severity of symptoms can overlap between the categories. For example, some people who have mild hemophilia may have bleeding problems almost as often or as severe as some people who have moderate hemophilia.

Severe hemophilia can cause serious bleeding problems in babies. Thus, children who have severe hemophilia usually are diagnosed during the first year of life. People who have milder forms of hemophilia may not be diagnosed until they're adults.

How Is Hemophilia Treated?

Treatment with Replacement Therapy

The main treatment for hemophilia is called replacement therapy. Concentrates of clotting factor VIII (for hemophilia A) or clotting factor IX (for hemophilia B) are slowly dripped or injected into a vein. These infusions help replace the clotting factor that's missing or low.

Clotting factor concentrates can be made from human blood. The blood is treated to prevent the spread of diseases, such as hepatitis. With the current methods of screening and treating donated blood, the risk of getting an infectious disease from human clotting factors is very small.

To further reduce the risk, you or your child can take clotting factor concentrates that aren't made from human blood. These are called recombinant clotting factors. Clotting factors are easy to store, mix, and use at home—it only takes about 15 minutes to receive the factor.

You may have replacement therapy on a regular basis to prevent bleeding. This is called preventive or prophylactic therapy. Or, you may only need replacement therapy to stop bleeding when it occurs. This use of the treatment, on an as-needed basis, is called demand therapy.

Demand therapy is less intensive and expensive than preventive therapy. However, there's a risk that bleeding will cause damage before you receive the demand therapy.

Complications of Replacement Therapy

Complications of replacement therapy include:

- Developing antibodies (proteins) that attack the clotting factor
- Developing viral infections from human clotting factors
- Damage to joints, muscles, or other parts of the body resulting from delays in treatment

Antibodies to the clotting factor. Antibodies can destroy the clotting factor before it has a chance to work. This is a very serious problem. It prevents the main treatment for hemophilia (replacement therapy) from working.

These antibodies, also called inhibitors, develop in about 20–30 percent of people who have severe hemophilia A. Inhibitors develop in 2–5 percent of people who have hemophilia B.

When antibodies develop, doctors may use larger doses of clotting factor or try different clotting factor sources. Sometimes the antibodies go away.

Researchers are studying new ways to deal with antibodies to clotting factors.

Viruses from human clotting factors. Clotting factors made from human blood can carry the viruses that cause HIV/AIDS and hepatitis. However, the risk of getting an infectious disease from human clotting factors is very small due to:

- careful screening of blood donors
- testing of donated blood products
- treating donated blood products with a detergent and heat to destroy viruses
- vaccinating people who have hemophilia for hepatitis A and B

Damage to joints, muscles, and other parts of the body. Delays in treatment can cause damage such as:

- Bleeding into a joint. If this happens many times, it can lead to changes in the shape of the joint and impair the joint's function.

- Swelling of the membrane around a joint.

- Pain, swelling, and redness of a joint.

- Pressure on a joint from swelling, which can destroy the joint.

Home Treatment with Replacement Therapy

You can do both preventive (ongoing) and demand (as-needed) replacement therapy at home. Many people learn to do the infusions at home for their child or for themselves. Home treatment has several advantages:

- You or your child can get quicker treatment when bleeding happens. Early treatment lowers the risk of complications.

- Fewer visits to the doctor or emergency room are needed.

- Home treatment costs less than treatment in a medical care setting.

- Home treatment helps children accept treatment and take responsibility for their own health.

Discuss options for home treatment with your doctor or your child's doctor. A doctor or other healthcare provider can teach you the steps and safety procedures for home treatment. Hemophilia treatment centers are another good resource for learning about home treatment.

Doctors can surgically implant vein access devices to make it easier for you to access a vein for treatment with replacement therapy. These devices can be helpful if treatment occurs often. However, infections can be a problem with these devices. Your doctor can help you decide whether this type of device is right for you or your child.

Other Types of Treatment

Desmopressin

Desmopressin (DDAVP) is a man-made hormone used to treat people who have mild hemophilia A. DDAVP isn't used to treat hemophilia B or severe hemophilia A.

DDAVP stimulates the release of stored factor VIII and von Willebrand factor; it also increases the level of these proteins in your blood. Von Willebrand factor carries and binds factor VIII, which can then stay in the bloodstream longer.

DDAVP usually is given by injection or as nasal spray. Because the effect of this medicine wears off if it's used often, the medicine is given only in certain situations. For example, you may take this medicine prior to dental work or before playing certain sports to prevent or reduce bleeding.

Antifibrinolytic Medicines

Antifibrinolytic medicines (including tranexamic acid and epsilon aminocaproic acid) may be used with replacement therapy. They're usually given as a pill, and they help keep blood clots from breaking down.

These medicines most often are used before dental work or to treat bleeding from the mouth or nose or mild intestinal bleeding.

Gene Therapy

Researchers are trying to find ways to correct the faulty genes that cause hemophilia. Gene therapy hasn't yet developed to the point that it's an accepted treatment for hemophilia. However, researchers continue to test gene therapy in clinical trials.

Treatment of a Specific Bleeding Site

Pain medicines, steroids, and physical therapy may be used to reduce pain and swelling in an affected joint. Talk with your doctor or pharmacist about which medicines are safe for you to take.

Which Treatment Is Best for You?

The type of treatment you or your child receives depends on several things, including how severe the hemophilia is, the activities you'll be doing, and the dental or medical procedures you'll be having.

- Mild hemophilia—Replacement therapy usually isn't needed for mild hemophilia. Sometimes, though, DDAVP is given to raise the body's level of factor VIII.

- Moderate hemophilia—You may need replacement therapy only when bleeding occurs or to prevent bleeding that could occur when doing certain activities. Your doctor also may recommend DDAVP prior to having a procedure or doing an activity that increases the risk of bleeding.

- Severe hemophilia—You usually need replacement therapy to prevent bleeding that could damage your joints, muscles, or other parts of your body. Typically, replacement therapy is given at home two or three times a week. This preventive therapy usually is started in patients at a young age and may need to continue for life.

For both types of hemophilia, getting quick treatment for bleeding is important. Quick treatment can limit damage to your body. If you or your child has hemophilia, learn to recognize signs of bleeding.

Other family members also should learn to watch for signs of bleeding in a child who has hemophilia. Children sometimes ignore signs of bleeding because they want to avoid the discomfort of treatment.

Living with Hemophilia

If you or your child has hemophilia, you can take steps to prevent bleeding problems.

Ongoing Care

If you have hemophilia, you can take steps to avoid complications. For example:

- Follow your treatment plan exactly as your doctor prescribes.

- Have regular checkups and vaccinations as recommended.

- Tell all of your healthcare providers—such as your doctor, dentist, and pharmacist—that you have hemophilia. You also may want to tell people like your employee health nurse, gym trainer, and sports coach about your condition.

- Have regular dental care. Dentists at the HTCs are experts in providing dental care for people who have hemophilia. If you see another dentist, tell him or her that you have hemophilia. The dentist can provide medicine that will reduce bleeding during dental work.

- Know the signs and symptoms of bleeding in joints and other parts of the body. Know when to call your doctor or go to the emergency room. For example, you'll need care if you have:

  - Heavy bleeding that can't be stopped or a wound that continues to ooze blood.

  - Any signs or symptoms of bleeding in the brain. Such bleeding is life threatening and requires emergency care.

  - Limited motion, pain, or swelling of any joint.

It's a good idea to keep a record of all previous treatments. Be sure to take this information with you to medical appointments and to the hospital or emergency room.

Section 39.4

Klinefelter Syndrome

This section includes text excerpted from "Klinefelter Syndrome (KS)," *Eunice Kennedy Shriver* National Institute of Child Health and Human Development (NICHD), October 25, 2013. Reviewed August 2016.

Klinefelter Syndrome (KS): Overview

KS describes a set of physical, language, and social development symptoms in males who have an extra X chromosome. Its main feature is infertility. Outward signs of KS can be subtle, so symptoms often are not recognized, and may not be treated in a timely manner.

Medical or Scientific Names

- Klinefelter syndrome

- 47, XXY

- XXY syndrome or condition

- XXY trisomy

- 47, XXY/46, XY or mosaic syndrome (rare variation)

- Poly-X Klinefelter syndrome, including the following rare variations:

    - 48, XXYY (or tetrasomy)

    - 48, XXXY (or tetrasomy)

    - 49, XXXXY (or pentasomy)

What Is Klinefelter Syndrome?

The term "Klinefelter syndrome," or KS, describes a set of features that can occur in a male who is born with an extra X chromosome in his cells. It is named after Dr. Henry Klinefelter, who identified the condition in the 1940s.

Usually, every cell in a male's body, except sperm and red blood cells, contains 46 chromosomes. The 45th and 46th chromosomes—the X and Y chromosomes—are sometimes called "sex chromosomes" because they determine a person's sex. Normally, males have one X and one Y chromosome, making them XY. Males with KS have an extra X chromosome, making them XXY.

KS is sometimes called "47, XXY" (47 refers to total chromosomes) or the "XXY condition." Those with KS are sometimes called "XXY males."

Some males with KS may have both XY cells and XXY cells in their bodies. This is called "mosaic." Mosaic males may have fewer symptoms of KS depending on the number of XY cells they have in their bodies and where these cells are located. For example, males who have normal XY cells in their testes may be fertile.

In very rare cases, males might have two or more extra X chromosomes in their cells, for instance XXXY or XXXXY, or an extra Y, such as XXYY. This is called poly-X Klinefelter syndrome, and it causes more severe symptoms.

How Many People Are Affected by or at Risk for Klinefelter Syndrome?

Researchers estimate that 1 male in about 500 newborn males has an extra X chromosome, making KS among the most common chromosomal disorders seen in all newborns. The likelihood of a third or fourth X is much rarer:

Table 39.2. Prevalence of Klinefelter syndrome variants

Number of extra X chromosomes	One (XXY)	Two (XXXY)	Three (XXXXY)
Number of newborn males with the condition	1 in 500	1 in 50,000	1 in 85,000 to 100,000

Scientists are not sure what factors increase the risk of KS. The error that produces the extra chromosome occurs at random, meaning the error is not hereditary or passed down from parent to child. Research suggests that older mothers might be slightly more likely to have a son with KS. However, the extra X chromosome in KS comes from the father about one-half of the time.

What Are Common Symptoms of Klinefelter Syndrome?

KS symptoms fall into these main categories:

- physical symptoms
- language and learning symptoms
- social and behavioral symptoms
- symptoms of Poly-X KS

Physical Symptoms

Many physical symptoms of KS result from low testosterone levels in the body. The degree of symptoms differs based on the amount of testosterone needed for a specific age or developmental stage and the amount of testosterone the body makes or has available.

During the first few years of life, when the need for testosterone is low, most XXY males do not show any obvious differences from typical male infants and young boys. Some may have slightly weaker muscles, meaning they might sit up, crawl, and walk slightly later than average. For example, on average, baby boys with KS do not start walking until age 18 months.

After age 5 years, when compared to typically developing boys, boys with KS may be slightly:

- taller
- fatter around the belly
- clumsier
- slower in developing motor skills, coordination, speed, and muscle strength

Puberty for boys with KS usually starts normally. But because their bodies make less testosterone than non-KS boys, their pubertal development may be disrupted or slow. In addition to being tall, KS boys may have:

- smaller testes and penis
- breast growth (about one-third of teens with KS have breast growth)

- less facial and body hair

- reduced muscle tone

- narrower shoulders and wider hips

- weaker bones, greater risk for bone fractures

- decreased sexual interest

- lower energy

- reduced sperm production

An adult male with KS may have these features:

- Infertility: Nearly all men with KS are unable to father a biolog-ically-related child without help from a fertility specialist.

- Small testes, with the possibility of testes shrinking slightly after the teen years

- Lower testosterone levels, which lead to less muscle, hair, and sexual interest and function

- Breasts or breast growth (called gynecomastia, pronounced GUY-nuh-kow-mast-ee-uh).

In some cases, breast growth can be permanent, and about 10% of XXY males need breast-reduction surgery.

Language and Learning Symptoms

Most males with KS have normal intelligence quotients (IQs) and successfully complete education at all levels. (IQ is a frequently used intelligence measure, but does not include emotional, creative, or other types of intelligence.)

KS males may experience some of the following learning and lan-guage-related challenges:

- A delay in learning to talk

- trouble using language to express their thoughts and needs

- trouble processing what they hear

- reading difficulties

By adulthood, most males with KS learn to speak and converse normally, although they may have a harder time doing work that involves extensive reading and writing.

Social and Behavioral Symptoms

Many of the social and behavioral symptoms in KS may result from the language and learning difficulties.

Boys with KS, compared to typically developing boys, tend to be:

- quieter

- less assertive or self-confident

- more anxious or restless

- less physically active

- more helpful and eager to please

- more obedient or more ready to follow directions

In the teenage years, boys with KS may feel their differences more strongly. As a result, these teen boys are at higher risk of depression, substance abuse, and behavioral disorders. Some teens might withdraw, feel sad, or act out their frustration and anger.

As adults, most men with KS have lives similar to those of men without KS. They successfully complete high school, college, and other levels of education. They have successful and meaningful careers and professions. They have friends and families.

Contrary to research findings published several decades ago, males with KS are no more likely to have serious psychiatric disorders or to get into trouble with the law.

Symptoms of Poly-X KS

Males with poly-X KS have more than one extra X chromosome, so their symptoms might be more pronounced than in males with KS. In childhood, they may also have seizures, crossed eyes, constipation, and recurrent ear infections. Poly-KS males might also show slight differences in other physical features.

Some common additional symptoms for several poly-X KS are listed below.

48, XXYY

- long legs

- little body hair

- lower IQ, average of 60 to 80 (normal IQ is 90 to 110)

- leg ulcers and other vascular disease symptoms
- extreme shyness, but also sometimes aggression and impulsiveness

48, XXXY (or tetrasomy)

- eyes set further apart
- flat nose bridge
- arm bones connected to each other in an unusual way
- short
- fifth (smallest) fingers curve inward (clinodactyly, pronounced KLAHY-noh-dak-tl-ee)
- lower IQ, average 40 to 60
- immature behavior

49, XXXXY (or pentasomy)

- low IQ, usually between 20 and 60
- small head
- short
- upward-slanted eyes
- heart defects, such as when the chambers do not form properly12
- high feet arches
- shy, but friendly
- difficulty with changing routines

What Are the Treatments for Symptoms in Klinefelter Syndrome?

It's important to remember that because symptoms can be mild, many males with KS are never diagnosed are treated.

The earlier in life that KS symptoms are recognized and treated, the more likely it is that the symptoms can be reduced or eliminated. It is especially helpful to begin treatment by early puberty. Puberty is a time of rapid physical and psychological change, and treatment can successfully limit symptoms. However, treatment can bring benefits at any age.

The type of treatment needed depends on the type of symptoms being treated.

- treating physical symptoms

- treating language and learning symptoms

- treating social and behavioral symptoms

Treating Physical Symptoms

- treatment for low testosterone

- treatment for enlarged breasts

- treatment for infertility

Treating Language and Learning Symptoms

- **Physical therapists** design activities and exercises to build motor skills and strength and to improve muscle control, posture, and balance.

- **Occupational therapists** help build skills needed for daily functioning, such as social and play skills, interaction and conversation skills, and job or career skills that match interests and abilities.

- **Behavioral therapists** help with specific social skills, such as asking other kids to play and starting conversations. They can also teach productive ways of handling frustration, shyness, anger, and other emotions that can arise from feeling "different."

- **Mental health therapists or counselors** help males with KS find ways to cope with feelings of sadness, depression, self-doubt, and low self-esteem. They can also help with substance abuse problems. These professionals can also help families deal with the emotions of having a son with KS.

- **Family therapists** provide counseling to a man with KS, his spouse, partner, or family. They can help identify relationship problems and help patients develop communication skills and understand other people's needs.

541

Treating Social and Behavioral Symptoms

Many of the professionals and methods for treating learning and language symptoms of the XXY condition are similar to or the same as the ones used to address social and behavioral symptoms.

For instance, boys with KS may need help with social skills and interacting in groups. Occupational or behavioral therapists might be able to assist with these skills. Some school districts and health centers might also offer these types of skill-building programs or classes.

In adolescence, symptoms such as lack of body hair could make XXY males uncomfortable in school or other social settings, and this discomfort can lead to depression, substance abuse, and behavioral problems or "acting out." They might also have questions about their masculinity or gender identity. In these instances, consulting a psychologist, counselor, or psychiatrist may be helpful.

Contrary to research results released decades ago, current research shows that XXY males are no more likely than other males to have serious psychiatric disorders or to get into trouble with the law.

How Do Healthcare Providers Diagnose Klinefelter Syndrome?

The only way to confirm the presence of an extra chromosome is by a karyotype test. A healthcare provider will take a small blood or skin sample and send it to a laboratory, where a technician inspects the cells under a microscope to find the extra chromosome. A karyotype test shows the same results at any time in a person's life.

Tests for chromosome disorders, including KS, may be done before birth. To obtain tissue or liquid for this test, a pregnant woman undergoes chorionic villus sampling or amniocentesis. These types of prenatal testing carry a small risk for miscarriage and are not routinely conducted unless the woman has a family history of chromosomal disorders, has other medical problems, or is above 35 years of age.

Section 39.5

Muscular Dystrophy

This section includes text excerpted from "Muscular Dystrophy,"
Eunice Kennedy Shriver National Institute of Child Health and
Human Development (NICHD), December 6, 2013.
Reviewed August 2016.

What Is Muscular Dystrophy?

Muscular dystrophy (MD) refers to a group of more than 30 inherited diseases that cause muscle weakness and muscle loss. Some forms of MD appear in infancy or childhood, while others may not appear until middle age or even later. In addition, the types of MD differ in the areas of the body they affect and in the severity of the symptoms. All forms of MD grow worse as the person's muscles get weaker. Most people with MD eventually lose their ability to walk.

What Causes Muscular Dystrophy?

MD is generally an inherited disease caused by gene mutations (changes in the DNA sequence) that affect proteins in muscles. In some cases, the mutation was not inherited from a person's parents but instead happened spontaneously. Such a mutation can then be inherited by the affected person's offspring.

Hundreds of genes are involved in making the proteins that affect muscles. Each type of MD is caused by a genetic mutation that is specific to that type. Some of the forms, like lamb-girdle and distal, are caused by defects in the same gene.

MD is not contagious and cannot be caused by injury or activity.

What Are the Types of Muscular Dystrophy?

There are more than 30 forms of muscular dystrophy (MD), with information on the primary types included in the table below.

Table 39.3. Types of Muscular Dystrophy (MD)

Form of MD	What It Is	Common Symptoms	How It Develops
Duchenne (DMD)	The most common and severe form of MD among children, DMD accounts for more than 50% of all cases. DMD is caused by a deficiency of dystrophin, a protein that helps strengthen muscle fibers and protect them from injury.	Weakness begins in the upper legs and pelvis. People with DMD may also: • Fall down a lot • Have trouble rising from a lying or sitting position • Waddle when walking • Have difficulty running and jumping • Have calf muscles that appear large because of fat accumulation	DMD appears typically in boys between ages 3 and 5 and progresses rapidly. Most people with DMD are unable to walk by age 12 and may later need a respirator to breathe. They usually die in their late teens or early 20s from heart trouble, respiratory complications, or infection.
Becker	Also caused by a deficiency of dystrophin, and with symptoms similar to those of DMD, Becker can progress slowly or quickly.	Patients with Becker MD may: • Walk on their tiptoes • Fall down a lot Have difficulty rising from the floor • Have cramping in their muscles	Becker MD appears primarily in males between ages 11 and 25. Some people may never need to use a wheelchair, while others lose the ability to walk during their teens, mid-30s, or later.
Myotonic	The most common adult form of MD, myotonic MD appears in two forms, type 1 and type 2. Type 1 is more common and is caused by an abnormally large number of repeats of a three-letter "word" (CTG) in genetic code. While most people have up to 37 repeats of CTG, people with myotonic can	Myotonic MD causes an inability to relax muscles following a sudden contraction. Other symptoms include: • Long, thin face and neck • Swallowing difficulties • Drooping eyelids, cataracts, and other vision problems • Baldness at the front of the scalp	Myotonic MD affects both men and women between ages 20 and 30.

Table 39.3. Continued

Form of MD	What It Is	Common Symptoms	How It Develops
	have up to 4,000. The number of repeats may reflect the severity of symptoms.	• Weight loss • Increased sweating • Drowsiness • Heart problems that may lead to death during the 30s or 40s • Irregular menstrual periods • Infertility • Impotence	
Congenital	About half of all U.S. cases with congenital MD are caused by a defect in the protein merosin, which surrounds muscle fibers. When caused by defects in other proteins, this type of MD may also affect the central nervous system.	People with congenital MD may: • Have problems with motor function and muscle control that appear at birth or during infancy • Develop chronic shortening of muscles or tendons around joints, which prevents joints from moving freely • Develop scoliosis (curvature of the spine) • Have trouble breathing and swallowing • Have foot deformities • Have intellectual disabilities	This form of MD appears at birth or by age 2. Congenital means "present from birth." Congenital MD affects both boys and girls, who often require support to sit or stand and may never learn to walk. Some patients die in infancy, but others live into adulthood with only mild disability.

Table 39.3. Continued

Form of MD	What It Is	Common Symptoms	How It Develops
Emery-Dreifuss	Affecting boys primarily, the two forms of Emery-Dreifuss MD are caused by defects in the proteins that surround the nucleus in cells.	Weakness begins in the upper arm and lower leg muscles. People with this form may also • Develop chronic shortening of muscles around joints (preventing them from moving freely), in the spine, ankles, knees, elbows, and back of the neck • Have elbows locked in a flexed position • Develop shoulder deterioration • Have a rigid spine • Walk on their toes • Experience mild weakness in their facial muscles	Symptoms usually begin by age 10 but can appear in patients up to their mid-20s. People with this form often develop heart problems by age 30, and they may die in mid-adulthood from progressive pulmonary or cardiac failure.
Facioscapulo-humeral (FSHD)	FSHD refers to the areas affected: the face (facio), the shoulders (scapulo), and the upper arms (humeral). Researchers don't know what gene causes FSHD. They do know where the defect occurs and that it affects specific muscle groups.	FSHD MD often appears first in the eyes (difficulty in opening and shutting) and mouth (inability to smile or pucker). Other symptoms may include • Muscle wasting that causes shoulders to appear slanted and shoulder blades to appear "winged" • Impaired reflexes only at the biceps and triceps	FSHD affects teen boys and girls typically but may occur as late as age 40. Most individuals have a normal life span, but symptoms can vary from mild to severely disabling.

Table 39.3. Continued

Form of MD	What It Is	Common Symptoms	How It Develops
		• Trouble swallowing, chewing, or speaking • Hearing problems • Swayback curve in the spine, called lordosis	
Limb-girdle	Affecting both males and females, different types of limb-girdle are caused by different gene mutations. Patients with limb-girdle inherit a defective gene from either parent, or, in the more severe form, the same defective gene from both parents.	Patients with limb-girdle MD may: • First develop weakness around the hips, which then spreads to the shoulders, legs, and neck • Fall down a lot • Have trouble rising from chairs, climbing stairs, or carrying things • Waddle when they walk • Have a rigid spine	This form of MD can appear in childhood but most often appears in adolescence or young adulthood. Limb-girdle can progress quickly or slowly, but most patients become severely disabled (with muscle damage and inability to walk) within 20 years of developing the disease.
Distal	Distal MDs refer to a group of diseases that affect the muscles of the forearms, hands, lower legs, and feet. They are caused by defects in the protein dysferlin and can occur in both men and women.	Distal MD may cause: • Inability to perform hand movements • Difficulty extending fingers • Trouble walking and climbing stairs • Inability to hop or stand on the heels	This form typically appears between ages 40 and 60. Distal MD is less severe and progresses more slowly than other forms of MD, but it can spread to other muscles. Patients may eventually need a ventilator.

Table 39.3. Continued

Form of MD	What It Is	Common Symptoms	How It Develops
Oculopharyngeal	This form occurs in both men and women, and it can be mild or severe. It is caused by a defect in a protein that binds to molecules that help make other proteins. It is common among Americans of French-Canadian descent, Jewish Ashkenazi, and Hispanics from the Southwest region.	Oculopharyngeal MD may cause: • Drooping eyelids and other vision problems • Swallowing problems • Muscle wasting and weakness in the neck, shoulders, and sometimes limbs • Heart problems	This form of MD typically appears in a person's 40s or 50s. Some people will eventually lose their ability to walk.

How Many People Are Affected by or Are at Risk of Muscular Dystrophy?

The incidence of MD in the United States varies, because different kinds of MD are rarer than others. The most common forms in children, Duchenne and Becker, affect approximately 1 in every 5,600 to 7,700 males ages 5 to 24. The most common adult form, type 1 myotonic MD, affects 1 in 8,000 worldwide.

What Are Common Symptoms of Muscular Dystrophy?

Muscle weakness that worsens over time is a common symptom of all forms of muscular dystrophy (MD). Each form of MD varies in the order in which symptoms occur and in the parts of the body that are affected.

How Is Muscular Dystrophy Diagnosed?

The first step in diagnosing MD is a visit with a healthcare provider for a physical exam. The healthcare provider will ask a series of questions about the patient's family history and medical history, including any problems affecting the muscles that the patient may be experiencing.

The healthcare provider may order tests to determine whether the problems are a result of MD and, if so, what form of this disorder. The tests may also rule out other problems that could cause muscle weakness, such as surgery, toxic exposure, medications, or other muscle diseases. These tests may include:

- **Blood tests** to measure levels of serum creatine kinase, an enzyme that is released into the bloodstream when muscle fibers are deteriorating, and serum aldolase, an enzyme that helps break down sugars into energy. Elevated levels of either of these enzymes can signal muscle weakness and indicate a need for additional testing.

- **Muscle biopsies,** which involve the removal of muscle tissue using a biopsy needle. The tissue is then examined under a microscope to provide information on the amount and level of the genes that may cause MD. Patients diagnosed by muscle biopsy typically require genetic testing as well to determine any mutations in their genes.

- **Genetic testing** to evaluate missing or repeated mutations in the dystrophin gene. A lack of the dystrophin gene can lead to a diagnosis of Duchenne or Becker MD. The test is important not only to confirm the MD diagnosis in males but also to determine whether women with a family history of Duchenne or Becker MD may be carriers.

- **Neurological tests** to rule out other nervous system disorders, to identify patterns of muscle weakness and wasting, to test reflexes and coordination, and to detect contractions.

- **Heart testing,** such as an electrocardiogram (ECG), to measure the rate and frequency of heartbeats. Some forms of MD cause heart problems, such as an irregular heartbeat.

- **Exercise assessments** to evaluate the patient's level of strength and respiratory function and to detect any increased rates of certain chemicals such as nitric oxide following exercise.

- **Imaging tests** such as magnetic resonance imaging (MRI) and ultrasound imaging. These painless tests use radio waves (MRI) and sound waves (ultrasound) to obtain pictures of the inside of the body and to examine muscle quality and bulk as well as the fatty replacement of muscle tissue.

What Are the Treatments for Muscular Dystrophy?

No treatment is currently available to stop or reverse any form of MD. Instead, certain therapies and medications aim to treat the various problems that result from MD and improve the quality of life for patients. These include the following:

Physical Therapy

Beginning physical therapy early can help keep muscles flexible and strong. A combination of physical activity and stretching exercises may be recommended.

Respiratory Therapy

Many people with MD do not realize they have little respiratory strength until they have difficulty coughing or an infection leads to pneumonia. Regular visits to a specialist early in the diagnosis of MD can help guide treatment before a respiratory problem occurs. Eventually, many MD patients require assisted ventilation.

Speech Therapy

MD patients who experience weakness in the facial and throat muscles may benefit from learning to slow the pace of their speech by pausing more between breaths and by using special communication equipment.

Occupational Therapy

As physical abilities change, occupational therapy can help patients with MD relearn these movements and abilities. Occupational therapy also teaches patients to use assistive devices such as wheelchairs and utensils.

Corrective Surgery

At various times and depending on the form of MD, many patients require surgery to treat the conditions that result from MD. People with myotonic MD may need a pacemaker to treat heart problems or surgery to remove cataracts, a clouding of the lens of the eye that blocks light from entering the eye.

Drug Therapy

Certain medications can help slow or control the symptoms of MD. These include the following:

- Glucocorticoids, such as prednisone. Studies show that daily treatment with prednisone can increase muscle strength, ability, and respiratory function and slow the progression of weakness. Side effects may include weight gain. Long-term use may result in brittle bones, cataracts, and high blood pressure. The NIH's Therapeutics for Rare and Neglected Diseases (TRND) Program is collaborating on a new glucocorticoid treatment called VBP15. Early clinical trial results show that the treatment may have the same positive results as prednisone, but without the side effects.

- Anticonvulsants. Typically taken for epilepsy, these drugs may help control seizures and some muscle spasms.

- Immunosuppressants. Commonly given to treat autoimmune diseases such as lupus and eczema, immunosuppressant drugs may help delay some damage to dying muscle cells.

- Antibiotics to treat respiratory infections.

Chapter 40

Breast Concerns in Men

Chapter Contents

Section 40.1—Breast Cancer in Men 554

Section 40.2—Gynecomastia 563

Section 40.1

Breast Cancer in Men

This section includes text excerpted from "Male Breast
Cancer Treatment (PDQ®)—Patient Version," National
Cancer Institute (NCI), July 18, 2016.

General Information about Male Breast Cancer

Male Breast Cancer Is a Disease in Which Malignant (Cancer) Cells Form in the Tissues of the Breast

Breast cancer may occur in men. Men at any age may develop breast
cancer, but it is usually detected (found) in men between 60 and 70
years of age. Male breast cancer makes up less than 1% of all cases
of breast cancer.

The following types of breast cancer are found in men:

- Infiltrating ductal carcinoma: Cancer that has spread beyond
  the cells lining ducts in the breast. Most men with breast cancer
  have this type of cancer.

- Ductal carcinoma in situ: Abnormal cells that are found in the
  lining of a duct; also called intraductal carcinoma.

- Inflammatory breast cancer: A type of cancer in which the breast
  looks red and swollen and feels warm.

- Paget disease of the nipple: A tumor that has grown from ducts
  beneath the nipple onto the surface of the nipple.

Lobular carcinoma in situ (abnormal cells found in one of the lobes
or sections of the breast), which sometimes occurs in women, has not
been seen in men.

Radiation Exposure, High Levels of Estrogen, and a Family History of Breast Cancer Can Increase a Man's Risk of Breast Cancer

Anything that increases your risk of getting a disease is called a
risk factor. Having a risk factor does not mean that you will get cancer;

not having risk factors doesn't mean that you will not get cancer. Talk with your doctor if you think you may be at risk. Risk factors for breast cancer in men may include the following:

- Being exposed to radiation.

- Having a disease linked to high levels of estrogen in the body, such as cirrhosis (liver disease) or Klinefelter syndrome (a genetic disorder.)

- Having several female relatives who have had breast cancer, especially relatives who have an alteration of the *BRCA2* gene.

Male Breast Cancer Is Sometimes Caused by Inherited Gene Mutations (Changes)

The genes in cells carry the hereditary information that is received from a person's parents. Hereditary breast cancer makes up about 5% to 10% of all breast cancer. Some mutated genes related to breast cancer are more common in certain ethnic groups. Men who have a mutated gene related to breast cancer have an increased risk of this disease.

There are tests that can detect (find) mutated genes. These genetic tests are sometimes done for members of families with a high risk of cancer.

Men with Breast Cancer Usually Have Lumps That Can Be Felt

Lumps and other signs may be caused by male breast cancer or by other conditions. Check with your doctor if you notice a change in your breasts.

Tests That Examine the Breasts Are Used to Detect (Find) and Diagnose Breast Cancer in Men

The following tests and procedures may be used:

- Physical exam and history
- Clinical breast exam (CBE)
- Ultrasound exam
- MRI (magnetic resonance imaging)
- Blood chemistry studies

- Biopsy
  - Fine-needle aspiration (FNA) biopsy
  - Core biopsy
  - Excisional biopsy

If Cancer Is Found, Tests Are Done to Study the Cancer Cells

Decisions about the best treatment are based on the results of these tests. The tests give information about:

- how quickly the cancer may grow
- how likely it is that the cancer will spread through the body
- how well certain treatments might work
- how likely the cancer is to recur (come back)

Tests include the following:

- Estrogen and progesterone receptor test
- HER2 test

Survival for Men with Breast Cancer Is Similar to Survival for Women with Breast Cancer

Survival for men with breast cancer is similar to that for women with breast cancer when their stage at diagnosis is the same. Breast cancer in men, however, is often diagnosed at a later stage. Cancer found at a later stage may be less likely to be cured.

Certain Factors Affect Prognosis (Chance of Recovery) and Treatment Options

The prognosis (chance of recovery) and treatment options depend on the following:

- the stage of the cancer (whether it is in the breast only or has spread to other places in the body)
- the type of breast cancer
- estrogen-receptor and progesterone-receptor levels in the tumor tissue

- whether the cancer is also found in the other breast

- the patient's age and general health

Stages of Male Breast Cancer

After Breast Cancer Has Been Diagnosed, Tests Are Done to Find out If Cancer Cells Have Spread within the Breast or to Other Parts of the Body

After breast cancer has been diagnosed, tests are done to find out if cancer cells have spread within the breast or to other parts of the body. This process is called staging. The information gathered from the staging process determines the stage of the disease. It is important to know the stage in order to plan treatment. Breast cancer in men is staged the same as it is in women. The spread of cancer from the breast to lymph nodes and other parts of the body appears to be similar in men and women.

The following tests and procedures may be used in the staging process:

There Are Three Ways That Cancer Spreads in the Body

Cancer can spread through tissue, the lymph system, and the blood:

- **Tissue.** The cancer spreads from where it began by growing into nearby areas.

- **Lymph system.** The cancer spreads from where it began by getting into the lymph system. The cancer travels through the lymph vessels to other parts of the body.

- **Blood.** The cancer spreads from where it began by getting into the blood. The cancer travels through the blood vessels to other parts of the body.

Cancer May Spread from Where It Began to Other Parts of the Body

When cancer spreads to another part of the body, it is called metastasis. Cancer cells break away from where they began (the primary tumor) and travel through the lymph system or blood.

- **Lymph system.** The cancer gets into the lymph system, travels through the lymph vessels, and forms a tumor (metastatic tumor) in another part of the body.

557

- **Blood.** The cancer gets into the blood, travels through the blood vessels, and forms a tumor (metastatic tumor) in another part of the body.

The metastatic tumor is the same type of cancer as the primary tumor. For example, if breast cancer spreads to the bone, the cancer cells in the bone are actually breast cancer cells. The disease is metastatic breast cancer, not bone cancer.

The Following Stages Are Used for Male Breast Cancer

This section describes the stages of breast cancer. The breast cancer stage is based on the results of testing that is done on the tumor and lymph nodes removed during surgery and other tests.

Stage 0 (carcinoma in situ)

There are 3 types of breast carcinoma in situ:

- Ductal carcinoma in situ (DCIS) is a noninvasive condition in which abnormal cells are found in the lining of a breast duct. The abnormal cells have not spread outside the duct to other tissues in the breast. In some cases, DCIS may become invasive cancer and spread to other tissues. At this time, there is no way to know which lesions could become invasive.

- Paget disease of the nipple is a condition in which abnormal cells are found in the nipple only.

- Lobular carcinoma in situ (LCIS) is a condition in which abnormal cells are found in the lobules of the breast. This condition has not been seen in men.

Stage I

- In stage I, cancer has formed. Stage I is divided into stages IA and IB.

- In stage IA, the tumor is 2 centimeters or smaller. Cancer has not spread outside the breast.

- In stage IB, small clusters of breast cancer cells (larger than 0.2 millimeter but not larger than 2 millimeters) are found in the lymph nodes and either:
    - no tumor is found in the breast or
    - the tumor is 2 centimeters or smaller

Stage II

Stage II is divided into stages IIA and IIB.

- In stage IIA
  - no tumor is found in the breast or the tumor is 2 centimeters or smaller. Cancer (larger than 2 millimeters) is found in 1 to 3 axillary lymph nodes or in the lymph nodes near the breastbone (found during a sentinel lymph node biopsy); or
  - the tumor is larger than 2 centimeters but not larger than 5 centimeters. Cancer has not spread to the lymph nodes.

- In stage IIB, the tumor is:
  - larger than 2 centimeters but not larger than 5 centimeters. Small clusters of breast cancer cells (larger than 0.2 millimeter but not larger than 2 millimeters) are found in the lymph nodes; or
  - larger than 2 centimeters but not larger than 5 centimeters. Cancer has spread to 1 to 3 axillary lymph nodes or to the lymph nodes near the breastbone (found during a sentinel lymph node biopsy); or
  - larger than 5 centimeters. Cancer has not spread to the lymph nodes.

Stage IIIA

In stage IIIA:

- no tumor is found in the breast or the tumor may be any size. Cancer is found in 4 to 9 axillary lymph nodes or in the lymph nodes near the breastbone (found during imaging tests or a physical exam); or

- the tumor is larger than 5 centimeters. Small clusters of breast cancer cells (larger than 0.2 millimeter but not larger than 2 millimeters) are found in the lymph nodes; or

- the tumor is larger than 5 centimeters. Cancer has spread to 1 to 3 axillary lymph nodes or to the lymph nodes near the breastbone (found during a sentinel lymph node biopsy).

Stage IIIB

In stage IIIB, the tumor may be any size and cancer has spread to the chest wall and/or to the skin of the breast and caused swelling or an ulcer. Also, cancer may have spread to:

- up to 9 axillary lymph nodes or

- the lymph nodes near the breastbone

Cancer that has spread to the skin of the breast may also be inflammatory breast cancer.

Stage IIIC

In stage IIIC, no tumor is found in the breast or the tumor may be any size. Cancer may have spread to the skin of the breast and caused swelling or an ulcer and/or has spread to the chest wall. Also, cancer has spread to:

- 10 or more axillary lymph nodes or

- lymph nodes above or below the collarbone or

- axillary lymph nodes and lymph nodes near the breastbone

Cancer that has spread to the skin of the breast may also be inflammatory breast cancer.

For treatment, stage IIIC breast cancer is divided into operable and inoperable stage IIIC.

Stage IV

In stage IV, cancer has spread to other organs of the body, most often the bones, lungs, liver, or brain.

Treatment Option Overview

There Are Different Types of Treatment for Men with Breast Cancer

Different types of treatment are available for men with breast cancer. Some treatments are standard (the currently used treatment), and some are being tested in clinical trials. A treatment clinical trial is a research study meant to help improve current treatments or obtain information on new treatments for patients with cancer. When clinical trials show that a new treatment is better than the standard treatment, the new treatment may become the standard treatment.

For some patients, taking part in a clinical trial may be the best treatment choice. Many of today's standard treatments for cancer are based on earlier clinical trials. Patients who take part in a clinical trial may receive the standard treatment or be among the first to receive a new treatment.

Patients who take part in clinical trials also help improve the way cancer will be treated in the future. Even when clinical trials do not lead to effective new treatments, they often answer important questions and help move research forward.

Some clinical trials only include patients who have not yet received treatment. Other trials test treatments for patients whose cancer has not gotten better. There are also clinical trials that test new ways to stop cancer from recurring (coming back) or reduce the side effects of cancer treatment.

Treatments Used to Treat Men with Breast Cancer

Surgery

Surgery for men with breast cancer is usually a modified radical mastectomy (removal of the breast, many of the lymph nodes under the arm, the lining over the chest muscles, and sometimes part of the chest wall muscles).

Breast-conserving surgery, an operation to remove the cancer but not the breast itself, is also used for some men with breast cancer. A lumpectomy is done to remove the tumor (lump) and a small amount of normal tissue around it. Radiation therapy is given after surgery to kill any cancer cells that are left.

Chemotherapy

Chemotherapy is a cancer treatment that uses drugs to stop the growth of cancer cells, either by killing the cells or by stopping them from dividing. When chemotherapy is taken by mouth or injected into a vein or muscle, the drugs enter the bloodstream and can reach cancer cells throughout the body (systemic chemotherapy). When chemotherapy is placed directly into the cerebrospinal fluid, an organ, or a body cavity such as the abdomen, the drugs mainly affect cancer cells in those areas (regional chemotherapy). The way the chemotherapy is given depends on the type and stage of the cancer being treated.

Hormone Therapy

Hormone therapy is a cancer treatment that removes hormones or blocks their action and stops cancer cells from growing. Hormones are substances made by glands in the body and circulated in the blood-stream. Some hormones can cause certain cancers to grow. If tests show that the cancer cells have places where hormones can attach (receptors), drugs, surgery, or radiation therapy is used to reduce the production of hormones or block them from working.

Radiation Therapy

Radiation therapy is a cancer treatment that uses high-energy X-rays or other types of radiation to kill cancer cells or keep them from growing. There are two types of radiation therapy:

- External radiation therapy uses a machine outside the body to send radiation toward the cancer.

- Internal radiation therapy uses a radioactive substance sealed in needles, seeds, wires, or catheters that are placed directly into or near the cancer.

The way the radiation therapy is given depends on the type and stage of the cancer being treated. External radiation therapy is used to treat male breast cancer.

Targeted Therapy

Targeted therapy is a type of treatment that uses drugs or other substances to identify and attack specific cancer cells without harming normal cells. Monoclonal antibody therapy is a type of targeted therapy used to treat men with breast cancer.

Monoclonal antibody therapy uses antibodies made in the laboratory from a single type of immune system cell. These antibodies can identify substances on cancer cells or normal substances that may help cancer cells grow. The antibodies attach to the substances and kill the cancer cells, block their growth, or keep them from spreading. Monoclonal antibodies are given by infusion. They may be used alone or to carry drugs, toxins, or radioactive material directly to cancer cells. Monoclonal antibodies are also used with chemotherapy as adjuvant therapy (treatment given after surgery to lower the risk that the cancer will come back).

Trastuzumab is a monoclonal antibody that blocks the effects of the growth factor protein HER2.

Section 40.2

Gynecomastia

What Is Gynecomastia?

Gynecomastia is a condition in which breast tissue forms in guys, usually due to normal hormonal changes during puberty. Hormones are chemicals produced by your body's glands. In a guy, hormones produced in the testicles are responsible for the physical changes that begin to take place during puberty—facial hair, muscle development, a deepening of the voice, and the lengthening of the penis, for example. Guys and girls produce both androgens (hormones that help develop and maintain male characteristics) and estrogen (a hormone that is responsible for most female characteristics).

Guys have mostly androgens in their systems, but they also have small amounts of estrogen. In girls, breast growth is caused by high levels of estrogen. Normally, when going through puberty, a guy's production of androgens increases significantly, whereas estrogen production remains low.

However, sometimes guys produce enough estrogen during puberty that some breast tissue develops. Breast tissue growth in guys can appear on one or both sides of the chest, and the breast area can feel tender. This doesn't mean you're turning into a girl or anything. It's just a minor change in your hormones as you begin to grow into adulthood.

How Common Is It?

It's estimated that about half of all males going through puberty experience some degree of gynecomastia in one or both breasts. Gynecomastia is almost always a temporary condition, and it's very unusual for the breasts to stay developed—they will eventually flatten out completely within a few months to a couple of years. It usually goes away on its own and no medical treatment or surgery is needed.

Even though it's just a temporary change for most teens, some guys with gynecomastia feel embarrassed or self-conscious about their appearance. Many guys find that wearing loose-fitting shirts helps make the condition less noticeable until the breast tissue shrinks over time. Surgical removal of the breast tissue is an option in some cases. If a guy finds his gynecomastia is bothering him, he can talk to a doctor about it.

Although the most common cause of gynecomastia is puberty, it can sometimes be caused by certain diseases or side effects of some medications. Using illegal drugs such as anabolic steroids, marijuana, or heroin can also disrupt hormonal balance and lead to gynecomastia.

There's also something called pseudogynecomastia (or false gynecomastia). This has nothing to do with puberty or hormones. It's just simply due to the fact that some guys have extra fat in the chest area, making it look like they have breasts. A doctor's exam can tell whether a guy has gynecomastia or pseudogynecomastia.

Chapter 41

Osteoporosis in Men

Osteoporosis is a disease that causes the skeleton to weaken and the bones to break. It poses a significant threat to millions of men in the United States.

Despite these compelling figures, surveys suggest that a majority of American men view osteoporosis solely as a "woman's disease." Moreover, among men whose lifestyle habits put them at increased risk, few recognize the disease as a significant threat to their mobility and independence.

Osteoporosis is called a "silent disease" because it progresses without symptoms until a fracture occurs. It develops less often in men than in women because men have larger skeletons, their bone loss starts later and progresses more slowly, and they have no period of rapid hormonal change and bone loss. However, in the past few years the problem of osteoporosis in men has been recognized as an important public health issue, particularly in light of estimates that the number of men above the age of 70 will continue to increase as life expectancy continues to rise.

What Causes Osteoporosis?

Bone is constantly changing—that is, old bone is removed and replaced by new bone. During childhood, more bone is produced than

This chapter includes text excerpted from "Osteoporosis in Men," National Institute of Arthritis and Musculoskeletal and Skin Diseases (NIAMS), June 2015.

removed, so the skeleton grows in both size and strength. For most people, bone mass peaks during the third decade of life. By this age, men typically have accumulated more bone mass than women. After this point, the amount of bone in the skeleton typically begins to decline slowly as removal of old bone exceeds formation of new bone.

Men in their fifties do not experience the rapid loss of bone mass that women do in the years following menopause. By age 65 or 70, however, men and women are losing bone mass at the same rate, and the absorption of calcium, an essential nutrient for bone health throughout life, decreases in both sexes. Excessive bone loss causes bone to become fragile and more likely to fracture.

Fractures resulting from osteoporosis most commonly occur in the hip, spine, and wrist, and can be permanently disabling. Hip fractures are especially dangerous. Perhaps because such fractures tend to occur at older ages in men than in women, men who sustain hip fractures are more likely than women to die from complications.

Causes of Secondary Osteoporosis in Men

- ankylosing spondylitis and rheumatoid arthritis
- anticonvulsant medications
- chronic obstructive pulmonary disease and asthma
- cystic fibrosis
- excessive alcohol consumption
- gastrointestinal disease
- glucocorticoid medications
- homocystinuria
- hypercalciuria
- hyperparathyroidism
- hypogonadism (low testosterone levels)
- immobilization
- neoplastic disease
- osteogenesis imperfecta
- other immunosuppressive drugs
- smoking

- systemic mastocytosis

- thyrotoxicosis

Primary and Secondary Osteoporosis

There are two main types of osteoporosis: primary and secondary. In cases of primary osteoporosis, either the condition is caused by age-related bone loss (sometimes called *senile osteoporosis*) or the cause is unknown (*idiopathic osteoporosis*). The term idiopathic osteoporosis is typically used only for men younger than 70 years old; in older men, age-related bone loss is assumed to be the cause.

The majority of men with osteoporosis have at least one (sometimes more than one) secondary cause. In cases of secondary osteoporosis, the loss of bone mass is caused by certain lifestyle behaviors, diseases, or medications. The most common causes of secondary osteoporosis in men include exposure to glucocorticoid medications, hypogonadism (low levels of testosterone), alcohol abuse, smoking, gastrointestinal disease, hypercalciuria, and immobilization.

Glucocorticoid medications. Glucocorticoids are steroid medications used to treat diseases such as asthma and rheumatoid arthritis. Bone loss is a very common side effect of these medications. The bone loss these medications cause may be due to their direct effect on bone, muscle weakness or immobility, reduced intestinal absorption of calcium, a decrease in testosterone levels, or, most likely, a combination of these factors.

When glucocorticoid medications are used on an ongoing basis, bone mass often decreases quickly and continuously, with most of the bone loss in the ribs and vertebrae. Therefore, people taking these medications should talk to their doctor about having a bone mineral density (BMD) test. Men should also be tested to monitor testosterone levels, as glucocorticoids often reduce testosterone in the blood.

A treatment plan to minimize loss of bone during long-term glucocorticoid therapy may include using the minimal effective dose, and discontinuing the drug or administering it through the skin, if possible. Adequate calcium and vitamin D intake is important, as these nutrients help reduce the impact of glucocorticoids on the bones. Other possible treatments include testosterone replacement and osteoporosis medication.

Hypogonadism. Hypogonadism refers to abnormally low levels of sex hormones. It is well known that loss of estrogen causes osteoporosis in women. In men, reduced levels of sex hormones may also cause osteoporosis.

Although it is natural for testosterone levels to decrease with age, there should not be a sudden drop in this hormone that is comparable to the drop in estrogen experienced by women at menopause. However, medications such as glucocorticoids (discussed above), cancer treatments (especially for prostate cancer), and many other factors can affect testosterone levels. Testosterone replacement therapy may be helpful in preventing or slowing bone loss. Its success depends on factors such as age and how long testosterone levels have been reduced. Also, it is not yet clear how long any beneficial effect of testosterone replacement will last. Therefore, doctors usually treat the osteoporosis directly, using medications approved for this purpose.

Research suggests that estrogen deficiency may also be a cause of osteoporosis in men. For example, estrogen levels are low in men with hypogonadism and may play a part in bone loss.

Osteoporosis has been found in some men who have rare disorders involving estrogen. Therefore, the role of estrogen in men is under active investigation.

Alcohol abuse. There is a wealth of evidence that alcohol abuse may decrease bone density and lead to an increase in fractures. Low bone mass is common in men who seek medical help for alcohol abuse.

In cases where bone loss is linked to alcohol abuse, the first goal of treatment is to help the patient stop, or at least reduce, his consumption of alcohol. More research is needed to determine whether bone lost to alcohol abuse will rebuild once drinking stops, or even whether further damage will be prevented. It is clear, though, that alcohol abuse causes many other health and social problems, so quitting is ideal. A treatment plan may also include a balanced diet with lots of calcium- and vitamin D-rich foods, a program of physical exercise, and smoking cessation.

What Are the Risk Factors for Men?

Several risk factors have been linked to osteoporosis in men:

- Chronic diseases that affect the kidneys, lungs, stomach, and intestines or alter hormone levels.
- Regular use of certain medications, such as glucocorticoids.
- Undiagnosed low levels of the sex hormone testosterone.

- Unhealthy lifestyle habits: smoking, excessive alcohol use, low calcium intake, and inadequate physical exercise.

- Age. The older you are, the greater your risk.

- Race. Caucasian men appear to be at particularly high risk, but all men can develop this disease.

Smoking. Bone loss is more rapid, and rates of hip and vertebral fracture are higher, among men who smoke, although more research is needed to determine exactly how smoking damages bone. Tobacco, nicotine, and other chemicals found in cigarettes may be directly toxic to bone, or they may inhibit absorption of calcium and other nutrients needed for bone health. Quitting is the ideal approach, as smoking is harmful in so many ways.

As with alcohol, it is not known whether quitting smoking leads to reduced rates of bone loss or to a gain in bone mass.

Gastrointestinal disorders. Several nutrients, including amino acids, calcium, magnesium, phosphorous, and vitamins D and K, are important for bone health. Diseases of the stomach and intestines can lead to bone disease when they impair absorption of these nutrients. In such cases, treatment for bone loss may include taking supplements to replenish these nutrients.

Hypercalciuria. Hypercalciuria is a disorder that causes too much calcium to be lost through the urine, which makes the calcium unavailable for building bone. Patients with hypercalciuria should talk to their doctor about having a BMD test and, if bone density is low, discuss treatment options.

Immobilization. Weight-bearing exercise is essential for maintaining healthy bones. Without it, bone density may decline rapidly. Prolonged bed rest (following fractures, surgery, spinal cord injuries, or illness) or immobilization of some part of the body often results in significant bone loss. It is crucial to resume weight-bearing exercise (such as walking, jogging, dancing, and lifting weights) as soon as possible after a period of prolonged bed rest. If this is not possible, you should work with your doctor to minimize other risk factors for osteoporosis.

How Is Osteoporosis Diagnosed in Men?

Osteoporosis can be effectively treated if it is detected before significant bone loss has occurred. A medical workup to diagnose osteoporosis will include a complete medical history, X-rays, and urine and blood tests. The doctor may also order a bone mineral density test. This test can identify osteoporosis, determine your risk for fractures (broken bones), and measure your response to osteoporosis treatment. The most widely recognized BMD test is called a central dual-energy X-ray absorptiometry, or central DXA test. It is painless a bit like having an X-ray, but with much less exposure to radiation. It can measure bone density at your hip and spine.

In men, the diagnosis is often not made until a fracture occurs or a man complains of back pain and sees his doctor. This makes it especially important for men to inform their doctors about risk factors for developing osteoporosis, loss of height or change in posture, a fracture, or sudden back pain.

What Treatments Are Available?

Once a man has been diagnosed with osteoporosis, his doctor may prescribe one of the medications approved by the U.S. Food and Drug Administration (FDA) for this disease. The treatment plan will also likely include the nutrition, exercise, and lifestyle guidelines for preventing bone loss. If bone loss is due to glucocorticoid use, the doctor may prescribe a medication approved to prevent or treat glucocorticoid-induced osteoporosis, monitor bone density and testosterone levels, and suggest using the minimum effective dose of glucocorticoid.

Other possible prevention or treatment approaches include calcium and/or vitamin D supplements and regular physical activity. If osteoporosis is the result of another condition (such as testosterone deficiency) or exposure to certain other medications, the doctor may design a treatment plan to address the underlying cause.

How Can Osteoporosis Be Prevented?

There have been fewer research studies on osteoporosis in men than in women. However, experts agree that all people should take the following steps to preserve their bone health:

- Avoid smoking, reduce alcohol intake, and increase your level of physical activity.

- Ensure a daily calcium intake that is adequate for your age.

- Ensure an adequate intake of vitamin D. Dietary vitamin D intake should be 600 IU (International Units) per day up to age 70. Men over age 70 should increase their uptake to 800 IU daily. The amount of vitamin D found in 1 quart of fortified milk and most multivitamins is 400 IU.

Table 41.1. Recommended Calcium and Vitamin D Intakes

Life-stage group	Calcium mg/day	Vitamin D IU/day
Infants 0 to 6 months	200	400
Infants 6 to 12 months	260	400
1 to 3 years old	700	600
4 to 8 years old	1,000	600
9 to 13 years old	1,300	600
14 to 18 years old	1,300	600
19 to 30 years old	1,000	600
31 to 50 years old	1,000	600
51- to 70-year-old males	1,000	600
>70 years old	1,200	800

- Engage in a regular regimen of weight-bearing exercises in which bones and muscles work against gravity. This might include walking, jogging, racquet sports, climbing stairs, team sports, weight training, and using resistance machines. A doctor should evaluate the exercise program of anyone already diagnosed with osteoporosis to determine if twisting motions and impact activities, such as those used in golf, tennis, or basketball, need to be curtailed.

- Discuss with your doctor the use of medications that are known to cause bone loss, such as glucocorticoids.

- Recognize and seek treatment for any underlying medical conditions that affect bone health.

Chapter 42

Sleep Apnea in Men

What Is Sleep Apnea?

Sleep apnea is a common disorder in which you have one or more pauses in breathing or shallow breaths while you sleep.

Breathing pauses can last from a few seconds to minutes. They may occur 30 times or more an hour. Typically, normal breathing then starts again, sometimes with a loud snort or choking sound.

Sleep apnea usually is a chronic (ongoing) condition that disrupts your sleep. When your breathing pauses or becomes shallow, you'll often move out of deep sleep and into light sleep.

As a result, the quality of your sleep is poor, which makes you tired during the day. Sleep apnea is a leading cause of excessive daytime sleepiness.

Other Names for Sleep Apnea

- Central sleep apnea
- Obstructive sleep apnea
- Sleep-disordered breathing

This chapter includes text excerpted from "Sleep Apnea," National Heart, Lung, and Blood Institute (NHLBI), July 10, 2012. Reviewed August 2016.

What Causes Sleep Apnea?

When you're awake, throat muscles help keep your airway stiff and open so air can flow into your lungs. When you sleep, these muscles relax, which narrows your throat.

Normally, this narrowing doesn't prevent air from flowing into and out of your lungs. But if you have sleep apnea, your airway can become partially or fully blocked because:

- Your throat muscles and tongue relax more than normal.

- Your tongue and tonsils (tissue masses in the back of your mouth) are large compared with the opening into your windpipe.

- You're overweight. The extra soft fat tissue can thicken the wall of the windpipe. This narrows the inside of the windpipe, which makes it harder to keep open.

- The shape of your head and neck (bony structure) may cause a smaller airway size in the mouth and throat area.

- The aging process limits your brain signals' ability to keep your throat muscles stiff during sleep. Thus, your airway is more likely to narrow or collapse.

Not enough air flows into your lungs if your airway is partially or fully blocked during sleep. As a result, loud snoring and a drop in your blood oxygen level can occur.

If the oxygen drops to a dangerous level, it triggers your brain to disturb your sleep. This helps tighten the upper airway muscles and open your windpipe. Normal breathing then starts again, often with a loud snort or choking sound.

Frequent drops in your blood oxygen level and reduced sleep quality can trigger the release of stress hormones. These hormones raise your heart rate and increase your risk for high blood pressure, heart attack, stroke, and arrhythmias (irregular heartbeats). The hormones also can raise your risk for, or worsen, heart failure.

Untreated sleep apnea also can lead to changes in how your body uses energy. These changes increase your risk for obesity and diabetes.

Who Is at Risk for Sleep Apnea?

Obstructive sleep apnea is a common condition. About half of the people who have this condition are overweight.

Men are more likely than women to have sleep apnea. Although the condition can occur at any age, the risk increases as you get older. A family history of sleep apnea also increases your risk for the condition.

People who have small airways in their noses, throats, or mouths are more likely to have sleep apnea. Small airways might be due to the shape of these structures or allergies or other conditions that cause congestion.

About half of the people who have sleep apnea also have high blood pressure. Sleep apnea also is linked to smoking, metabolic syndrome, diabetes, and risk factors for stroke and heart failure.

Race and ethnicity might play a role in the risk of developing sleep apnea. However, more research is needed.

What Are the Signs and Symptoms of Sleep Apnea?

Major Signs and Symptoms

One of the most common signs of obstructive sleep apnea is loud and chronic (ongoing) snoring. Pauses may occur in the snoring. Choking or gasping may follow the pauses.

The snoring usually is loudest when you sleep on your back; it might be less noisy when you turn on your side. You might not snore every night. Over time, however, the snoring can happen more often and get louder.

You're asleep when the snoring or gasping happens. You likely won't know that you're having problems breathing or be able to judge how severe the problem is. A family member or bed partner often will notice these problems before you do.

Not everyone who snores has sleep apnea.

Another common sign of sleep apnea is fighting sleepiness during the day, at work, or while driving. You may find yourself rapidly falling asleep during the quiet moments of the day when you're not active. Even if you don't have daytime sleepiness, talk with your doctor if you have problems breathing during sleep.

Other Signs and Symptoms

Others signs and symptoms of sleep apnea include:

- morning headaches
- memory or learning problems and not being able to concentrate
- feeling irritable, depressed, or having mood swings or personality changes

575

- waking up frequently to urinate

- dry mouth or sore throat when you wake up

How Is Sleep Apnea Diagnosed?

Doctors diagnose sleep apnea based on medical and family histories, a physical exam, and sleep study results. Your primary care doctor may evaluate your symptoms first. He or she will then decide whether you need to see a sleep specialist.

Sleep specialists are doctors who diagnose and treat people who have sleep problems. Examples of such doctors include lung and nerve specialists and ear, nose, and throat specialists. Other types of doctors also can be sleep specialists.

Medical and Family Histories

If you think you have a sleep problem, consider keeping a sleep diary for 1 to 2 weeks. Bring the diary with you to your next medical appointment.

Write down when you go to sleep, wake up, and take naps. Also write down how much you sleep each night, how alert and rested you feel in the morning, and how sleepy you feel at various times during the day. This information can help your doctor figure out whether you have a sleep disorder.

At your appointment, your doctor will ask you questions about how you sleep and how you function during the day.

Your doctor also will want to know how loudly and often you snore or make gasping or choking sounds during sleep. Often you're not aware of such symptoms and must ask a family member or bed partner to report them.

Let your doctor know if anyone in your family has been diagnosed with sleep apnea or has had symptoms of the disorder.

Many people aren't aware of their symptoms and aren't diagnosed.

If you're a parent of a child who may have sleep apnea, tell your child's doctor about your child's signs and symptoms.

Physical Exam

Your doctor will check your mouth, nose, and throat for extra or large tissues. Children who have sleep apnea might have enlarged tonsils. Doctors may need only a physical exam and medical history to diagnose sleep apnea in children.

Adults who have sleep apnea may have an enlarged uvula or soft palate. The uvula is the tissue that hangs from the middle of the back of your mouth. The soft palate is the roof of your mouth in the back of your throat.

Sleep Studies

Sleep studies are tests that measure how well you sleep and how your body responds to sleep problems. These tests can help your doctor find out whether you have a sleep disorder and how severe it is. Sleep studies are the most accurate tests for diagnosing sleep apnea.

There are different kinds of sleep studies. If your doctor thinks you have sleep apnea, he or she may recommend a polysomnogram (PSG) or a home-based portable monitor.

Polysomnogram

A PSG is the most common sleep study for diagnosing sleep apnea. This study records brain activity, eye movements, heart rate, and blood pressure.

A PSG also records the amount of oxygen in your blood, air movement through your nose while you breathe, snoring, and chest movements. The chest movements show whether you're making an effort to breathe.

PSGs often are done at sleep centers or sleep labs. The test is painless. You'll go to sleep as usual, except you'll have sensors attached to your scalp, face, chest, limbs, and a finger. The staff at the sleep center will use the sensors to check on you throughout the night.

A sleep specialist will review the results of your PSG to see whether you have sleep apnea and how severe it is. He or she will use the results to plan your treatment.

Your doctor also may use a PSG to find the best setting for you on a CPAP (continuous positive airway pressure) machine. CPAP is the most common treatment for sleep apnea. A CPAP machine uses mild air pressure to keep your airway open while you sleep.

If your doctor thinks that you have sleep apnea, he or she may schedule a split-night sleep study. During the first half of the night, your sleep will be checked without a CPAP machine. This will show whether you have sleep apnea and how severe it is.

If the PSG shows that you have sleep apnea, you'll use a CPAP machine during the second half of the split-night study. The staff at the sleep center will adjust the flow of air from the CPAP machine to find the setting that works best for you.

Home-Based Portable Monitor

Your doctor may recommend a home-based sleep test with a portable monitor. The portable monitor will record some of the same information as a PSG. For example, it may record:

- the amount of oxygen in your blood

- air movement through your nose while you breathe

- your heart rate

- chest movements that show whether you're making an effort to breathe

A sleep specialist may use the results from a home-based sleep test to help diagnose sleep apnea. He or she also may use the results to decide whether you need a full PSG study in a sleep center.

How Is Sleep Apnea Treated?

Sleep apnea is treated with lifestyle changes, mouthpieces, breathing devices, and surgery. Medicines typically aren't used to treat the condition.

The goals of treating sleep apnea are to:

- Restore regular breathing during sleep

- Relieve symptoms such as loud snoring and daytime sleepiness

Treatment may improve other medical problems linked to sleep apnea, such as high blood pressure. Treatment also can reduce your risk for heart disease, stroke, and diabetes.

If you have sleep apnea, talk with your doctor or sleep specialist about the treatment options that will work best for you.

Lifestyle changes and/or mouthpieces may relieve mild sleep apnea. People who have moderate or severe sleep apnea may need breathing devices or surgery.

If you continue to have daytime sleepiness despite treatment, your doctor may ask whether you're getting enough sleep. (Adults should get at least 7 to 8 hours of sleep; children and teens need more.

If treatment and enough sleep don't relieve your daytime sleepiness, your doctor will consider other treatment options.

Lifestyle Changes

If you have mild sleep apnea, some changes in daily activities or habits might be all the treatment you need.

- Avoid alcohol and medicines that make you sleepy. They make it harder for your throat to stay open while you sleep.

- Lose weight if you're overweight or obese. Even a little weight loss can improve your symptoms.

- Sleep on your side instead of your back to help keep your throat open. You can sleep with special pillows or shirts that prevent you from sleeping on your back.

- Keep your nasal passages open at night with nasal sprays or allergy medicines, if needed. Talk with your doctor about whether these treatments might help you.

- If you smoke, quit. Talk with your doctor about programs and products that can help you quit smoking.

Mouthpieces

A mouthpiece, sometimes called an oral appliance, may help some people who have mild sleep apnea. Your doctor also may recommend a mouthpiece if you snore loudly but don't have sleep apnea.

A dentist or orthodontist can make a custom-fit plastic mouthpiece for treating sleep apnea. (An orthodontist specializes in correcting teeth or jaw problems.) The mouthpiece will adjust your lower jaw and your tongue to help keep your airways open while you sleep.

If you use a mouthpiece, tell your doctor if you have discomfort or pain while using the device. You may need periodic office visits so your doctor can adjust your mouthpiece to fit better.

Breathing Devices

CPAP (continuous positive airway pressure) is the most common treatment for moderate to severe sleep apnea in adults. A CPAP machine uses a mask that fits over your mouth and nose, or just over your nose.

The machine gently blows air into your throat. The pressure from the air helps keep your airway open while you sleep.

Treating sleep apnea may help you stop snoring. But not snoring doesn't mean that you no longer have sleep apnea or can stop using CPAP. Your sleep apnea will return if you stop using your CPAP machine or don't use it correctly.

Usually, a technician will come to your home to bring the CPAP equipment. The technician will set up the CPAP machine and adjust it based on your doctor's prescription. After the initial setup, you may need to have the CPAP adjusted from time to time for the best results.

CPAP treatment may cause side effects in some people. These side effects include a dry or stuffy nose, irritated skin on your face, dry mouth, and headaches. If your CPAP isn't adjusted properly, you may get stomach bloating and discomfort while wearing the mask.

If you're having trouble with CPAP side effects, work with your sleep specialist, his or her nursing staff, and the CPAP technician. Together, you can take steps to reduce the side effects.

For example, the CPAP settings or size/fit of the mask might need to be adjusted. Adding moisture to the air as it flows through the mask or using nasal spray can help relieve a dry, stuffy, or runny nose.

There are many types of CPAP machines and masks. Tell your doctor if you're not happy with the type you're using. He or she may suggest switching to a different type that might work better for you.

People who have severe sleep apnea symptoms generally feel much better once they begin treatment with CPAP.

Surgery

Some people who have sleep apnea might benefit from surgery. The type of surgery and how well it works depend on the cause of the sleep apnea.

Surgery is done to widen breathing passages. It usually involves shrinking, stiffening, or removing excess tissue in the mouth and throat or resetting the lower jaw.

Surgery to shrink or stiffen excess tissue is done in a doctor's office or a hospital. Shrinking tissue may involve small shots or other treatments to the tissue. You may need a series of treatments to shrink the excess tissue. To stiffen excess tissue, the doctor makes a small cut in the tissue and inserts a piece of stiff plastic.

Surgery to remove excess tissue is done in a hospital. You're given medicine to help you sleep during the surgery. After surgery, you may have throat pain that lasts for 1 to 2 weeks.

Surgery to remove the tonsils, if they're blocking the airway, might be helpful for some children. Your child's doctor may suggest waiting some time to see whether these tissues shrink on their own. This is common as small children grow.

Living with Sleep Apnea

Sleep apnea can be very serious. However, following an effective treatment plan often can improve your quality of life quite a bit.

Treatment can improve your sleep and relieve daytime sleepiness. Treatment also might lower your risk for high blood pressure, heart disease, and other health problems linked to sleep apnea.

Treatment may improve your overall health and happiness as well as your quality of sleep (and possibly your family's quality of sleep).

Chapter 43

Male Pattern Baldness

Androgenetic alopecia (AGA) is a common form of hair loss in both men and women. In men, this condition is also known as male-pattern baldness. Hair is lost in a well-defined pattern, beginning above both temples. Over time, the hairline recedes to form a characteristic "M" shape. Hair also thins at the crown (near the top of the head), often progressing to partial or complete baldness.

AGA in men has been associated with several other medical conditions including coronary heart disease and enlargement of the prostate. Additionally, prostate cancer, disorders of insulin resistance (such as diabetes and obesity), and high blood pressure (hypertension) have been related to androgenetic alopecia.

Frequency

AGA is a frequent cause of hair loss in both men and women. This form of hair loss affects an estimated 50 million men and 30 million women in the United States. Androgenetic alopecia can start as early as a person's teens and risk increases with age; more than 50 percent of men over age 50 have some degree of hair loss.

Genetic Changes

A variety of genetic and environmental factors likely play a role in causing AGA. Although researchers are studying risk factors that may

This chapter includes text excerpted from "Androgenetic Alopecia," Genetics Home Reference (GHR), National Institute of Health (NIH), August 2015.

contribute to this condition, most of these factors remain unknown. Researchers have determined that this form of hair loss is related to hormones called androgens, particularly an androgen called dihydrotestosterone. Androgens are important for normal male sexual development before birth and during puberty. Androgens also have other important functions in both males and females, such as regulating hair growth and sex drive.

Hair growth begins under the skin in structures called follicles. Each strand of hair normally grows for 2 to 6 years, goes into a resting phase for several months, and then falls out. The cycle starts over when the follicle begins growing a new hair. Increased levels of androgens in hair follicles can lead to a shorter cycle of hair growth and the growth of shorter and thinner strands of hair. Additionally, there is a delay in the growth of new hair to replace strands that are shed.

Although researchers suspect that several genes play a role in androgenetic alopecia, variations in only one gene, *AR*, have been confirmed in scientific studies. The *AR* gene provides instructions for making a protein called an androgen receptor. Androgen receptors allow the body to respond appropriately to dihydrotestosterone and other androgens. Studies suggest that variations in the *AR* gene lead to increased activity of androgen receptors in hair follicles. It remains unclear, however, how these genetic changes increase the risk of hair loss in men and women with androgenetic alopecia.

Researchers continue to investigate the connection between AGA and other medical conditions, such as coronary heart disease and prostate cancer in men. They believe that some of these disorders may be associated with elevated androgen levels, which may help explain why they tend to occur with androgen-related hair loss. Other hormonal, environmental, and genetic factors that have not been identified also may be involved.

Inheritance Pattern

The inheritance pattern of AGA is unclear because many genetic and environmental factors are likely to be involved. This condition tends to cluster in families, however, and having a close relative with patterned hair loss appears to be a risk factor for developing the condition.

Other Names for This Condition

- androgenic alopecia

- female pattern baldness
- male pattern alopecia
- male pattern baldness
- pattern baldness

Chapter 44

Mental Health Concerns in Men

Chapter Contents

Section 44.1—Depression 588

Section 44.2—Posttraumatic Stress Disorder 593

Section 44.3—Schizophrenia 600

Section 44.1

Depression

This section includes text excerpted from "Depression,"
National Institute of Mental Health (NIMH), May 2016.

Depression (major depressive disorder or clinical depression) is a
common but serious mood disorder. It causes severe symptoms that
affect how you feel, think, and handle daily activities, such as sleeping,
eating, or working. To be diagnosed with depression, the symptoms
must be present for at least two weeks.

Some forms of depression are slightly different, or they may develop
under unique circumstances, such as:

- **Persistent depressive disorder** (also called dysthymia) is a
  depressed mood that lasts for at least two years. A person diagnosed with persistent depressive disorder may have episodes of
  major depression along with periods of less severe symptoms,
  but symptoms must last for two years to be considered persistent depressive disorder.

- **Psychotic depression** occurs when a person has severe depression plus some form of psychosis, such as having disturbing false
  fixed beliefs (delusions) or hearing or seeing upsetting things
  that others cannot hear or see (hallucinations). The psychotic
  symptoms typically have a depressive "theme," such as delusions
  of guilt, poverty, or illness.

- **Seasonal affective disorder** is characterized by the onset of
  depression during the winter months, when there is less natural
  sunlight. This depression generally lifts during spring and sum-
  mer. Winter depression, typically accompanied by social withdrawal, increased sleep, and weight gain, predictably returns
  every year in seasonal affective disorder.

- **Bipolar disorder** is different from depression, but it is included
  in this list is because someone with bipolar disorder experiences episodes of extremely low moods that meet the criteria
  for major depression (called "bipolar depression"). But a person

with bipolar disorder also experiences extreme high—euphoric or irritable—moods called "mania" or a less severe form called "hypomania."

Examples of other types of depressive disorders newly added to the diagnostic classification of *Diagnostic and Statistical Manual of Mental Disorders* (DSM-5) include disruptive mood dysregulation disorder (diagnosed in children and adolescents) and premenstrual dysphoric disorder (PMDD).

Signs and Symptoms

If you have been experiencing some of the following signs and symptoms most of the day, nearly every day, for at least two weeks, you may be suffering from depression:

- persistent sad, anxious, or "empty" mood
- feelings of hopelessness, or pessimism
- irritability
- feelings of guilt, worthlessness, or helplessness
- loss of interest or pleasure in hobbies and activities
- decreased energy or fatigue
- moving or talking more slowly
- feeling restless or having trouble sitting still
- difficulty concentrating, remembering, or making decisions
- difficulty sleeping, early-morning awakening, or oversleeping
- appetite and/or weight changes
- thoughts of death or suicide, or suicide attempts
- aches or pains, headaches, cramps, or digestive problems without a clear physical cause and/or that do not ease even with treatment

Not everyone who is depressed experiences every symptom. Some people experience only a few symptoms while others may experience many. Several persistent symptoms in addition to low mood are required for a diagnosis of major depression, but people with only a few—but distressing—symptoms may benefit from treatment of their "subsyndromal" depression. The severity and frequency of symptoms and how long they last will vary depending on the individual and his or her particular illness. Symptoms may also vary depending on the stage of the illness.

Risk Factors

Depression is one of the most common mental disorders in the United States. Current research suggests that depression is caused by a combination of genetic, biological, environmental, and psychological factors.

Depression can happen at any age, but often begins in adulthood. Depression is now recognized as occurring in children and adolescents, although it sometimes presents with more prominent irritability than low mood. Many chronic mood and anxiety disorders in adults begin as high levels of anxiety in children.

Depression, especially in midlife or older adults, can co-occur with other serious medical illnesses, such as diabetes, cancer, heart disease, and Parkinson disease. These conditions are often worse when depression is present. Sometimes medications taken for these physical illnesses may cause side effects that contribute to depression. A doctor experienced in treating these complicated illnesses can help work out the best treatment strategy.

Risk factors include:

- personal or family history of depression
- major life changes, trauma, or stress
- certain physical illnesses and medications

Treatment and Therapies

Depression, even the most severe cases, can be treated. The earlier that treatment can begin, the more effective it is. Depression is usually treated with medications, psychotherapy, or a combination of the two. If these treatments do not reduce symptoms, electroconvulsive therapy (ECT) and other brain stimulation therapies may be options to explore.

Quick Tip: No two people are affected the same way by depression and there is no "one-size-fits-all" for treatment. It may take some trial and error to find the treatment that works best for you.

Medications

Antidepressants are medicines that treat depression. They may help improve the way your brain uses certain chemicals that control mood or stress. You may need to try several different anti-depressant medicines before finding the one that improves your symptoms and has manageable side effects. A medication that has helped you or a close family member in the past will often be considered.

Antidepressants take time—usually 2 to 4 weeks—to work, and often, symptoms such as sleep, appetite, and concentration problems improve before mood lifts, so it is important to give medication a chance before reaching a conclusion about its effectiveness. If you begin taking antidepressants, do not stop taking them without the help of a doctor. Sometimes people taking antidepressants feel better and then stop taking the medication on their own, and the depression returns. When you and your doctor have decided it is time to stop the medication, usually after a course of 6 to 12 months, the doctor will help you slowly and safely decrease your dose. Stopping them abruptly can cause withdrawal symptoms.

You may have heard about an herbal medicine called St. John's wort. Although it is a top-selling botanical product, the U.S. Food and Drug Administration (FDA) has not approved its use as an over-the-counter or prescription medicine for depression, and there are serious concerns about its safety (it should never be combined with a prescription antidepressant) and effectiveness. Do not use St. John's wort before talking to your healthcare provider. Other natural products sold as dietary supplements, including omega-3 fatty acids and S-adenosylmethionine (SAMe), remain under study but have not yet been proven safe and effective for routine use.

Please Note: In some cases, children, teenagers, and young adults under 25 may experience an increase in suicidal thoughts or behavior when taking antidepressants, especially in the first few weeks after starting or when the dose is changed. This warning from the FDA also says that patients of all ages taking antidepressants should be watched closely, especially during the first few weeks of treatment.

Psychotherapies

Several types of psychotherapy (also called "talk therapy" or, in a less specific form, counseling) can help people with depression. Examples of evidence-based approaches specific to the treatment of depression include cognitive-behavioral therapy (CBT), interpersonal therapy (IPT), and problem-solving therapy.

Brain Stimulation Therapies

If medications do not reduce the symptoms of depression, electro-convulsive therapy (ECT) may be an option to explore. Based on the latest research:

- ECT can provide relief for people with severe depression who have not been able to feel better with other treatments.

- Electroconvulsive therapy can be an effective treatment for depression. In some severe cases where a rapid response is necessary or medications cannot be used safely, ECT can even be a first-line intervention.

- Once strictly an inpatient procedure, today ECT is often performed on an outpatient basis. The treatment consists of a series of sessions, typically three times a week, for two to four weeks.

- ECT may cause some side effects, including confusion, disorientation, and memory loss. Usually these side effects are short-term, but sometimes memory problems can linger, especially for the months around the time of the treatment course. Advances in ECT devices and methods have made modern ECT safe and effective for the vast majority of patients. Talk to your doctor and make sure you understand the potential benefits and risks of the treatment before giving your informed consent to undergoing ECT.

- ECT is not painful, and you cannot feel the electrical impulses. Before ECT begins, a patient is put under brief anesthesia and given a muscle relaxant. Within one hour after the treatment session, which takes only a few minutes, the patient is awake and alert.

Other more recently introduced types of brain stimulation therapies used to treat medicine-resistant depression include repetitive transcranial magnetic stimulation (rTMS) and vagus nerve stimulation (VNS). Other types of brain stimulation treatments are under study.

If you think you may have depression, start by making an appointment to see your doctor or healthcare provider. This could be your primary care practitioner or a health provider who specializes in diagnosing and treating mental health conditions.

Beyond Treatment: Things You Can Do

Here are other tips that may help you or a loved one during treatment for depression:

- Try to be active and exercise.

- Set realistic goals for yourself.

- Try to spend time with other people and confide in a trusted friend or relative.

- Try not to isolate yourself, and let others help you.

- Expect your mood to improve gradually, not immediately.

- Postpone important decisions, such as getting married or divorced, or changing jobs until you feel better. Discuss decisions with others who know you well and have a more objective view of your situation.

- Continue to educate yourself about depression.

Section 44.2

Posttraumatic Stress Disorder

This section includes text excerpted from "Posttraumatic Stress Disorder," National Institute of Mental Health (NIMH), February 2016.

Posttraumatic stress disorder (PTSD) is a disorder that develops in some people who have experienced a shocking, scary, or dangerous event.

It is natural to feel afraid during and after a traumatic situation. Fear triggers many split-second changes in the body to help defend against danger or to avoid it. This "fight-or-flight" response is a typical reaction meant to protect a person from harm. Nearly everyone will experience a range of reactions after trauma, yet most people recover from initial symptoms naturally. Those who continue to experience problems may be diagnosed with PTSD. People who have PTSD may feel stressed or frightened even when they are not in danger.

Signs and Symptoms

Not every traumatized person develops ongoing (chronic) or even short-term (acute) PTSD. Not everyone with PTSD has been through a dangerous event. Some experiences, like the sudden, unexpected death of a loved one, can also cause PTSD. Symptoms usually begin early, within 3 months of the traumatic incident, but sometimes they begin years afterward. Symptoms must last more than a month and be severe enough to interfere with relationships or work to be considered PTSD. The course of the illness varies. Some people recover within 6 months, while others have symptoms that last much longer. In some people, the condition becomes chronic.

A doctor who has experience helping people with mental illnesses, such as a psychiatrist or psychologist, can diagnose PTSD.

To be diagnosed with PTSD, an adult must have all of the following for at least 1 month:

- at least one re-experiencing symptom

- at least one avoidance symptom

- at least two arousal and reactivity symptoms

- at least two cognition and mood symptoms

Re-experiencing symptoms include:

- flashbacks—reliving the trauma over and over, including physical symptoms like a racing heart or sweating

- bad dreams

- frightening thoughts

Re-experiencing symptoms may cause problems in a person's everyday routine. The symptoms can start from the person's own thoughts and feelings. Words, objects, or situations that are reminders of the event can also trigger re-experiencing symptoms.

Avoidance symptoms include:

- staying away from places, events, or objects that are reminders of the traumatic experience

- avoiding thoughts or feelings related to the traumatic event

Things that remind a person of the traumatic event can trigger avoidance symptoms. These symptoms may cause a person to change his or her personal routine. For example, after a bad car accident, a person who usually drives may avoid driving or riding in a car.

Arousal and reactivity symptoms include:

- being easily startled

- feeling tense or "on edge"

- having difficulty sleeping

- having angry outbursts

Arousal symptoms are usually constant, instead of being triggered by things that remind one of the traumatic events. These symptoms can make the person feel stressed and angry. They may make it hard to do daily tasks, such as sleeping, eating, or concentrating.

Cognition and mood symptoms include:

- trouble remembering key features of the traumatic event

- negative thoughts about oneself or the world

- distorted feelings like guilt or blame

- loss of interest in enjoyable activities

Cognition and mood symptoms can begin or worsen after the traumatic event, but are not due to injury or substance use. These symptoms can make the person feel alienated or detached from friends or family members.

It is natural to have some of these symptoms after a dangerous event. Sometimes people have very serious symptoms that go away after a few weeks. This is called acute stress disorder, or ASD. When the symptoms last more than a month, seriously affect one's ability to function, and are not due to substance use, medical illness, or anything except the event itself, they might be PTSD. Some people with PTSD don't show any symptoms for weeks or months. PTSD is often accompanied by depression, substance abuse, or one or more of the other anxiety disorders.

Do Children React Differently than Adults?

Children and teens can have extreme reactions to trauma, but their symptoms may not be the same as adults. In very young children (less than 6 years of age), these symptoms can include:

- wetting the bed after having learned to use the toilet

- forgetting how to or being unable to talk

- acting out the scary event during playtime

- Being unusually clingy with a parent or other adult

Older children and teens are more likely to show symptoms similar to those seen in adults. They may also develop disruptive, disrespectful, or destructive behaviors. Older children and teens may feel guilty for not preventing injury or deaths. They may also have thoughts of revenge.

Risk Factors

Anyone can develop PTSD at any age. This includes war veterans, children, and people who have been through a physical or sexual assault, abuse, accident, disaster, or many other serious events. According to the National Center for PTSD, about 7 or 8 out of every 100 people will experience PTSD at some point in their lives. Women are more likely to develop PTSD than men, and genes may make some people more likely to develop PTSD than others.

Not everyone with PTSD has been through a dangerous event. Some people develop PTSD after a friend or family member experiences danger or harm. The sudden, unexpected death of a loved one can also lead to PTSD.

Why Do Some People Develop PTSD and Other People Do Not?

It is important to remember that not everyone who lives through a dangerous event develops PTSD. In fact, most people will not develop the disorder.

Many factors play a part in whether a person will develop PTSD. Some examples are listed below. Risk factors make a person more likely to develop PTSD. Other factors, called resilience factors, can help reduce the risk of the disorder.

Risk Factors and Resilience Factors for PTSD

Some factors that increase risk for PTSD include:

- living through dangerous events and traumas
- getting hurt
- seeing another person hurt, or seeing a dead body
- childhood trauma
- feeling horror, helplessness, or extreme fear
- having little or no social support after the event

- dealing with extra stress after the event, such as loss of a loved one, pain and injury, or loss of a job or home

- having a history of mental illness or substance abuse

Some resilience factors that may reduce the risk of PTSD include:

- seeking out support from other people, such as friends and family

- finding a support group after a traumatic event

- learning to feel good about one's own actions in the face of danger

- having a positive coping strategy, or a way of getting through the bad event and learning from it

- being able to act and respond effectively despite feeling fear

Researchers are studying the importance of these and other risk and resilience factors, including genetics and neurobiology. With more research, someday it may be possible to predict who is likely to develop PTSD and to prevent it.

Treatments and Therapies

The main treatments for people with PTSD are medications, psychotherapy ("talk" therapy), or both. Everyone is different, and PTSD affects people differently so a treatment that works for one person may not work for another. It is important for anyone with PTSD to be treated by a mental health provider who is experienced with PTSD. Some people with PTSD need to try different treatments to find what works for their symptoms.

If someone with PTSD is going through an ongoing trauma, such as being in an abusive relationship, both of the problems need to be addressed. Other ongoing problems can include panic disorder, depression, substance abuse, and feeling suicidal.

Medications

The most studied medications for treating PTSD include antidepressants, which may help control PTSD symptoms such as sadness, worry, anger, and feeling numb inside. Antidepressants and other medications may be prescribed along with psychotherapy. Other medications may be helpful for specific PTSD symptoms. For example, although it is not currently U.S. Food and Drug Administration (FDA) approved, research has shown that Prazosin may be helpful with sleep problems, particularly nightmares, commonly experienced by people with PTSD.

Doctors and patients can work together to find the best medication or medication combination, as well as the right dose.

Psychotherapy

Psychotherapy (sometimes called "talk therapy") involves talking with a mental health professional to treat a mental illness. Psychotherapy can occur one-on-one or in a group. Talk therapy treatment for PTSD usually lasts 6 to 12 weeks, but it can last longer. Research shows that support from family and friends can be an important part of recovery.

Many types of psychotherapy can help people with PTSD. Some types target the symptoms of PTSD directly. Other therapies focus on social, family, or job-related problems. The doctor or therapist may combine different therapies depending on each person's needs.

Effective psychotherapies tend to emphasize a few key components, including education about symptoms, teaching skills to help identify the triggers of symptoms, and skills to manage the symptoms. One helpful form of therapy is called cognitive behavioral therapy, or CBT. CBT can include:

- **Exposure therapy.** This helps people face and control their fear. It gradually exposes them to the trauma they experienced in a safe way. It uses imagining, writing, or visiting the place where the event happened. The therapist uses these tools to help people with PTSD cope with their feelings.

- **Cognitive restructuring.** This helps people make sense of the bad memories. Sometimes people remember the event differently than how it happened. They may feel guilt or shame about something that is not their fault. The therapist helps people with PTSD look at what happened in a realistic way.

There are other types of treatment that can help as well. People with PTSD should talk about all treatment options with a therapist. Treatment should equip individuals with the skills to manage their symptoms and help them participate in activities that they enjoyed before developing PTSD.

How Talk Therapies Help People Overcome PTSD

Talk therapies teach people helpful ways to react to the frightening events that trigger their PTSD symptoms. Based on this general goal, different types of therapy may:

- Teach about trauma and its effects.

- Use relaxation and anger-control skills.

- Provide tips for better sleep, diet, and exercise habits.

- Help people identify and deal with guilt, shame, and other feelings about the event.

- Focus on changing how people react to their PTSD symptoms. For example, therapy helps people face reminders of the trauma.

Beyond Treatment: How Can I Help Myself?

It may be very hard to take that first step to help yourself. It is important to realize that although it may take some time, with treatment, you can get better. If you are unsure where to go for help, ask your family doctor. You can also check NIMH's Help for Mental Illnesses page or search online for "mental health providers," "social services," "hotlines," or "physicians" for phone numbers and addresses. An emergency room doctor can also provide temporary help and can tell you where and how to get further help.

To help yourself while in treatment:

- Talk with your doctor about treatment options.

- Engage in mild physical activity or exercise to help reduce stress.

- Set realistic goals for yourself.

- Break up large tasks into small ones, set some priorities, and do what you can as you can.

- Try to spend time with other people, and confide in a trusted friend or relative. Tell others about things that may trigger symptoms.

- Expect your symptoms to improve gradually, not immediately.

- Identify and seek out comforting situations, places, and people.

Caring for yourself and others is especially important when large numbers of people are exposed to traumatic events (such as natural disasters, accidents, and violent acts).

Section 44.3

Schizophrenia

This section includes text excerpted from "Schizophrenia," National Institute of Mental Health (NIMH), December 4, 2015.

What Is Schizophrenia?

Schizophrenia is a chronic and severe disorder that affects how a person thinks, feels, and acts. Although schizophrenia is not as common as other mental disorders, it can be very disabling. Approximately 7 or 8 individuals out of 1,000 will have schizophrenia in their lifetime.

People with the disorder may hear voices or see things that aren't there. They may believe other people are reading their minds, controlling their thoughts, or plotting to harm them. This can be scary and upsetting to people with the illness and make them withdrawn or extremely agitated. It can also be scary and upsetting to the people around them.

People with schizophrenia may sometimes talk about strange or unusual ideas, which can make it difficult to carry on a conversation. They may sit for hours without moving or talking. Sometimes people with schizophrenia seem perfectly fine until they talk about what they are really thinking.

Families and society are impacted by schizophrenia too. Many people with schizophrenia have difficulty holding a job or caring for themselves, so they may rely on others for help. Stigmatizing attitudes and beliefs about schizophrenia are common and sometimes interfere with people's willingness to talk about and get treatment for the disorder.

People with schizophrenia may cope with symptoms throughout their lives, but treatment helps many to recover and pursue their life goals. Researchers are developing more effective treatments and using new research tools to understand the causes of schizophrenia. In the years to come, this work may help prevent and better treat the illness.

What Are the Symptoms of Schizophrenia?

The symptoms of schizophrenia fall into three broad categories: positive, negative, and cognitive symptoms.

Positive Symptoms

Positive symptoms are psychotic behaviors not generally seen in healthy people. People with positive symptoms may "lose touch" with some aspects of reality. For some people, these symptoms come and go. For others, they stay stable over time. Sometimes they are severe, and at other times hardly noticeable. The severity of positive symptoms may depend on whether the individual is receiving treatment. Positive symptoms include the following:

Hallucinations are sensory experiences that occur in the absence of a stimulus. These can occur in any of the five senses (vision, hearing, smell, taste, or touch). "Voices" (auditory hallucinations) are the most common type of hallucination in schizophrenia. Many people with the disorder hear voices. The voices can either be internal, seeming to come from within one's own mind, or they can be external, in which case they can seem to be as real as another person speaking. The voices may talk to the person about his or her behavior, command the person to do things, or warn the person of danger. Sometimes the voices talk to each other, and sometimes people with schizophrenia talk to the voices that they hear. People with schizophrenia may hear voices for a long time before family and friends notice the problem.

Other types of hallucinations include seeing people or objects that are not there, smelling odors that no one else detects, and feeling things like invisible fingers touching their bodies when no one is near.

Delusions are strongly held false beliefs that are not consistent with the person's culture. Delusions persist even when there is evidence that the beliefs are not true or logical. People with schizophrenia can have delusions that seem bizarre, such as believing that neighbors can control their behavior with magnetic waves. They may also believe that people on television are directing special messages to them, or that radio stations are broadcasting their thoughts aloud to others. These are called "delusions of reference."

Sometimes they believe they are someone else, such as a famous historical figure. They may have paranoid delusions and believe that others are trying to harm them, such as by cheating, harassing, poisoning, spying on, or plotting against them or the people they care about. These beliefs are called "persecutory delusions."

Thought disorders are unusual or dysfunctional ways of thinking. One form is called "disorganized thinking." This is when a person has trouble organizing his or her thoughts or connecting them logically. He or she may talk in a garbled way that is hard to understand. This is often called "word salad." Another form is called "thought blocking." This is when a person stops speaking abruptly in the middle of a thought. When asked why he or she stopped talking, the person may say that it felt as if the thought had been taken out of his or her head. Finally, a person with a thought disorder might make up meaningless words, or "neologisms."

Movement disorders may appear as agitated body movements. A person with a movement disorder may repeat certain motions over and over. In the other extreme, a person may become catatonic. Catatonia is a state in which a person does not move and does not respond to others. Catatonia is rare today, but it was more common when treatment for schizophrenia was not available.

Negative Symptoms

Negative symptoms are associated with disruptions to normal emotions and behaviors. These symptoms are harder to recognize as part of the disorder and can be mistaken for depression or other conditions. These symptoms include the following:

- "flat affect" (reduced expression of emotions via facial expression or voice tone)
- reduced feelings of pleasure in everyday life
- difficulty beginning and sustaining activities
- reduced speaking

People with negative symptoms may need help with everyday tasks. They may neglect basic personal hygiene.

This may make them seem lazy or unwilling to help themselves, but the problems are symptoms caused by schizophrenia.

Cognitive Symptoms

For some people, the cognitive symptoms of schizophrenia are subtle, but for others, they are more severe and patients may notice changes in their memory or other aspects of thinking. Similar to negative symptoms, cognitive symptoms may be difficult to recognize as part of the disorder. Often, they are detected only when specific tests are performed. Cognitive symptoms include the following:

- poor "executive functioning" (the ability to understand information and use it to make decisions)

- trouble focusing or paying attention

- problems with "working memory" (the ability to use information immediately after learning it)

Poor cognition is related to worse employment and social outcomes and can be distressing to individuals with schizophrenia.

When Does Schizophrenia Start, and Who Gets It?

Schizophrenia affects slightly more males than females. It occurs in all ethnic groups around the world. Symptoms such as hallucinations and delusions usually start between ages 16 and 30. Males tend to experience symptoms a little earlier than females. Most commonly, schizophrenia occurs in late adolescence and early adulthood. It is uncommon to be diagnosed with schizophrenia after age 45. Schizophrenia rarely occurs in children, but awareness of childhood-onset schizophrenia is increasing.

It can be difficult to diagnose schizophrenia in teens. This is because the first signs can include a change of friends, a drop in grades, sleep problems, and irritability—behaviors that are common among teens. A combination of factors can predict schizophrenia in up to 80 percent of youth who are at high risk of developing the illness. These factors include isolating oneself and withdrawing from others, an increase in unusual thoughts and suspicions, and a family history of psychosis. This pre-psychotic stage of the disorder is called the "prodromal" period.

Are People with Schizophrenia Violent?

Most people with schizophrenia are not violent. In fact, most violent crimes are not committed by people with schizophrenia. People with schizophrenia are much more likely to harm themselves than others. Substance abuse may increase the chance a person will become violent. The risk of violence is greatest when psychosis is untreated and decreases substantially when treatment is in place.

Schizophrenia and Suicide

Suicidal thoughts and behaviors are very common among people with schizophrenia. People with schizophrenia die earlier than people without a mental illness, partly because of the increased suicide risk.

It is hard to predict which people with schizophrenia are more likely to die by suicide, but actively treating any co-existing depressive symptoms and substance abuse may reduce suicide risk. People who take their antipsychotic medications as prescribed are less likely to attempt suicide than those who do not. If someone you know is talking about or has attempted suicide, help him or her find professional help right away or call 911.

Schizophrenia and Substance Use Disorders

Substance use disorders occur when frequent use of alcohol and/ or drugs interferes with a person's health, family, work, school, and social life. Substance use is the most common co-occurring disorder in people with schizophrenia, and the complex relationships between substance use disorders and schizophrenia have been extensively studied. Substance use disorders can make treatment for schizophrenia less effective, and individuals are also less likely to engage in treatment for their mental illness if they are abusing substances. It is commonly believed that people with schizophrenia who also abuse substances are trying to "self-medicate" their symptoms, but there is little evidence that people begin to abuse substances in response to symptoms or that abusing substances reduces symptoms.

Nicotine is the most common drug abused by people with schizophrenia. People with schizophrenia are much more likely to smoke than people without a mental illness, and researchers are exploring whether there is a biological basis for this. There is some evidence that nicotine may temporarily alleviate a subset of the cognitive deficits commonly observed in schizophrenia, but these benefits are outweighed by the detrimental effects of smoking on other aspects of cognition and general health. Bupropion has been found to be effective for smoking cessation in people with schizophrenia. Most studies find that reducing or stopping smoking does not make schizophrenia symptoms worse.

Cannabis (marijuana) is also frequently abused by people with schizophrenia, which can worsen health outcomes. Heavy cannabis use is associated with more severe and earlier onset of schizophrenia symptoms, but research has not yet definitively determined whether cannabis directly causes schizophrenia.

Drug abuse can increase rates of other medical illnesses (such as hepatitis, heart disease, and infectious disease) as well as suicide, trauma, and homelessness in people with schizophrenia.

It is generally understood that schizophrenia and substance use disorders have strong genetic risk factors. While substance use disorder and a family history of psychosis have individually been identified as risk factors for schizophrenia, it is less well understood if and how these factors are related.

When people have both schizophrenia and a substance abuse disorder, their best chance for recovery is a treatment program that integrates the schizophrenia and substance abuse treatment.

What Causes Schizophrenia?

Research has identified several factors that contribute to the risk of developing schizophrenia.

Genes and Environment

Scientists have long known that schizophrenia sometimes runs in families. The illness occurs in less than 1 percent of the general population, but it occurs in 10 percent of people who have a first-degree relative with the disorder, such as a parent, brother, or sister. People who have second-degree relatives (aunts, uncles, grandparents, or cousins) with the disease also develop schizophrenia more often than the general population. The risk is highest for an identical twin of a person with schizophrenia. He or she has a 40 to 65 percent chance of developing the disorder. Although these genetic relationships are strong, there are many people who have schizophrenia who don't have a family member with the disorder and, conversely, many people with one or more family members with the disorder who do not develop it themselves.

Scientists believe that many different genes contribute to an increased risk of schizophrenia, but that no single gene causes the disorder by itself. In fact, recent research has found that people with schizophrenia tend to have higher rates of rare genetic mutations. These genetic differences involve hundreds of different genes and probably disrupt brain development in diverse and subtle ways.

Research into various genes that are related to schizophrenia is ongoing, so it is not yet possible to use genetic information to predict who will develop the disease. Despite this, tests that scan a person's genes can be bought without a prescription or a health professional's advice. Ads for the tests suggest that with a saliva sample, a company can determine if a client is at risk for developing specific diseases, including schizophrenia. However, scientists don't yet know all of the gene variations that contribute to schizophrenia and those that are known raise the risk only by very small amounts. Therefore, these "genome scans" are unlikely to provide a complete picture of a person's risk for developing a mental disorder like schizophrenia.

In addition, it certainly takes more than genes to cause the disorder. Scientists think that interactions between genes and aspects of the individual's environment are necessary for schizophrenia to develop. Many environmental factors may be involved, such as exposure to viruses or malnutrition before birth, problems during birth, and other, not yet known, psychosocial factors.

Different Brain Chemistry and Structure

Scientists think that an imbalance in the complex, interrelated chemical reactions of the brain involving the neurotransmitters dopamine and glutamate, and possibly others, plays a role in schizophrenia. Neurotransmitters are substances that brain cells use to communicate with each other. Scientists are learning more about how brain chemistry is related to schizophrenia.

Also, the brain structures of some people with schizophrenia are slightly different than those of healthy people. For example, fluid-filled cavities at the center of the brain, called ventricles, are larger in some people with schizophrenia. The brains of people with the illness also tend to have less gray matter, and some areas of the brain may have less or more activity.

These differences are observed when brain scans from a group of people with schizophrenia are compared with those from a group of people without schizophrenia. However, the differences are not large enough to identify individuals with the disorder and are not currently used to diagnose schizophrenia.

Studies of brain tissue after death also have revealed differences in the brains of people with schizophrenia. Scientists have found small changes in the location or structure of brain cells that are formed before birth. Some experts think problems during brain development before birth may lead to faulty connections. The problem may not show up in a person until puberty. The brain undergoes major changes during puberty, and these changes could trigger psychotic symptoms in people who are vulnerable due to genetics or brain differences. Scientists have learned a lot about schizophrenia, but more research is needed to help explain how it develops.

How Is Schizophrenia Treated?

Because the causes of schizophrenia are still unknown, treatments focus on eliminating the symptoms of the disease. Treatments include antipsychotic medications and various psychosocial treatments. Research on "coordinated specialty care," where a case manager, the patient, and a medication and psychosocial treatment team work together, has shown promising results for recovery.

Antipsychotic Medications

Antipsychotic medications have been available since the mid-1950s. The older types are called conventional or typical antipsychotics.

In the 1990s, new antipsychotic medications were developed. These new medications are called second-generation or atypical antipsychotics.

What Are the Side Effects?

Some people have side effects when they start taking medications. Most side effects go away after a few days. Others are persistent but can often be managed successfully. People who are taking antipsychotic medications should not drive until they adjust to their new medication. Side effects of many antipsychotics include:

- drowsiness

- dizziness when changing positions

- blurred vision

- rapid heartbeat

- sensitivity to the sun

- skin rashes

Atypical antipsychotic medications can cause major weight gain and changes in a person's metabolism. This may increase a person's risk of getting diabetes and high cholesterol. A doctor should monitor a person's weight, glucose levels, and lipid levels regularly while the individual is taking an atypical antipsychotic medication.

Typical antipsychotic medications can cause side effects related to physical movement, such as:

- rigidity

- persistent muscle spasms

- tremors

- restlessness

Doctors and individuals should work together to choose the right medication, medication dose, and treatment plan, which should be based on a person's individual needs and medical situation.

Long-term use of typical antipsychotic medications may lead to a condition called tardive dyskinesia (TD). TD causes muscle movements a person can't control. The movements commonly happen around the mouth. TD can range from mild to severe, and in some people the problem cannot be cured. Sometimes people with TD recover partially or fully after they stop taking the medication.

TD happens to fewer people who take the atypical antipsychotics, but some people may still get TD. People who think that they might have TD should check with their doctor before stopping their medication.

How Are Antipsychotic Medications Taken, and How Do People Respond to Them?

Antipsychotic medications are usually taken daily in pill or liquid form. Some antipsychotics are injections that are given once or twice a month.

Symptoms of schizophrenia, such as feeling agitated and having hallucinations, usually improve within days after starting antipsychotic treatment. Symptoms like delusions usually improve within a few weeks. After about 6 weeks, many people will experience improvement in their symptoms. Some people will continue to have some symptoms, but usually medication helps to keep the symptoms from getting very intense.

However, people respond in different ways to antipsychotic medications, and no one can tell beforehand how a person will respond. Sometimes a person needs to try several medications before finding the right one. Doctors and patients can work together to find the best medication or medication combination, as well as the right dose.

Most people will have one or more periods of relapse—their symptoms come back or get worse. Usually, relapses happen when people stop taking their medication or when they take it less often than prescribed.

Some people stop taking the medication because they feel better or they may feel they don't need it anymore. But no one should stop taking an antipsychotic medication without first talking to his or her doctor. Medication should be gradually tapered off, never stopped suddenly.

How Do Antipsychotic Medications Interact with Other Medications?

Antipsychotic medications can produce unpleasant or dangerous side effects when taken with certain other medications. For this reason, all doctors treating a patient need to be aware of all the medications that person is taking. Doctors need to know about prescription and over-the-counter medicine, vitamins, minerals, and herbal supplements. People also need to discuss any alcohol or street drug use with their doctor.

Psychosocial Treatments

Psychosocial treatments can help people with schizophrenia who are already stabilized. Psychosocial treatments help individuals deal with the everyday challenges of their illness, such as difficulty with communication, work, and forming and keeping relationships. Learning and using coping skills to address these problems helps people with schizophrenia to pursue their life goals, such as attending school or work. Individuals who participate in regular psychosocial treatment are less likely to have relapses or be hospitalized.

Illness Management Skills

People with schizophrenia can take an active role in managing their own illness. Once they learn basic facts about schizophrenia and its treatment, they can make informed decisions about their care. If they know how to watch for the early warning signs of relapse and make a plan to respond, patients can learn to prevent relapses. Patients can also use coping skills to deal with persistent symptoms.

Rehabilitation

Rehabilitation emphasizes social and vocational training to help people with schizophrenia participate fully in their communities. Because schizophrenia usually develops during the critical career-development years (ages 18 to 35), the career and life trajectories for individuals with schizophrenia are usually interrupted and they need to learn new skills to get their work life back on track. Rehabilitation programs can include employment services, money management counseling, and skills training to maintain positive relationships.

Family Education and Support

Family education and support teaches relatives or interested individuals about schizophrenia and its treatment and strengthens their capacity to aid in their loved one's recovery.

Cognitive Behavioral Therapy

Cognitive behavioral therapy (CBT) is a type of psychotherapy that focuses on changing unhelpful patterns of thinking and behavior. The CBT therapist teaches people with schizophrenia how to test the reality of their thoughts and perceptions, how to "not listen" to their voices, and how to manage their symptoms overall. CBT can help reduce the severity of symptoms and reduce the risk of relapse. CBT can be delivered individually or in groups.

Self-Help Groups

In self-help groups for people with schizophrenia, group members support and comfort each other and share information on helpful coping strategies and services. Professional therapists usually are not involved. People in self-help groups know that others are facing the same problems, which can help everyone feel less isolated and more connected.

How Can You Help a Person with Schizophrenia?

Family and friends can help their loved one with schizophrenia by supporting their engagement in treatment and pursuit of their recovery goals. Positive communication approaches will be most helpful. It can be difficult to know how to respond to someone with schizophrenia who makes strange or clearly false statements. Remember that these beliefs or hallucinations seem very real to the person. It is not helpful to say they are wrong or imaginary. But going along with the delusions is not helpful, either. Instead, calmly say that you see things differently. Tell them that you acknowledge that everyone has the right to see things his or her own way. In addition, it is important to understand that schizophrenia is a biological illness. Being respectful, supportive, and kind without tolerating dangerous or inappropriate behavior is the best way to approach people with this disorder.

Chapter 45

Alcohol, Tobacco, and Drug Use in Men

Chapter Contents

Section 45.1—Alcohol: Frequently Asked Questions 612

Section 45.2—Smoking: Harmful Effects and
Benefits of Quitting 617

Section 45.3—Quitting Smoking 625

Section 45.4—Smokeless Tobacco 628

Section 45.5—Drugs: What You Should Know 630

Section 45.6—Anabolic Steroid Use 633

Section 45.1

Alcohol: Frequently Asked Questions

This section includes text excerpted from "Alcohol
and Public Health," Centers for Disease Control and
Prevention (CDC), February 29, 2016.

What Is Alcohol?

Ethyl alcohol, or ethanol, is an intoxicating ingredient found in
beer, wine, and liquor. Alcohol is produced by the fermentation of
yeast, sugars, and starches.

How Does Alcohol Affect a Person?

Alcohol affects every organ in the body. It is a central nervous system depressant that is rapidly absorbed from the stomach and small
intestine into the bloodstream. Alcohol is metabolized in the liver by
enzymes; however, the liver can only metabolize a small amount of
alcohol at a time, leaving the excess alcohol to circulate throughout
the body. The intensity of the effect of alcohol on the body is directly
related to the amount consumed.

Why Do Some People React Differently to Alcohol than Others?

Individual reactions to alcohol vary, and are influenced by many
factors; such as:

- age
- gender
- race or ethnicity
- physical condition (weight, fitness level, etc)
- amount of food consumed before drinking
- how quickly the alcohol was consumed
- use of drugs or prescription medicines
- family history of alcohol problems

What Is a Standard Drink in the United States?

A standard drink is equal to 14.0 grams (0.6 ounces) of pure alcohol. Generally, this amount of pure alcohol is found in

- 12-ounces of beer (5% alcohol content).

- 8-ounces of malt liquor (7% alcohol content).

- 5-ounces of wine (12% alcohol content).

- 1.5-ounces or a "shot" of 80-proof (40% alcohol content) distilled spirits or liquor (e.g., gin, rum, vodka, whiskey).

Is Beer or Wine Safer to Drink than Liquor?

No. One 12-ounce beer has about the same amount of alcohol as one 5-ounce glass of wine, or 1.5-ounce shot of liquor. It is the amount of alcohol consumed that affects a person most, not the type of alcoholic drink.

What Does Moderate Drinking Mean?

According to the *Dietary Guidelines for Americans*, moderate alcohol consumption is defined as having up to 2 drinks per day for men. This definition is referring to the amount consumed on any single day and is not intended as an average over several days. However, the *Dietary Guidelines* do not recommend that individuals who do not drink alcohol start drinking for any reason.

Is It Safe to Drink Alcohol and Drive?

No. Alcohol use slows reaction time and impairs judgment and coordination, which are all skills needed to drive a car safely. The more alcohol consumed, the greater the impairment.

What Does It Mean to Be above the Legal Limit for Drinking?

The legal limit for drinking is the alcohol level above which an individual is subject to legal penalties (e.g., arrest or loss of a driver's license).

- Legal limits are measured using either a blood alcohol test or a breathalyzer.

- Legal limits are typically defined by state law, and may vary based on individual characteristics, such as age and occupation.

All states in the United States have adopted 0.08% (80 mg/dL) as the legal limit for operating a motor vehicle for drivers aged 21 years or older. However, drivers younger than 21 are not allowed to operate a motor vehicle with any level of alcohol in their system.

Note: Legal limits do not define a level below which it is safe to operate a vehicle or engage in some other activity. Impairment due to alcohol use begins to occur at levels well below the legal limit.

How Do I Know If It's Okay to Drink?

According to the 2015–2020 *Dietary Guidelines for Americans*, some people should not drink alcoholic beverages at all, including:

- Anyone younger than age 21.

- Individuals who are driving, planning to drive, or are participating in other activities requiring skill, coordination, and alertness.

- Individuals taking certain prescription or over-the-counter medications that can interact with alcohol.

- Individuals with certain medical conditions.

- Persons recovering from alcoholism or are unable to control the amount they drink.

What Is Excessive Alcohol Use?

Excessive alcohol use includes binge drinking, heavy drinking, any alcohol use by people under the age 21 minimum legal drinking age, and any alcohol use by pregnant women.

What Is Binge Drinking?

According to the National Institute on Alcohol Abuse and Alcoholism (NIAAA) binge drinking is defined as a pattern of alcohol consumption that brings the blood alcohol concentration (BAC) level to 0.08% or more. This pattern of drinking usually corresponds to 5 or more drinks on a single occasion for men or 4 or more drinks on a single occasion for women, generally within about 2 hours.

What Do You Mean by Heavy Drinking?

For men, heavy drinking is typically defined as consuming 15 drinks or more per week. For women, heavy drinking is typically defined as consuming 8 drinks or more per week.

What Is the Difference between Alcoholism and Alcohol Abuse?

Alcohol abuse is a pattern of drinking that results in harm to one's health, interpersonal relationships, or ability to work. Manifestations of alcohol abuse include the following:

• Failure to fulfill major responsibilities at work, school, or home.

• Drinking in dangerous situations, such as drinking while driving or operating machinery.

• Legal problems related to alcohol, such as being arrested for drinking while driving or for physically hurting someone while drunk.

• Continued drinking despite ongoing relationship problems that are caused or worsened by drinking.

• Long-term alcohol abuse can turn into alcohol dependence.

Dependency on alcohol, also known as alcohol addiction and alcoholism, is a chronic disease. The signs and symptoms of alcohol dependence include—

• A strong craving for alcohol.

• Continued use despite repeated physical, psychological, or interpersonal problems.

• The inability to limit drinking.

What Does It Mean to Get Drunk?

"Getting drunk" or intoxicated is the result of consuming excessive amounts of alcohol. Binge drinking typically results in acute intoxication.

Alcohol intoxication can be harmful for a variety of reasons, including—

• Impaired brain function resulting in poor judgment, reduced reaction time, loss of balance and motor skills, or slurred speech.

- Dilation of blood vessels causing a feeling of warmth but resulting in rapid loss of body heat.

- Increased risk of certain cancers, stroke, and liver diseases (e.g., cirrhosis), particularly when excessive amounts of alcohol are consumed over extended periods of time.

- Increased risk of motor-vehicle traffic crashes, violence, and other injuries.

Coma and death can occur if alcohol is consumed rapidly and in large amounts.

How Do I Know If I Have a Drinking Problem?

Drinking is a problem if it causes trouble in your relationships, in school, in social activities, or in how you think and feel. If you are concerned that either you or someone in your family might have a drinking problem, consult your personal healthcare provider.

What Can I Do If I or Someone I Know Has a Drinking Problem?

Consult your personal healthcare provider if you feel you or someone you know has a drinking problem. Other resources include the National Drug and Alcohol Treatment Referral Routing Service available at 1-800-662-HELP (1-800-662-4357). This service can provide you with information about treatment programs in your local community and allow you to speak with someone about alcohol problems.

What Health Problems Are Associated with Excessive Alcohol Use?

Excessive drinking both in the form of heavy drinking or binge drinking, is associated with numerous health problems, including—

- Chronic diseases such as liver cirrhosis (damage to liver cells); pancreatitis (inflammation of the pancreas); various cancers, including liver, mouth, throat, larynx (the voice box), and esophagus; high blood pressure; and psychological disorders.

- Unintentional injuries, such as motor-vehicle traffic crashes, falls, drowning, burns and firearm injuries.

- Violence, such as child maltreatment, homicide, and suicide.
- Alcohol abuse or dependence.

I'm Young. Is Drinking Bad for My Health?

Yes. Studies have shown that alcohol use by youth and young adults increases the risk of both fatal and nonfatal injuries. Research has also shown that youth who use alcohol before age 15 are six times more likely to become alcohol dependent than adults who begin drinking at age 21. Other consequences of youth alcohol use include increased risky sexual behaviors, poor school performance, and increased risk of suicide and homicide.

Section 45.2

Smoking: Harmful Effects and Benefits of Quitting

This section contains text excerpted from the following sources:
Text beginning with the heading "Health Effects" is excerpted from
"Health Effects," Smokefree.gov, National Cancer Institute (NCI),
June 29, 2016; Text beginning with the heading "Benefits of
Quitting" is excerpted from "Benefits of Quitting," Smokefree.gov,
National Cancer Institute (NCI), June 29, 2016.

Health Effects

Smoking harms nearly every organ of the body. Some of these harmful effects are immediate.

Brain

Addiction. Nicotine from cigarettes is as addictive as heroin. Nicotine addiction is hard to beat because it changes your brain. The brain develops extra nicotine receptors to accommodate the large doses of nicotine from tobacco. When the brain stops getting the nicotine it's used to, the result is nicotine withdrawal. You may feel anxious, irritable, and have strong cravings for nicotine.

Head and Face

Ears

Hearing loss. Smoking reduces the oxygen supply to the cochlea, a snail-shaped organ in the inner ear. This may result in permanent damage to the cochlea and mild to moderate hearing loss.

Eyes

Blindness and night vision. Smoking causes physical changes in the eyes that can threaten your eyesight. Nicotine from cigarettes restricts the production of a chemical necessary for you to be able to see at night. Also, smoking increases your risk of developing cataracts and macular degeneration (both can lead to blindness).

Mouth

Cavities. Smoking takes a toll on your mouth. Smokers have more oral health problems than non-smokers, like mouth sores, ulcers and gum disease. You are more likely to have cavities and lose your teeth at a younger age. You are also more likely to get cancers of the mouth and throat.

Face

Smoker's face. Smoking can cause your skin to be dry and lose elasticity, leading to wrinkles and stretch marks. Your skin tone may become dull and grayish. By your early 30s, wrinkles can begin to appear around your mouth and eyes, adding years to your face.

Heart

Stressed Heart

Smoking raises your blood pressure and puts stress on your heart. Over time, stress on the heart can weaken it, making it less able to pump blood to other parts of your body. Carbon monoxide from inhaled cigarette smoke also contributes to a lack of oxygen, making the heart work even harder. This increases the risk of heart disease, including heart attacks.

Sticky Blood

Smoking makes your blood thick and sticky. The stickier the blood, the harder your heart must work to move it around your body. Sticky blood is also more likely to form blood clots that block blood flow to your heart, brain, and legs. Over time, thick, sticky blood damages the delicate lining of your blood vessels. This damage can increase your risk for a heart attack or stroke.

Fatty Deposits

Smoking increases the cholesterol and unhealthy fats circulating in the blood, leading to unhealthy fatty deposits. Over time, cholesterol, fats, and other debris build up on the walls of your arteries. This buildup narrow-no-jss the arteries and blocks normal blood flow to the heart, brain, and legs. Blocked blood flow to the heart or brain can cause a heart attack or stroke. Blockage in the blood vessels of your legs could result in the amputation of your toes or feet.

Lungs

Scarred Lung

Smoking causes inflammation in the small airways and tissues of your lungs. This can make your chest feel tight or cause you to wheeze or feel short of breath. Continued inflammation builds up scar tissue, which leads to physical changes to your lungs and airways that can make breathing hard. Years of lung irritation can give you a chronic cough with mucus.

Emphysema

Smoking destroys the tiny air sacs, or alveoli, in the lungs that allow oxygen exchange. When you smoke, you are damaging some of those air sacs. Alveoli don't grow back, so when you destroy them, you have permanently destroyed part of your lungs. When enough alveoli are destroyed, the disease emphysema develops. Emphysema causes severe shortness of breath and can lead to death.

Cilia and Respiratory Infections

Your airways are lined with tiny brush like hairs, called cilia. The cilia sweep out mucus and dirt so your lungs stay clear. Smoking temporarily paralyzes and even kills cilia. This makes you more at risk for infection. Smokers get more colds and respiratory infections than non-smokers.

DNA

Cancer

Your body is made up of cells that contain genetic material, or DNA, that acts as an "instruction manual" for cell growth and function. Every single puff of a cigarette causes damages to your DNA. When DNA is damaged, the "instruction manual" gets messed up, and the cell can begin growing out of control and create a cancer tumor. Your body tries to repair the damage that smoking does to your DNA, but over time, smoking can wear down this repair system and lead to cancer (like lung cancer). One-third of all cancer deaths are caused by tobacco.

Stomach and Hormones

Belly

Bigger belly. Smokers have bigger bellies and less muscle than non-smokers. They are more likely to develop type 2 diabetes, even if they don't smoke every day. Smoking also makes it harder to control diabetes once you already have it. Diabetes is a serious disease that can lead to blindness, heart disease, kidney failure, and amputations.

Erectile Dysfunction

Failure to Launch

Smoking increases the risk of erectile dysfunction—the inability to get or keep and erection. Toxins from cigarette smoke can also damage the genetic material in sperm, which can cause infertility or genetic defects in your children.

Blood and the Immune System

High White Blood Cell Count

When you smoke, the number of white blood cells (the cells that defend your body from infections) stays high. This is a sign that your body is under stress—constantly fighting against the inflammation and damage caused by tobacco. A high white blood cell count is like a signal from your body, letting you know you've been injured. White blood cell counts that stay elevated for a long time are linked with an increased risk of heart attacks, strokes, and cancer.

Longer to Heal

Nutrients, minerals, and oxygen are all supplied to the tissue through the blood stream. Nicotine causes blood vessels to tighten, which decreases levels of nutrients supplied to wounds. As a result, wounds take longer to heal. Slow wound healing increases the risk of infection after an injury or surgery and painful skin ulcers can develop, causing the tissue to slowly die.

Weakened Immune System

Cigarette smoke contains high levels of tar and other chemicals, which can make your immune system less effective at fighting off infections. This means you're more likely to get sick. Continued weakening of the immune system can make you more vulnerable to autoimmune diseases like rheumatoid arthritis and multiple sclerosis. It also decreases your body's ability to fight off cancer!

Muscles and Bones

Tired Muscles

Muscle deterioration. When you smoke, less blood and oxygen flow to your muscles, making it harder to build muscle. The lack of oxygen also makes muscles tire more easily. Smokers have more muscle aches and pains than non-smokers.

More Broken Bones

Ingredients in cigarette smoke disrupt the natural cycle of bone health. Your body is less able to form healthy new bone tissue, and it breaks down existing bone tissue more rapidly. Over time, smoking leads to a thinning of bone tissue and loss of bone density. This causes bones to become weak and brittle. Compared to non-smokers, smokers have a higher risk of bone fractures, and their broken bones take longer to heal.

Benefits of Quitting

Quitting smoking can help most of the major parts of your body: from your brain to your DNA.

Brain

Broken Addiction Cycle

Quitting smoking can re-wire your brain and help break the cycle of addiction. The large number of nicotine receptors in your brain will return to normal levels after about a month of being quit.

Head and Face

Sharp Hearing

Quitting smoking will keep your hearing sharp. Remember, even mild hearing loss can cause problems (like not hearing directions correctly and doing a task wrong).

Better Vision

Quitting smoking will improve your night vision and help preserve your overall vision by stopping the damage that smoking does to your eyes.

Clean Mouth

Nobody likes a dirty mouth. After a few days without cigarettes, your smile will be brighter. Quitting smoking now will keep your mouth healthy for years to come.

Clear Skin

Quitting smoking is better than anti-aging lotion. Quitting can help clear up blemishes and protect your skin from premature aging and wrinkling.

Heart

Decreased Heart Risks

Smoking is the leading cause of heart attacks and heart disease. But many of these heart risks can be reversed simply by quitting smoking. Quitting can lower your blood pressure and heart rate almost immediately. Your risk of a heart attack declines within 24 hours.

Thin Blood

When you quit smoking, your blood will become thinner and less likely to form dangerous blood clots. Your heart will also have less work to do, because it will be able to move the blood around your body more easily.

Lower Cholesterol

Quitting smoking will not get rid of the fatty deposits that are already there. But it will lower the levels of cholesterol and fats circulating in your blood, which will help to slow the buildup of new fatty deposits in your arteries.

Lungs

Stop Lung Damage

Scarring of the lungs is not reversible. That is why it is important to quit smoking before you do permanent damage to your lungs. Within two weeks of quitting, you might notice it's easier to walk up the stairs because you may be less short of breath. Don't wait until later; quit today!

Prevent Emphysema

There is no cure for emphysema. But quitting when you are young, before you have done years of damage to the delicate air sacs in your lungs, will help protect you from developing emphysema later.

Return of Cilia

Cilia start to regrow and re-gain normal function very quickly after you quit smoking. They are one of the first things in your body to heal. People sometimes notice that they cough more than usual when they first quit smoking. This is a sign that the cilia are coming back to life. But you're more likely to fight off colds and infections when you're cilia are working properly.

DNA

Lower Cancer Risk

Quitting smoking will prevent new DNA damage from happening and can even help repair the damage that has already been done. Quitting smoking immediately is the best way to lower your risk of getting cancer.

Stomach and Hormones

Smaller Belly

Quitting smoking will reduce your belly fat and lower your risk of diabetes. If you already have diabetes, quitting can help you keep your blood sugar levels in check.

Erectile Dysfunction

Sexual Healing

If you quit smoking now, you can lower your chances of erectile dysfunction and improve your chances of having a healthy sexual life.

Blood and the Immune System

Normal White Blood Cell Count

When you quit smoking, your body will begin to heal from the injuries that smoking caused. Eventually, your white blood cell counts will return to normal and will no longer be on the defensive.

Proper Healing

Quitting smoking will improve blood flow to wounds, allowing important nutrients, minerals, and oxygen to reach the wound and help it heal properly.

Stronger Immune System

When you quit smoking, your immune system is no longer exposed to tar and nicotine. It will become stronger, and you will be less likely to get sick.

Muscles and Bones

Strong Muscles

Quitting smoking will help increase the availability of oxygen in your blood, and your muscles will become stronger and healthier.

Stronger Bones

Quitting smoking can reduce your risk of fractures, both now and later in life. Keep your bones strong and healthy by quitting now.

Section 45.3

Quitting Smoking

This section includes text excerpted from "Quitting Smoking," Centers for Disease Control and Prevention (CDC), February 17, 2016.

What You Need to Know about Quitting Smoking

- Tobacco use can lead to tobacco/nicotine dependence and serious health problems. Quitting smoking greatly reduces the risk of developing smoking-related diseases.

- Tobacco/nicotine dependence is a condition that often requires repeated treatments, but there are helpful treatments and resources for quitting.

- Smokers can and do quit smoking. In fact, there are more former smokers than current smokers.

Nicotine Dependence

- Most smokers become addicted to nicotine, a drug that is found naturally in tobacco.

- More people in the United States are addicted to nicotine than to any other drug. Research suggests that nicotine may be as addictive as heroin, cocaine, or alcohol.

- Quitting smoking is hard and may require several attempts. People who stop smoking often start again because of withdrawal symptoms, stress, and weight gain.

- Nicotine withdrawal symptoms may include:
  - Feeling irritable, angry, or anxious
  - Having trouble thinking
  - Craving tobacco products
  - Feeling hungrier than usual

Health Benefits of Quitting

Tobacco smoke contains a deadly mix of more than 7,000 chemicals; hundreds are harmful, and about 70 can cause cancer. Smoking increases the risk for serious health problems, many diseases, and death.

People who stop smoking greatly reduce their risk for disease and early death. Although the health benefits are greater for people who stop at earlier ages, there are benefits at any age. You are never too old to quit.

Stopping smoking is associated with the following health benefits:

- Lowered risk for lung cancer and many other types of cancer.

- Reduced risk for heart disease, stroke, and peripheral vascular disease (narrowing of the blood vessels outside your heart).

- Reduced heart disease risk within 1 to 2 years of quitting.

- Reduced respiratory symptoms, such as coughing, wheezing, and shortness of breath. While these symptoms may not disappear, they do not continue to progress at the same rate among people who quit compared with those who continue to smoke.

- Reduced risk of developing some lung diseases (such as chronic obstructive pulmonary disease, also known as COPD, one of the leading causes of death in the United States).

Smokers' Attempts to Quit

Percentage of adult daily cigarette smokers who stopped smoking for more than 1 day in 2012 because they were trying to quit:

- More than 4 out of 10 (42.7%) of all adult smokers

- Nearly 5 out of 10 (48.5%) smokers aged 18–24 years

- More than 4 out of 10 (46.8%) smokers aged 25–44 years

- Nearly 4 out of 10 (38.8%) smokers aged 45–64 years

- More than 3 out of 10 (34.6%) smokers aged 65 years or older

Ways to Quit Smoking

Most former smokers quit without using one of the treatments that scientific research has shown can work. However,

the following treatments are proven to be effective for smokers who want help to quit:

- Brief help by a doctor (such as when a doctor takes 10 minutes or less to give a patient advice and assistance about quitting)

- Individual, group, or telephone counseling

- Behavioral therapies (such as training in problem solving)

- Treatments with more person-to-person contact and more intensity (such as more or longer counseling sessions)

- Programs to deliver treatments using mobile phones

Medications for quitting that have been found to be effective include the following:

- Nicotine replacement products

  - Over-the-counter (nicotine patch [which is also available by prescription], gum, lozenge)

  - Prescription (nicotine patch, inhaler, nasal spray)

- Prescription non-nicotine medications: bupropion SR (Zyban®),6 varenicline tartrate (Chantix®)

Counseling and medication are both effective for treating tobacco dependence, and using them together is more effective than using either one alone.

- More information is needed about quitting for people who smoke cigarettes and also use other types of tobacco.

Section 45.4

Smokeless Tobacco

This section includes text excerpted from "Smoking and Tobacco Use," Centers for Disease Control and Prevention (CDC), February 18, 2016.

What Is Smokeless Tobacco?

Smokeless tobacco:

- Is not burned

- Includes tobacco that can be sucked or chewed

- Can be spit or swallowed, depending on the product

- Can be spitless, depending on the product

- Contains nicotine and is addictive

- May appeal to youth because it comes in flavors such as cinnamon, berry, vanilla, and apple

Types of smokeless tobacco:

- Chewing tobacco (loose leaf, plug, or twist and may come in flavors)

- Snuff (moist, dry, or in packets [U.S. snus])

- Dissolvables (lozenges, sticks, strips, orbs)

Overview

Smokeless tobacco is associated with many health problems. Using smokeless tobacco:

- Can lead to nicotine addiction

- Causes cancer of the mouth, esophagus (the passage that connects the throat to the stomach), and pancreas (a gland that helps with digestion and maintaining proper blood sugar levels)

- Is associated with diseases of the mouth
- Can cause nicotine poisoning in children
- May increase the risk for death from heart disease and stroke

Addiction to Smokeless Tobacco

- Smokeless tobacco contains nicotine, which is highly addictive.
- Because young people who use smokeless tobacco can become addicted to nicotine, they may be more likely to also become cigarette smokers.

Smokeless Tobacco and Cancer

- Many smokeless tobacco products contain cancer-causing chemicals.
  - The most harmful chemicals are tobacco-specific nitrosamines, which form during the growing, curing, fermenting, and aging of tobacco. The amount of these chemicals varies by product.
  - The higher the levels of these chemicals, the greater the risk for cancer.
  - Other chemicals found in tobacco can also cause cancer. These include:
  - A radioactive element (polonium-210) found in tobacco fertilizer
  - Chemicals formed when tobacco is cured with heat (polynuclear aromatic hydrocarbons—also known as polycyclic aromatic hydrocarbons)
  - Harmful metals (arsenic, beryllium, cadmium, chromium, cobalt, lead, nickel, mercury)
- Smokeless tobacco causes cancer of the mouth, esophagus, and pancreas.

Smokeless Tobacco and Oral Disease

- Smokeless tobacco can cause white or gray patches inside the mouth (leukoplakia) that can lead to cancer.
- Smokeless tobacco can cause gum disease, tooth decay, and tooth loss.

Other Risks

- Using smokeless tobacco increases the risk for death from heart disease and stroke.

- Smokeless tobacco can cause nicotine poisoning in children.

- Additional research is needed to examine long-term effects of newer smokeless tobacco products, such as dissolvables and U.S. snus.

Section 45.5

Drugs: What You Should Know

Medicines Are Legal Drugs

If you've ever been sick and had to take medicine, you already know about one kind of drugs. Medicines are legal drugs, meaning doctors are allowed to prescribe them for patients, stores can sell them, and people are allowed to buy them. But it's not legal, or safe, for people to use these medicines any way they want or to buy them from people who are selling them illegally.

Cigarettes and Alcohol

Cigarettes and alcohol are two other kinds of legal drugs. (In the United States, adults 18 and older can buy cigarettes and those 21 and older can buy alcohol.) But smoking and excessive drinking are not healthy for adults and are off limits for kids.

Illegal Drugs

When people talk about a "drug problem," they usually mean abusing legal drugs or using illegal drugs, such as marijuana, ecstasy, cocaine, LSD, crystal meth, and heroin. (Marijuana is generally an illegal drug, but some states allow doctors to recommend it to adults for certain illnesses.)

Why Are Illegal Drugs Dangerous?

Illegal drugs aren't good for anyone, but they are particularly bad for a kid or teen whose body is still growing. Illegal drugs can damage the brain, heart, and other important organs. Cocaine, for instance, can cause a heart attack—even in a kid or teen.

While using drugs, people are also less able to do well in school, sports, and other activities. It's often harder to think clearly and make good decisions. People can do dumb or dangerous things that could hurt them—or other people—when they use drugs.

Why Do People Use Illegal Drugs?

Sometimes kids and teens try drugs to fit in with a group of friends. Or they might be curious or just bored. Someone may use illegal drugs for many reasons, but often because they help the person escape from reality for a while. A drug might—temporarily—make someone who is sad or upset feel better or forget about problems. But this escape lasts only until the drug wears off.

Drugs don't solve problems, of course. And using drugs often causes other problems on top of the problems the person had in the first place. Somebody who uses drugs can become dependent on them, or **addicted**. This means that the person's body becomes so accustomed to having this drug that he or she can't function well without it.

Once someone is addicted, it's very hard to stop taking drugs. Stopping can cause withdrawal symptoms, such as vomiting (throwing up), sweating, and tremors (shaking). These sick feelings continue until the person's body gets adjusted to being drug free again.

Table 45.1. Drugs with Street Names

Drugs	Street Names	Common Ways Taken
Cocaine	Blow, Bump, C, Candy, Charlie, Coke, Crack, Flake, Rock, Snow, Toot	Snorted, smoked, injected
GHB	G, Georgia Home Boy, Goop, Grievous Bodily Harm, Liquid Ecstasy, Liquid X, Soap, Scoop	Swallowed (often combined with alcohol or other beverages)

Table 45.1. Continued

Drugs	Street Names	Common Ways Taken
Heroin	Brown sugar, China White, Dope, H, Horse, Junk, Skag, Skunk, Smack, White Horse	Injected, smoked, snorted
Inhalants	Poppers, snappers, whippets, laughing gas	Inhaled through the nose or mouth
Ketamine	Cat Valium, K, Special K, Vitamin K	Injected, snorted, smoked (powder added to tobacco or marijuana cigarettes), swallowed
LSD	Acid, Blotter, Blue Heaven, Cubes, Microdot, Yellow Sunshine	Swallowed, absorbed through mouth tissues (paper squares)
Marijuana (Cannabis)	Blunt, Bud, Dope, Ganja, Grass, Green, Herb, Joint, Mary Jane, Pot, Reefer, Sinsemilla, Skunk, Smoke, Trees, Weed; Hashish: Boom, Gangster, Hash, Hemp	Smoked, eaten (mixed in food or brewed as tea)
Methamphetamine	Crank, Chalk, Crystal, Fire, Glass, Go Fast, Ice, Meth, Speed	Swallowed, snorted, smoked, injected
Cough/Cold Medicines (DXM)	Robotripping, Robo, Triple C	Swallowed
Rohypnol (Flunitrazepam)	Circles, Date Rape Drug, Forget Pill, Forget-Me Pill, La Rocha, Lunch Money, Mexican Valium, Mind Eraser, Pingus, R2, Reynolds, Rib, Roach, Roach 2, Roaches, Roachies, Roapies, Rochas Dos, Roofies, Rope, Rophies, Row-Shay, Ruffies, Trip-and-Fall, Wolfies	Swallowed (as a pill or as dissolved in a drink), snorted

Commonly Abused Drugs Charts, National Institute on Drug Abuse (NIDA), April 2016.

Section 45.6

Anabolic Steroid Use

This section includes text excerpted from "Anabolic Steroids,"
National Institute on Drug Abuse (NIDA), March 6, 2016.

What Are Anabolic Steroids?

Anabolic steroids are synthetic variations of the male sex hormone testosterone. The proper term for these compounds is *anabolic-andro-genic steroids*. "Anabolic" refers to muscle building, and "androgenic" refers to increased male sex characteristics. Some common names for anabolic steroids are Gear, Juice, Roids, and Stackers.

Healthcare providers can prescribe steroids to treat hormonal issues, such as delayed puberty. Steroids can also treat diseases that cause muscle loss, such as cancer and AIDS. But some athletes and bodybuilders abuse these drugs to boost performance or improve their physical appearance.

How Do People Abuse Anabolic Steroids?

People who abuse anabolic steroids usually take them orally or inject them into the muscles. These doses may be 10 to 100 times higher than doses prescribed to treat medical conditions. Steroids are also applied to the skin as a cream, gel, or patch. Some athletes and others who abuse steroids believe that they can avoid unwanted side effects or maximize the drugs' effects by taking them in ways that include:

- cycling—taking doses for a period of time, stopping for a time, and then restarting

- stacking—combining two or more different types of steroids

- pyramiding—slowly increasing the dose or frequency of abuse, reaching a peak amount, and then gradually tapering off

There is no scientific evidence that any of these practices reduce the harmful medical consequences of these drugs.

How Do Anabolic Steroids Affect the Brain?

Anabolic steroids work differently from other drugs of abuse; they do not have the same shortterm effects on the brain. The most important difference is that steroids do not trigger rapid increases in the brain chemical dopamine, which causes the "high" that drives people to abuse other substances. However, long-term steroid abuse can act on some of the same brain pathways and chemicals—including dopamine, serotonin, and opioid systems—that are affected by other drugs. This may result in a significant effect on mood and behavior.

Short-Term Effects

- Abuse of anabolic steroids may lead to mental problems, such as:

- paranoid (extreme, unreasonable)

- jealousy extreme irritability

- *delusions*—false beliefs or ideas

- impaired judgment

Extreme mood swings can also occur, including "roid rage"—angry feelings and behavior that may lead to violence.

What Are Other Health Effects of Anabolic Steroids?

Aside from mental problems, steroid use commonly causes severe acne. It also causes the body to swell, especially in the hands and feet.

Long-Term Effects

Anabolic steroid abuse may lead to serious, even permanent, health problems such as:

- kidney problems or failure

- liver damage

- enlarged heart, high blood pressure, and changes in blood cholesterol, all of which increase the risk of stroke and heart attack, even in young people

Several other effects are:

- In men:

  - shrinking testicles

- decreased sperm count
- baldness
- development of breasts
- increased risk for prostate cancer
- In teens:
  - stunted growth (when high hormone levels from steroids signal to the body to stop bone growth too early)
  - stunted height (if teens use steroids before their growth spurt)

Some of these physical changes, such as shrinking sex organs in men, can add to mental side effects such as mood disorders.

Are Anabolic Steroids Addictive?

Even though anabolic steroids do not cause the same high as other drugs, they can lead to addiction. Studies have shown that animals will self-administer steroids when they have the chance, just as they do with other addictive drugs. People may continue to abuse steroids despite physical problems, high costs to buy the drugs, and negative effects on their relationships. These behaviors reflect steroids' addictive potential. Research has further found that some steroid users turn to other drugs, such as opioids, to reduce sleep problems and irritability caused by steroids.

People who abuse steroids may experience withdrawal symptoms when they stop use, including:

- mood swings
- fatigue
- restlessness
- loss of appetite
- sleep problems
- decreased sex drive
- steroid cravings

One of the more serious withdrawal symptoms is depression, which can sometimes lead to suicide attempts.

How Can People Get Treatment for Anabolic Steroid Addiction?

Some people seeking treatment for anabolic steroid addiction have found behavioral therapy to be helpful. More research is needed to identify the most effective treatment options.

In certain cases of severe addiction, patients have taken medicines to help treat symptoms of withdrawal. For example, healthcare providers have prescribed anti-depressants to treat depression and pain medicines for headaches and muscle and joint pain. Other medicines have been used to help restore the patient's hormonal system.

Chapter 46

Violence Against Men

Chapter Contents

Section 46.1—Myths and Realities of Domestic
     Abuse Against Men 638

Section 46.2—Sexual Assault of Men 641

Section 46.1

Myths and Realities of Domestic Abuse Against Men

"Myths and Realities of Domestic Abuse against Men,"
© 2017 Omnigraphics. Reviewed August 2016.

Domestic or intimate partner abuse can be defined as a pattern of behaviors—including physical and sexual violence, verbal and emotional abuse, or stalking—used by one partner in a relationship to coerce, intimidate, and gain power and control over the other partner. When most people think about domestic violence or intimate partner abuse, they envision a male perpetrating abuse against a female victim. This is the scenario that is most often presented in the media.

In reality, however, domestic abuse can and does affect men as well as women. Studies have shown that one in every seven men in the United States has been the victim of physical violence by an intimate partner, while one in every ten men has experienced rape or stalking by an intimate partner. Experts believe that these figures underrepresent the true extent of the problem, though, because male victims are less likely to report incidents of domestic violence or seek support for intimate partner abuse.

The topic of domestic abuse against men is surrounded by cultural myths and stereotypes. It is important to examine these myths with a critical eye in order to understand the reality of the problem and ensure that services and support are available for men who need help. Some of the common myths of domestic abuse against men include the following:

- **Any man who allows himself to be the victim of abuse must be weak.**

  The cultural image of manliness leads many people to believe that a "real" man would fight back rather than submit to abuse, especially from a woman. In reality, male victims of domestic abuse often have many reasons for not defending themselves against an intimate partner's assaults. Some have been taught that it is wrong for a man to strike a woman, no matter the circumstances. Others restrain themselves because they realize that their superior size and strength means that they could cause serious physical harm to their partner if they fought back. Finally, some men worry that any actions taken to protect themselves could be misinterpreted and cause them to be arrested as the perpetrator of the abuse.

- **In a domestic dispute, the bigger, stronger person is always the aggressor.**

Many people assume that women cannot be perpetrators of domestic abuse because they are usually smaller and weaker than their male partners. In reality, though, physical size and strength has no bearing on whether a person will be an abuser or a victim of abuse. Many strong people are nonviolent, while even small, frail people can use threats, intimidation, or weapons to coerce or gain power over an intimate partner.

- **Men should not express feelings or share details of their personal lives.**

From an early age, many boys are taught that it is not "manly" to cry, express emotions, or talk openly about their problems. As a result, they grow up believing that their only choice in confronting a difficult situation is to "suck it up" and deal with it on their own. For men who find themselves in abusive relationships, this ingrained attitude may prevent them from acknowledging the abuse or seeking help.

- **Domestic abuse against men is not as serious as domestic abuse against women.**

Some people tend to treat domestic abuse against men as a joke or fail to take it seriously. While the media tends to portray female victims sympathetically, male victims are often treated with scorn, sarcasm, or snide remarks. But domestic abuse is no laughing matter in any situation and can have serious consequences for victims. In fact, studies show that male victims of intimate partner violence are significantly more likely to report physical and mental health problems than non-victims.

- **Intimate partner abuse does not impact children in the home.**

Some people believe that children do not notice domestic abuse or at least do not suffer lasting effects from it. But domestic violence is a learned behavior, and witnessing abuse in the home increases the likelihood that children will eventually choose violent partners or become abusers themselves. In addition, intimate partner abuse creates a climate of fear and insecurity in the home that may lead children to develop behavioral problems or addiction issues as they get older.

- **If a man is really being abused, he can simply leave the relationship.**

  Many people assume that men face fewer obstacles to leaving an abusive relationship than women, who are more likely to be financially dependent on their abusive partners. But leaving an abusive relationship can be extremely difficult, and it requires money, transportation, housing, and support. Male victims may have many concerns that prevent them from leaving, including fear for the safety of their children; worry that they will be prevented from seeing their children; love and commitment to their partner; a belief that their partner will change; embarrassment about their situation; or confusion about where to go or how to get help. Some men worry that trying to leave will only make the situation worse, since incidents of domestic violence tend to become more severe if the victim attempts to get out of the relationship.

- **There are plenty of shelters and support services available for male victims.**

  Although domestic violence programs must provide services to all victims of abuse in order to receive federal funding, many organizations and shelters are focused on helping women. In fact, some male victims of intimate partner abuse are turned away from women's shelters and referred to local homeless shelters. In addition, few support groups are available to male survivors of domestic violence, and those that are available tend to be aimed at GLBT (gay, lesbian, bisexual, and transsexual) people rather than straight men. Support groups are an important part of the healing process, offering survivors an opportunity to share information and experiences with one another. Men who experience domestic violence need access to such services in order to understand that—despite cultural myths and stereotypes to the contrary—they are not alone.

References

1. "Common Myths about Intimate Partner Abuse against Men," Domestic Abuse Hotline for Men and Women, 2012.
2. "Men Can Be Victims of Abuse Too," National Domestic Violence Hotline, July 22, 2014.

Section 46.2

Sexual Assault of Men

This section includes text excerpted from "Men and Sexual Trauma,"
U.S. Department of Veterans Affairs (VA), April 18, 2016.

At least 1 out of every 10 (or 10%) of men in our country have suffered from trauma as a result of sexual assault. Like women, men who experience sexual assault may suffer from depression, posttraumatic stress disorder (PTSD), and other emotional problems as a result. However, because men and women have different life experiences due to their different gender roles, emotional symptoms following trauma can look different in men than they do in women.

Who Are the Perpetrators of Male Sexual Assault?

- Those who sexually assault men or boys differ in a number of ways from those who assault only females.

- Boys are more likely than girls to be sexually abused by strangers or by authority figures in organizations such as schools, the church, or athletics programs.

- Those who sexually assault males usually choose young men and male adolescents (the average age is 17 years old) as their victims and are more likely to assault many victims, compared to those who sexually assault females.

- Perpetrators often assault young males in isolated areas where help is not readily available. For instance, a perpetrator who assaults males may pick up a teenage hitchhiker on a remote road or find some other way to isolate his intended victim.

- As is true about those who assault and sexually abuse women and girls, most perpetrators of males are men. Specifically, men are perpetrators in about 86 out of every 100 (or 86%) of male victimization cases.

- Despite popular belief that only gay men would sexually assault men or boys, most male perpetrators identify themselves as heterosexuals and often have consensual sexual relationships with women.

What Are Some Symptoms Related to Sexual Trauma in Boys and Men?

Particularly when the assailant is a woman, the impact of sexual assault upon men may be downplayed by professionals and the public. However, men who have early sexual experiences with adults report problems in various areas at a much higher rate than those who do not.

Emotional Disorders

Men and boys who have been sexually assaulted are more likely to suffer from PTSD, anxiety disorders, and depression than those who have never been abused sexually.

Substance Abuse

Men who have been sexually assaulted have a high incidence of alcohol and drug use. For example, the probability for alcohol problems in adulthood is about 80 out of every 100 (or 80%) for men who have experienced sexual abuse, as compared to 11 out of every 100 (or 11%) for men who have never been sexually abused.

Risk Taking Behavior

Exposure to sexual trauma can lead to risk-taking behavior during adolescence, such as running away and other delinquent behaviors. Having been sexually assaulted also makes boys more likely to engage in behaviors that put them at risk for contracting HIV (such as having sex without using condoms).

Help for Men Who Have Been Sexually Assaulted

Men who have been assaulted often feel stigmatized, which can be the most damaging aspect of the assault. It is important for men to discuss the assault with a caring and unbiased support person, whether that person is a friend, clergyman, or clinician. However, it is vital that this person be knowledgeable about sexual assault and men.

A local rape crisis center may be able to refer men to mental-health practitioners who are well-informed about the needs of male sexual assault victims. If you are a man who has been assaulted and you suffer from any of these difficulties, please seek help from a mental-health professional who has expertise working with men who have been sexually assaulted.

Chapter 47

A Guy's Guide to Body Image

The Truth about Guys

Many people think of guys as being carefree when it comes to their appearance. But the reality is that a lot of guys spend plenty of time in front of the mirror. It's a fact—some guys care just as much as girls do about their appearance.

You may hear a lot about being a tough guy, but how often do you hear that being a guy is tough? Guys might think that they shouldn't worry about how they look, but body image can be a real problem for them. Unlike girls, guys are less likely to talk to friends and relatives about their bodies and how they're developing. Without support from friends and family, they may develop a negative self-image.

The good news is that self-image and body image can be changed.

Why Is Body Image Important?

Body image is a person's opinions, thoughts, and feelings about his or her own body and physical appearance. Having a positive body image means feeling pretty satisfied with the way you look, appreciating your body for its capabilities and accepting its imperfections.

Body image is part of someone's total self-image. So how a guy feels about his body can affect how he feels about himself. If he gets too focused on not liking the way he looks, a guy's self-esteem can take a hit and his confidence can slide.

How Puberty Affects Body Image

Although body image is just one part of our self-image, during the teen years, and especially during puberty, it can be easy for a guy's whole self-image to be based on how his body looks. That's because our bodies are changing so much during this time that they can become the main focus of our attention.

A change in your body can be tough to deal with emotionally— mainly because, well, your body is yours and you have become used to it.

Some guys don't feel comfortable in their changing bodies and can feel as if they don't know who they are anymore. Being the only guy whose voice is changing or who's growing body hair (or the only guy who isn't) can also make some guys feel self-conscious for a while.

Some guys go into puberty not feeling too satisfied with their body or appearance to begin with. They may have wrestled with body image even before puberty started (for example, battles with weight or dissatisfaction with height). For them, puberty may add to their insecurities.

It Could Be in Your Genes

It can be tough to balance what you expect to happen to your body with what actually does happen. Lots of guys can have high expectations for puberty, thinking they'll develop quickly or in a certain way.

The best way to approach your own growth and development is to not assume you'll be a certain way. Look at everyone in your family— uncles, grandfathers, and even female relatives—to get an idea of the kinds of options your genes may have in store for you.

When Everyone Else Seems Bigger

Not everyone's body changes at the same time or even at the same pace. It can be tough if all of your friends have already matured physically and are taller and more muscular. Most guys eventually catch up in terms of growth, although some will always be taller or more muscular than others—it's in their genes.

It's natural to observe friends and classmates and notice the different ways they're growing and developing. Guys often compare themselves with other guys in certain settings, and one of the most common is the locker room. Whether at a local gym or getting ready for a game at school, time in the locker room can be daunting for any guy.

Try to keep in mind in these situations that you aren't alone if you feel you don't "measure up." Many guys feel exactly the same way about their own bodies—even those whose physiques you envy. Just knowing that almost everyone else will go through the same thing can make all the difference.

You could try talking to a trusted male adult—maybe a coach, a doctor, a teacher, or your dad. Chances are they went through similar experiences and had some of the same feelings and apprehensions when their bodies were changing.

Picture Perfect?

Guys put enough pressure on themselves, but what about the pressure society puts on them to be perfect?

It used to be that only girls felt the pressure of picture-perfect images, but these days the media emphasis on men's looks creates a sense of pressure for guys, too. And sometimes (actually, many times) that "as-advertised" body is just not attainable. The men you see in those pictures may not even be real. Magazines and ad agencies often alter photographs of models, either by airbrushing the facial and muscular features, or by putting a good-looking face on someone else's buff body.

Building a Better Body Image

So in the face of all the pressure society places on guys—and guys place on themselves—what can you do to fuel a positive body image? Here are some ideas:

- **Recognize your strengths.** Different physical attributes and body types are good for different things—and sometimes the things you did well as a kid can change during puberty. What does your body do well? Maybe your speed, flexibility, strength, or coordination leads you to excel at a certain sport. Or perhaps you have non-sports skills, like drawing, painting, singing, playing a musical instrument, writing, or acting. Just exploring talents that you feel good about can help your self-esteem and how you think of yourself.

- **A good body doesn't always translate into athletic success.** Too often, the way guys see their body image is closely associated with their performance on a sports field or in the gym. The upside to this is that if you're good at a team sport, you might have a pretty good view of your body. But what if you don't like team sports or you got cut from a team you really wanted to make? In these cases, it helps to look at individual accomplishments.

If you don't like team sports, that's OK. Find another form of physical activity that gets you going. Depending on your interests and where you live, that may be mountain biking, rock climbing, yoga, dancing, or jogging. This will help you stay in shape and help you to appreciate skills you may not have realized you had in a team environment.

If you like team sports but didn't make a particular team, don't let it get you down. Use this as an opportunity to discover what you're good at, not to lament what you aren't best at. Maybe try out for another team—so soccer wasn't for you, but maybe cross-country running will be. Or, continue to practice the sport you were cut from and try again next year. The people around you probably won't remember that you didn't make the team—not being picked is a much bigger deal to you than it was to them.

- **Look into starting a strength training program.** Exercise can help you look good and feel good about yourself. Good physiques don't just happen—they take hard work, regular workouts, and a healthy diet. There's no need to work out obsessively. A healthy routine can be as simple as exercising 20 minutes to an hour 3 days a week. Another benefit to working out properly is that it can boost your mood—lifting weights can lift your spirits.

- **Don't trash your body, respect it!** To help improve your view of your body, take care of it. Smoking and other things you know to be harmful will take a toll after a while. Treating yourself well over time results in a healthier, stronger body—and that contributes to a better body image. Practicing good grooming habits—regular showering; taking care of your teeth, hair, and skin; wearing clean clothes, etc—also can help you build a positive body image.

- **Be yourself.** Your body is just one part of who you are—along with your talent for comedy, a quick wit, or all the other things that make you unique. Your talents, skills, and beliefs are just as much a part of you as the casing they come in. So try not to let minor imperfections take over.

While it's important to have a positive body image, getting too focused on body image and appearance can cause a guy to overlook the other positive parts of himself. If you're like most guys who take care of their bodies and wear clothes that look good, you probably look great to others. You just might not be aware of that if you're too busy being self-critical.

Chapter 48

Body Dysmorphic Disorder

What Is Body Dysmorphic Disorder?

Body dysmorphic disorder (BDD) is a condition that involves **obsessions**, which are distressing thoughts that repeatedly intrude into a person's awareness. With BDD, the distressing thoughts are about perceived appearance flaws.

People with BDD might focus on what they think is a facial flaw, but they can also worry about other body parts, such as short legs, breast size, or body shape. Just as people with eating disorders obsess about their weight, those with BDD become obsessed over an aspect of their appearance. They may worry their hair is thin, their face is scarred, their eyes aren't exactly the same size, their nose is too big, or their lips are too thin.

BDD has been called "imagined ugliness" because the appearance issues the person is obsessing about usually are so small that others don't even notice them. Or, if others do notice them, they consider them minor. But for someone with BDD, the concerns feel very real, because the obsessive thoughts distort and magnify any tiny imperfection.

Because of the distorted body image caused by BDD, a person might believe that he or she is too horribly ugly or disfigured to be seen.

Text in this chapter is excerpted from "Body Dysmorphic Disorder," © 1995–2016. The Nemours Foundation/KidsHealth®. Reprinted with permission.

Behaviors That Are Part of Body Dysmorphic Disorder

Besides obsessions, BDD also involves compulsions and avoidance behaviors.

A **compulsion** is something a person does to try to relieve the tension caused by the obsessive thoughts. For example, someone with obsessive thoughts that her nose is horribly ugly might check her appearance in the mirror, apply makeup, or ask someone many times a day whether her nose looks ugly. These types of checking, fixing, and asking are compulsions.

Somebody with obsessions usually feels a strong or irresistible urge to do compulsions because they can provide temporary relief from the terrible distress. The compulsions seem like the only way to escape bad feelings caused by bad thoughts. Compulsive actions often are repeated many times a day, taking up lots of time and energy.

Avoidance behaviors are also a part of BDD. A person might stay home or cover up to avoid being seen by others. Avoidance behaviors also include things like not participating in class or socializing, or avoiding mirrors.

With BDD, a pattern of obsessive thoughts, compulsive actions, and avoidance sets in. Even though the checking, fixing, asking, and avoiding seem to relieve terrible feelings, the relief is just temporary. In reality, the more someone performs compulsions or avoids things, the stronger the pattern of obsessions, compulsions, and avoidance becomes.

After a while, it takes more and more compulsions to relieve the distress caused by the bad thoughts. A person with BDD doesn't want to be preoccupied with these thoughts and behaviors, but with BDD it can seem impossible to break the pattern.

What Causes Body Dysmorphic Disorder?

Although the exact cause of BDD is still unclear, experts believe it is related to problems with serotonin, one of the brain's chemical neurotransmitters. Poor regulation of serotonin also plays a role in obsessive compulsive disorder (OCD) and other anxiety disorders, as well as depression.

Some people may be more prone to problems with serotonin balance, including those with family members who have problems with anxiety or depression. This may help explain why some people develop BDD but others don't.

Cultural messages can also play a role in BDD by reinforcing somebody's concerns about appearance. Critical messages or unkind teasing about appearance as someone is growing up may also contribute to a person's sensitivity to BDD. But while cultural messages, criticism, and teasing might harm someone's body image, these things alone usually do not result in BDD.

It's hard to know exactly how common BDD is because most people with BDD are unwilling to talk about their concerns or seek help. But compared with those who feel somewhat dissatisfied with their appearance, very few people have true BDD. BDD usually begins in the teen years, and if it's not treated, can continue into adulthood.

How Body Dysmorphic Disorder Can Affect a Person's Life

Sometimes people with BDD feel ashamed and keep their concerns secret. They may think that others will consider them vain or superficial.

Other people might become annoyed or irritated with somebody's obsessions and compulsions about appearance. They don't understand BDD or what the person is going through. As a result, those with BDD may feel misunderstood, unfairly judged, or alone. Because they avoid contact with others, they may have few friends or activities to enjoy.

It's extremely upsetting to be tormented by thoughts about appearance imperfections. These thoughts intrude into a person's awareness throughout the day and are hard to ignore. People with mild to moderate symptoms of BDD usually spend a great deal of time grooming themselves in the morning. Throughout the day, they may frequently check their appearance in mirrors or windows. In addition, they may repeatedly seek reassurance from people around them that they look OK.

Although people with mild BDD usually continue to go to school, the obsessions can interfere with their daily lives. For example, someone might measure or examine the "flawed" body part repeatedly or spend large sums of money and time on makeup to cover the problem.

Some people with BDD hide from others, and avoid going places because of fear of being seen. Spending so much time and energy on appearance concerns robs a person of pleasure and happiness, and of opportunities for fun and socializing.

People with severe symptoms may drop out of school, quit their jobs, or refuse to leave their homes. Many people with BDD also develop depression. Those with the most severe BDD might even consider or attempt suicide.

Many people with BDD seek the help of a dermatologist or cosmetic surgeon to try to correct appearance flaws. But dermatology treatments or plastic surgery don't change the BDD. Those who find cosmetic surgeons willing to perform surgery are often not satisfied with the results. They may find that even though their appearance has changes, the obsessive thinking is still present, and they begin to focus on some other imperfection.

Getting Help for Body Dysmorphic Disorder

If you or someone you know has BDD, the first step is recognizing what might be causing the distress. Many times, people with BDD are so focused on their appearance that they believe the answer lies in correcting how they look, not with their thoughts.

The real problem with BDD lies in the obsessions and compulsions, which distort body image, making someone feel ugly. Because people with BDD believe what they're perceiving is true and accurate, sometimes the most challenging part of overcoming the disorder is being open to new ideas about what might help.

BDD can be treated by an experienced mental health professional. Usually, the treatment involves a type of talk therapy called cognitive-behavioral therapy. This approach helps to correct the pattern that's causing the body image distortion and the extreme distress.

In cognitive behavioral therapy, a therapist helps a person to examine and change faulty beliefs, resist compulsive behaviors, and face stressful situations that trigger appearance concerns. Sometimes doctors prescribe medication along with the talk therapy.

Treatment for BDD takes time, hard work, and patience. It helps if a person has the support of a friend or loved one. If someone with BDD is also dealing with depression, anxiety, feeling isolated or alone, or other life situations, the therapy can address those issues, too.

BDD, like other obsessions, can interfere with a person's life, robbing it of pleasure and draining energy. An experienced psychologist or psychiatrist who is knowledgeable about BDD can help break the grip of the disorder so that a person can fully enjoy life.

Chapter 49

Male Menopause

What Is Male Menopause?

Male menopause refers to a decline in male hormone levels that occurs due to the aging process. Since men aged 50 or older often undergo a drop in testosterone production, this condition is also known as androgen (testosterone) decline, andropause, or simply low testosterone.

Testosterone is a hormone that is found in both men and women. In men, it is produced in the testes and is responsible for the development of male sex organs before birth, brings about changes during puberty, plays a role in sex drive and sperm production, fuels physical and mental energy, and helps maintain muscle mass.

Although menopause affects men at about the same age as women, it is not the same as female menopause. In women, menopause occurs as ovulation ends and hormone production drops off quickly. In men, however, hormone production declines at a slower rate, and this may lead to only slight changes in the way the testes function.

What Are Its Symptoms?

Male menopause can lead to physical, sexual, and psychological problems that may worsen as the person ages.

"Male Menopause," © 2017 Omnigraphics. Reviewed August 2016.

These problems can include:

- lack of energy
- decreased muscle mass
- feelings of physical weakness
- insomnia or other sleep disorders
- increased body fat
- decreased libido
- erectile dysfunction
- infertility
- lowered self-confidence
- decreased motivation
- difficulty concentrating
- depression

Other less common symptoms may include reduced testicle size, tender or enlarged breasts, hot flashes, loss of body hair, and in rare cases osteoporosis.

How Is It Diagnosed?

A doctor will generally diagnose male menopause by asking about symptoms and performing a physical examination. During this conversation, it is vital that the patient inform the doctor fully about issues like sexual problems. Blood tests may be ordered to measure testosterone levels, and in some cases other tests may be required to rule out medical issues that may contribute to this condition.

How Is It Treated?

Symptoms of male menopause are commonly treated through lifestyle changes, such as eating a healthier diet, getting more sleep and regular exercise, and reducing stress. Antidepressants and therapy may be prescribed if the individual is suffering from depression.

Testosterone replacement therapy may also be suggested to help alleviate such symptoms as fatigue, decreased libido, and depression. Much like hormone replacement therapy for women, treatment using synthetic hormones is controversial and comes with potential risks and side effects. For instance, in an individual with prostate cancer, synthetic hormones may cause an increase in the growth of cancer cells. If a doctor suggests hormone replacement therapy, it is advisable to consider both the positives and negatives of this treatment option thoroughly before making a decision.

References

1. Krans, Brian. "What Is Male Menopause?" Healthline Media, March 8, 2016.

2. Derrer, David T. "Male Menopause," WebMD, LLC, August 17, 2014.

Part Five

Additional Help and Information

Chapter 52

Glossary of Men's Health Terms

abdominal ultrasound: A procedure used to examine the organs in the abdomen.

ablation: The removal or destruction of a body part or tissue or its function.

abstinence: Not having sexual intercourse.

active surveillance: Closely watching a patient's condition but not giving treatment unless there are changes in test results.

addiction: A chronic, relapsing disease, characterized by compulsive drug seeking and use accompanied by neurochemical and molecular changes in the brain.

adjuvant therapy: Treatment given after the main treatment to help cure a disease.

allergy: An abnormally high sensitivity to certain substances, such as pollens or foods.

alopecia: The lack or loss of hair from areas of the body where hair is usually found.

anemia: A condition in which the number of red blood cells is less than normal, resulting in less oxygen carried to the body's cells.

This glossary contains terms excerpted from documents produced by several sources deemed reliable.

aneurysm: A weak or thin spot on an artery wall that has stretched or ballooned out from the wall and filled with blood, or damage to an artery leading to pooling of blood between the layers of the blood vessel walls.

antiandrogen: A substance that prevents cells from making or using androgens (hormones that play a role in the formation of male sex characteristics).

antibiotic: A drug that can destroy or prevent the growth of bacteria.

anticoagulants: A drug therapy used to prevent the formation of blood clots that can become lodged in cerebral arteries and cause strokes.

antiretroviral therapy: The recommended treatment for HIV infection.

artery: Any of the thick-walled blood vessels that carry blood away from the heart to other parts of the body.

atherosclerosis: A blood vessel disease characterized by deposits of lipid material on the inside of the walls of large to medium-sized arteries which make the artery walls thick, hard, brittle, and prone to breaking.

axillary lymph node: A lymph node in the armpit region that drains lymph from the breast and nearby areas.

basal cell: A small, round cell found in the lower part (or base) of the epidermis, the outer layer of the skin.

biopsy: To remove cells or tissues from the body for testing and examination under a microscope.

calories: The energy provided by food/nutrients.

carcinoma: Cancer that begins in the skin or in tissues that line or cover internal organs.

chlamydia: A common sexually transmitted disease caused by the bacterium Chlamydia trachomatis.

cholangiocarcinoma: A rare type of cancer that develops in cells that line the bile ducts in the liver.

cholesterol: A waxy substance, produced naturally by the liver and also found in foods, that circulates in the blood and helps maintain tissues and cell membranes.

cocaine: A highly addictive stimulant drug derived from the coca plant that produces profound feelings of pleasure.

condom: A thin rubber sheath worn on a man's penis during sexual intercourse to block semen from coming in contact with the inside of the vagina.

depression: A disorder marked by sadness, inactivity, difficulty with thinking and concentration, significant increase or decrease in appetite and time spent sleeping, feelings of dejection and hopelessness, and, sometimes, suicidal thoughts or an attempt to commit suicide.

diabetes: A condition characterized by high blood glucose, resulting from the body's inability to use blood glucose for energy.

dialysis: The process of filtering wastes from the blood artificially.

diuretic: A chemical that stimulates the production of urine.

dopamine: A neurotransmitter present in regions of the brain that regulate movement, emotion, motivation, and the feeling of pleasure.

edema: The swelling of a cell that results from the influx of large amounts of water or fluid into the cell.

emphysema: A disease that affects the tiny air sacs in the lungs.

gallstone: Solid material that forms in the gallbladder or common bile duct. Gallstones are made of cholesterol or other substances found in the gallbladder.

gene: The basic unit of heredity. Genes play a role in how high a person's risk is for certain diseases.

gene therapy: Treatment that changes a gene. Gene therapy is used to help the body fight cancer. It also can be used to make cancer cells more sensitive to treatment.

genital warts: A sexually transmitted disease caused by the human papillomavirus.

germ cell tumor: A type of tumor that begins in the cells that give rise to sperm or eggs.

hemorrhagic stroke: Sudden bleeding into or around the brain.

hormone: A substance that stimulates the function of a gland.

human immunodeficiency virus (HIV): The virus that causes AIDS, which is the most advanced stage of HIV infection.

human papillomavirus: The virus that causes human papillomavirus infection, the most common sexually transmitted infection.

hypertension: Characterized by persistently high arterial blood pressure defined as a measurement greater than or equal to 140 mm/Hg systolic pressure over 90 mm/Hg diastolic pressure.

imaging: In medicine, a process that makes pictures of areas inside the body.

immune system: The complex group of organs and cells that defends the body against infections and other diseases.

immunosuppressant: A drug given to stop the natural responses of the body's immune system.

incontinence: The inability to control urination.

injection drug use: A method of illicit drug use. The drugs are injected directly into the body into a vein, into a muscle, or under the skin with a needle and syringe.

intracerebral hemorrhage: Occurs when a vessel within the brain leaks blood into the brain.

invasive cancer: Cancer that has spread beyond the layer of tissue in which it developed and is growing into surrounding, healthy tissues.

ischemia: A loss of blood flow to tissue, caused by an obstruction of the blood vessel, usually in the form of plaque stenosis or a blood clot.

jaundice: A condition in which the skin and the whites of the eyes become yellow, urine darkens, and the color of stool becomes lighter than normal.

leukoplakia: An abnormal patch of white tissue that forms on mucous membranes in the mouth and other areas of the body. It may become cancer.

lipoprotein: Small globules of cholesterol covered by a layer of protein; produced by the liver.

lobe: A portion of an organ, such as the liver, lung, breast, thyroid, or brain.

lupus: A chronic inflammatory disease that occurs when the body's immune system attacks its own tissues and organs.

lymph nodes: Small glands that help the body fight infection and disease. They filter a fluid called lymph and contain white blood cells.

magnetic resonance imaging: A type of imaging involving the use of magnetic fields to detect subtle changes in the water content of tissues.

medical test: Tests designed to rule out or avoid disease.

melanoma: A form of cancer that begins in melanocytes (cells that make the pigment melanin).

metabolism: Metabolism refers to all of the processes in the body that make and use energy, such as digesting food and nutrients and removing waste through urine and feces.

monoclonal antibody: A type of protein made in the laboratory that can bind to substances in the body, including tumor cells.

mutation: Any change in the DNA of a cell. Mutations may be caused by mistakes during cell division, or they may be caused by exposure to DNA-damaging agents in the environment.

needle biopsy: The removal of tissue or fluid with a needle for examination under a microscope.

neoplasm: An abnormal mass of tissue that results when cells divide more than they should or do not die when they should.

nonseminoma: A group of testicular cancers that begin in the germ cells (cells that give rise to sperm).

obstruction: A clog or blockage that prevents liquid from flowing easily.

oncologist: A doctor who specializes in treating cancer. Some oncologists specialize in a particular type of cancer treatment.

opioid: A natural or synthetic psychoactive chemical that binds to opioid receptors in the brain and body.

opportunistic infection: An infection that occurs more frequently or is more severe in people with weakened immune systems, such as people with HIV or people receiving chemotherapy, than in people with healthy immune systems.

outpatient surgery: A procedure in which the patient is not required to stay overnight in a hospital.

pancreas: A large gland that helps digest food and also makes some important hormones.

pap test: A procedure in which cells and secretions are collected from inside and around the cervix for examination under a microscope.

positron emission tomography (PET) scan: In a PET scan, the patient is given radioactive glucose (sugar) through a vein. A scanner then tracks the glucose in the body.

plaque: Fatty cholesterol deposits found along the inside of artery walls that lead to atherosclerosis and stenosis of the arteries.

prognosis: A prediction of the probable outcome of a disease.

psychosis: A mental disorder characterized by delusional or disordered thinking detached from reality; symptoms often include hallucinations.

pubic lice: Also called crab lice or crabs, pubic lice are parasitic insects found primarily in the pubic or genital area of humans.

radiation: The emission of energy in waves or particles. Often used to treat cancer cells.

recurrence: When cancer comes back after a period when no cancer could be found.

relapse: Return of the manifestations of a disease after an interval of improvement.

resection: Surgery to remove tissue, an organ, or part of an organ.

scabies: An infestation of the skin by the human itch mite (Sarcoptes scabiei var. hominis). The most common symptoms of scabies are intense itching and a pimple-like skin rash.

scrotum: The sac of skin that contains the testes.

semen: The fluid, containing sperm, which comes out of the penis during sexual excitement.

serotonin: A neurotransmitter used in widespread parts of the brain, which is involved in sleep, movement and emotions.

sexually transmitted disease: An infectious disease that spreads from person to person during sexual contact.

spermicide: A topical preparation or substance used during sexual intercourse to kill sperm.

stage: How much cancer is in the body and how far it has spread.

stroke: A stroke occurs when blood flow to your brain stops.

subarachnoid hemorrhage: Bleeding within the meninges, or outer membranes, of the brain into the clear fluid that surrounds the brain.

testes: The male reproductive glands where sperm are produced.

thrombosis: The formation of a blood clot in one of the cerebral arteries of the head or neck that stays attached to the artery wall until it grows large enough to block blood flow.

transient ischemic attack: A short-lived stroke that lasts from a few minutes up to twenty-four hours; often called a mini-stroke.

transmission: The spread of disease from one person to another.

trichomoniasis: A sexually transmitted disease caused by a parasite.

triglycerides: A type of fat in your blood, triglycerides can contribute to the hardening and narrowing of your arteries if levels are too high.

ulcer: An open lesion on the surface of the skin or a mucosal surface, caused by superficial loss of tissue, usually with inflammation.

ultrasound: A type of test in which sound waves too high to hear are aimed at a structure to produce an image of it.

urinalysis: A test of a urine sample that can reveal many problems of the urinary tract and other body systems.

urinary tract: The path that urine takes as it leaves the body. It includes the kidneys, ureters, bladder, and urethra.

vaccine: A substance meant to help the immune system respond to and resist disease.

virus: A microscopic infectious agent that requires a living host cell in order to replicate.

weight control: This refers to achieving and maintaining a healthy weight with healthy eating and physical activity.

Chapter 54

Directory of Resources That Provide Information about Men's Health

General

Eunice Kennedy Shriver
National Institute of Child Health and Human Development (NICHD)
Information Resource Center
P.O. Box 3006
Rockville, MD 20847
Toll-Free: 800-370-2943
Toll-Free TTY: 888-320-6942
Toll-Free Fax: 866-760-5947
Website: www.nichd.nih.gov
E-mail: NICHDInformation
ResourceCenter@mail.nih.gov

National Human Genome Research Institute (NHGRI)
National Institutes of Health
31 Center Dr., 9000 Rockville Pike
Bldg. 31 Rm. 4B09 MSC 2152
Bethesda, MD 20892-2152
Phone: 301-402-0911
Fax: 301-402-2218
Website: www.genome.gov

National Institute of Diabetes and Digestive and Kidney Diseases (NIDDK)
31 Center Dr.
Bldg. 31, Rm. 9A06 MSC 2560
Bethesda, MD 20892-2560
Phone: 301-496-3583
Website: www2.niddk.nih.gov

Resources in this chapter were compiled from several sources deemed reliable; all contact information was verified and updated in August 2016.

669

Occupational Safety and Health Administration (OSHA)
200 Constitution Ave., N.W.
Rm. No. N3626
Washington, DC 20210
800-321-6742 (OSHA)
Website: www.OSHA.gov

U.S. Department of Health and Human Services (HHS)
200 Independence Ave., S.W.
Washington, D.C. 20201
Toll-Free: 877-696-6775
Website: www.hhs.gov

U.S. Food and Drug Administration (FDA)
10903 New Hampshire Ave.
Silver Spring, MD 20993
Toll-Free: 888-INFO-FDA
(888-463-6332)
Website: www.fda.gov
E-mail: DRUGINFO@fda.hhs.gov

Cancer

American Cancer Society (ACS)
250 Williams St. N.W.
Atlanta, GA, 30303
Toll-Free: 800-227-2345
Website: www.cancer.org

American Childhood Cancer Organization (ACCO)
P.O. Box 498
Kensington, MD 20895
Toll-Free: 855-858-2226
Website: www.acco.org
E-mail: staff@acco.org

Cancer Care
275 Seventh Ave., 22nd Fl.
New York, NY 10001
Toll-Free: 800-813-4673
Website: www.cancercare.org
E-mail: info@cancercare.org

Colorectal Cancer Control Program (CRCCP)
4770 Buford Hwy N.E.
Atlanta, GA 30341
Toll-Free: 800-232-4636
Fax: 888-232-6348
Website: www.cdc.gov/cancer/crccp
E-mail: cdcinfo@cdc.gov

National Cancer Institute (NCI)
9609 Medical Center Dr.
BG 9609 MSC 9760
Bethesda, MD 20892-9760
Toll-Free: 800-4-CANCER
(800-422-6237)
Toll-Free TTY: 800-332-8615
Website: www.cancer.gov
E-mail: cancergovstaff@mail.nih.gov

Drug Abuse

National Council on Alcoholism and Drug Dependence, Inc. (NCADD)
217 Bdwy. Ste. 712
New York, NY 10007
Toll-Free Hope Line:
800-NCACALL (800-622-2255)
Phone: 212-269-7797
Fax: 212-269-7510
Website: www.ncadd.org
E-mail: national@ncadd.org

National Institute on Drug Abuse (NIDA)
6001 Executive Blvd.
Rm. 5213, MSC 9561
Bethesda, MD 20892-9561
Website: www.drugabuse.gov
E-mail: media@nida.nih.gov

Substance Abuse and Mental Health Services Administration (SAMHSA)
5600 Fishers Lane
Rockville, MD 20857
Toll-Free: 877-SAMHSA-7
(877-726-4727)
Fax: 240-221-4292
Website: www.samhsa.gov

Eating Disorders

The Academy for Eating Disorders (AED)
12100 Sunset Hills Rd.
Ste. 130
Reston, VA 20190
Phone: 703-234-4079
Fax: 703-435-4390
Website: www.aedweb.org
E-mail: info@aedweb.org

The Alliance for Eating Disorders Awareness ("The Alliance")
1649 Forum Pl.
Ste. 2
West Palm Beach, FL 33401
Toll-Free: 866-662-1235
Phone: 561-841-0900
Website: www.
allianceforeatingdisorders.com
E-mail: info@
allianceforeatingdisorders.com

The Binge Eating Disorder Association (BEDA)
637 Emerson Pl.
Severna Park, MD 21146
Toll-Free: 855-855-BEDA
(855-855-2332)
Fax: 410-741-3037
Website: bedaonline.com
E-mail: lizabeth@bedaonline.com

The British Columbia Eating Disorders Association (BCEDA)
526 Michigan St.
Victoria, BC, V8V 1S2
Canada
Phone: 250-383-2755
Website: webhome.idirect.
com/~bceda

Center for Eating Disorders (CED)
111 N. First St.
Ste. 2
Ann Arbor, MI 48104
Phone: 734-668-8585
Fax: 734-668-2645
Website: www.center4ed.org
E-mail: info@center4ed.org

Heart Disease

American Association of Cardiovascular and Pulmonary Rehabilitation (AACVPR)
330 N. Wabash Ave., Ste. 2000
Chicago, IL 60611
Phone: 312-321-5146
Fax: 312-673-6924
Website: www.aacvpr.org
E-mail: aacvpr@aacvpr.org

American Heart Association (AHA)
7272 Greenville Ave.
Dallas, TX 75231
Toll-Free: 800-AHA-USA-1
(800-242-8721)
Phone: 214-570-5978
Fax: 214-706-1551
Website: www.heart.org

Cardiovascular Research Foundation (CRF)
1700 Bdwy.
9th Fl.
New York, NY 10019
Phone: 646-434-4500
Website: www.crf.org
E-mail: info@crf.org

Heart Rhythm Society (HRS)
1325 G St. N.W.
Ste. 400
Washington, DC 20005
Phone: 202-464-3400
Fax: 202-464-3401
Website: www.hrsonline.org
E-mail: info@HRSonline.org

National Heart, Lung, and Blood Institute (NHLBI)
NHLBI Health Information Center
P.O. Box 30105
Bethesda, MD 20824-0105
Phone: 301-592-8573
TTY: 240-629-3255
Fax: 301-592-8563
Website: www.nhlbi.nih.gov
E-mail: nhlbiinfo@rover.nhlbi.nih.gov

Liver Disease

American Liver Foundation (ALF)
39 Broadway, Ste. 2700
New York, NY 10006
Toll-Free: 800-GO-LIVER
(800-465-4837)
Phone: 212-668-1000
Fax: 212-483-8179
Website: www.liverfoundation.org

Hepatitis Foundation International (HFI)
8121 Georgia Ave.
Ste. 350
Silver Spring, MD 20910
Toll-Free: 800-891-0707
Phone: 301-565-9410
Website: www.hepatitisfoundation.org
E-mail: info@hepatitisfoundation.org

United Network for Organ Sharing (UNOS)
700 N. 4th St.
Richmond, VA 23219
Toll-Free: 888-894-6361
Phone: 804-782-4800
Website: www.unos.org
E-mail: patientservices@unos.org

Mental Health Issues

Depression and Bipolar Support Alliance (DBSA)
55 E. Jackson Blvd., Ste. 490
Chicago, IL 60604
Toll-free: 800-826-3632
Fax: 312-642-7243
Website: www.dbsalliance.org

National Institute of Mental Health (NIMH)
6001 Executive Blvd.
Rm. 6200 MSC 9663
Bethesda, MD 20892-9663
Toll-Free: 866-615-6464
Phone: 301-443-4513
Toll-Free TTY: 866-415-8051
TTY: 301-443-8431
Fax: 301-443-4279
Website: www.nimh.nih.gov
E-mail: nimhinfo@nih.gov

Prostate and Urological Disorders

The American Urological Association Foundation
1000 Corporate Blvd.
Linthicum, MD 21090
Toll-Free: 800-828-7866
Phone: 410-689-3700
Fax: 410-689-3998
Website: www.urologyhealth.org
E-mail: info@
UrologyCareFoundation.org

National Kidney and Urologic Diseases Information Clearinghouse (NKUDIC)
3 Information Way
Bethesda, MD 20892
Toll-Free: 800-891-5390
Toll-Free TTY: 866-569-1162
Fax: 301–634–0176
Website: www.kidney.niddk.nih.gov
E-mail: nkdep@info.niddk.nih.gov

Prostatitis Foundation (PF)
1063 30th St.
Smithshire, IL 61478
Phone: 309-325-7184
Fax: 309-325-7189
Website: www.prostatitis.org
E-mail: info@prostatitis.org

Sexually Transmitted Diseases

AIDS Healthcare Foundation (AHF)
6255 W. Sunset Blvd.
21st Fl.
Los Angeles, CA 90028
Toll-Free: 800-263-0067
Phone: 323-860-5200
Website: www.aidshealth.org

Gay Men's Health Crisis (GMHC)
446 W. 33rd St.
New York, NY 10001-2601
Phone: 212-367-1000
Website: www.gmhc.org
E-mail: webmaster@gmhc.org

Sexuality Information and Education Council of the United States (SIECUS)
1012 14th St. N.W.
Ste. 1108
Washington, DC 20005
Phone: 202-265-2405
Fax: 202-462-2340
Website: www.siecus.org
E-mail: kromines@siecus.org

Suicide

American Association of Suicidology (AAS)

5221 Wisconsin Ave., N.W.
Washington, DC 20015
Toll-Free: 800-273-TALK
(800-273-8255)
Phone: 202-237-2280
Fax: 202-237-2282
Website: www.suicidology.org

Suicide Prevention Resource Center (SPRC)

43 Foundry Ave.
Waltham, MA 02453-8313
Toll-Free: 877-GET-SPRC
(877-438-7772)
TTY: 617-964-5448
Fax: 617-969-9186
Website: www.sprc.org
E-mail: info@sprc.org

Index

Index

Page numbers followed by 'n' indicate a footnote. Page numbers in *italics* indicate a table or illustration.

A

"A Guy's Guide to Body Image" (The Nemours Foundation/KidsHealth®) 645n
abdominal aortic aneurysm screening, overview 39–41
abdominal lymph node dissection *see* lymphadenectomy
abdominal ultrasound
  defined 661
  inguinal hernias tests 398
ablation, defined 661
ablation therapy, primary liver cancer 236
abnormality
  cryptorchidism 415
  kidney stones 350
  testicular self-examination 34
abstinence
  defined 661
  sexually transmitted diseases 473
The Academy for Eating Disorders (AED), contact 671
ACE inhibitors
  chronic kidney disease 225

ACE inhibitors, *continued*
  heart attack 195
  heart failure 174
acetaminophen (Tylenol), hepatitis B 490
action plan, heart attack 197
active surveillance
  defined 661
  prostate cancer 307
acupuncture
  hepatitis B 489
  prostatitis 437
addiction
  alcohol 615
  anabolic steroids 636
  defined 661
  gender 5
  smoking 622
adjuvant therapy
  defined 661
  penile cancer 298
  testicular cancer 322
"Adult Primary Liver Cancer Treatment (PDQ®)–Patient Version" (NCI) 229n
aerobic activity
  blood pressure 43
  physical activity for adults 113

African Americans
  diabetes 166
  fire injuries 273
  gonorrhea 486
  heart disease 16
  high blood pressure 42
  occupational injuries 275
  unintentional drowning 285
Agency for Healthcare Research and
  Quality (AHRQ)
  publication
        staying healthy 36n
aggressive driving, overview 246–8
"Aggressive Driving"
  (Omnigraphics) 246n
AHRQ *see* Agency for Healthcare
  Research and Quality
AIDS
  anabolic steroids 633
  chlamydia 477
  overview 203–9
AIDS Healthcare Foundation (AHF),
  contact 673
"Aim for a Healthy Weight"
  (NHLBI) 82n
Alagille syndrome, cirrhosis 142
Alaska Natives
  cancer statistics 124
  fire injuries 273
  heart disease 16
albumin, depicted *224*
alcohol abuse
  alcoholism 615
  heart failure 171
  osteoporosis 568
  premature ejaculation 442
"Alcohol and Public Health" (CDC) 612n
alcohol dependent 617
alcohol-impaired driving 257
alcohol poisoning, short-term health
  risks 12
alcohol-related liver disease,
  cirrhosis 141
alcohol use
  cirrhosis 145
  drowning 286
  liver cancer 230
  osteoporosis 569
  overview 10–4

alfuzosin
  tabulated *426*
  urinary incontinence 358
allergy
  defined 661
  epididymitis 390
  flu vaccine 64
  sleep apnea 579
The Alliance for Eating Disorders
  Awareness ("The Alliance"),
  contact 671
alopecia
  defined 661
alpha-blockers
  tabulated *426*
  urgency incontinence 358
Alzheimer disease
  overview 127–32
  urgency incontinence 353
"Alzheimer's Disease Fact Sheet"
  (NIA) 127n
American Association of
  Cardiovascular and Pulmonary
  Rehabilitation (AACVPR),
  contact 671
American Association of Suicidology
  (AAS), contact 674
American Cancer Society (ACS),
  contact 670
American Childhood Cancer
  Organization (ACCO), contact 670
American Heart Association (AHA),
  contact 672
American Indians
  diabetes 166
  fire injuries 273
  heart disease 16
American Liver Foundation (ALF),
  contact 672
The American Urological Association
  Foundation, contact 673
amphetamines, substance abuse 19
anabolic steroids
  gynecomastia 564
  overview 633–6
"Anabolic Steroids" (NIDA) 633n
anal sex
  chlamydia 476
  gonorrhea 487

anal sex, *continued*
  HIV 205
  male circumcision 366
  safe sex 468
"Androgenetic Alopecia" (GHR) 583n
anemia
  chronic kidney disease 225
  defined 661
  healthy muscles 109
  prostate cancer 302
  scabies 499
anesthesia
  inguinal hernia 398
  kidney stones 347
  prostatitis 433
  urgency incontinence 360
  varicocele 419
  vasectomy 456
aneurysm
  defined 662
  stroke 332
angina
  coronary heart disease 182
  heart attack 198
  high cholesterol 70
angiogram, heart disease 15
angioplasty
  coronary heart disease 186
  heart attack 195
  stroke 331
antiandrogen
  defined 662
  prostate cancer 310
antibiotic, defined 662
antibiotic medications
  balanitis 368
  chronic obstructive pulmonary
    disease 157
  cirrhosis 147
  kidney stones 351
  pneumonia 221
antibodies
  flu vaccine 65
  hemophilia 531
  HIV 207
  syphilis 504
anticoagulants
  defined 662
  heart attack 195

antidepressant medications,
  premature ejaculation 444
antimicrobial
  epididymitis 389
  trichomoniasis 508
antimuscarinics, urgency
  incontinence 358
antipsychotics, schizophrenia 607
antiretroviral therapy (ART)
  defined 662
  HIV 203
apixiban (Eliquis), heart attack 200
apnea *see* sleep apnea
Aricept (donepezil), Alzheimer
  disease 132
arrhythmia
  described 184
  heart failure 171
  sleep apnea 574
ART *see* antiretroviral therapy
artery, defined 662
artificial urinary sphincter (AUS),
  urgency incontinence 360
asalprostadil, erectile dysfunction 442
ascites, cirrhosis 143
Asian Americans, hepatitis B 136
aspirin
  colorectal cancer 163
  heart attacks 199–201
  hepatitis B 490
  prostatitis 436
assistive devices, muscular
  dystrophy 551
asthma
  chronic obstructive pulmonary
    disease 151
  flu 217
  nasal spray vaccine 64
  osteoporosis 566
atherosclerosis
  cholesterol screening 44
  defined 662
  depicted *179*
  erectile dysfunction 440
  stroke 327
AUS *see* artificial urinary sphincter
autoimmune disorders
  Peyronie disease 376
  multiple sclerosis 6

Avodart (dutasteride)
   prostatitis 436
   tabulated *426*
axillary lymph node
   male breast cancer 559
   defined 662

B

balanced diet
   healthy muscles 107
   osteoporosis 568
balanitis, overview 367–9
"Balanitis" (Omnigraphics) 367n
bariatric surgery, weight-loss 101
barium enema, colorectal cancer 49
basal cell
   defined 662
   skin cancer 30
"Basics about Diabetes" (CDC) 165n
behavioral therapy, anabolic steroid
   addiction 636
"Benefits of Physical Activity"
   (NHLBI) 115n
"Benefits of Quitting" (NCI) 617n
benign prostatic hyperplasia (BPH)
   overview 422–7
   prostate cancer 302
   prostate cancer screening 54
   urinary incontinence 352
beta blockers
   cirrhosis 147
   heart failure 174
   heart attack 195
bile
   cirrhosis 140
   liver cancer 231
bile duct stones, cirrhosis 148
binge drinking, alcohol 11
The Binge Eating Disorder
   Association (BEDA), contact 671
biofeedback
   prostatitis 437
   urgency incontinence 358
biologic therapy
   penile cancer 299
   prostate cancer 314
biopsy
   cirrhosis 146

biopsy, *continued*
   defined 662
   liver cancer 233
   male breast cancer 559
   penile cancer 293
   prostate screening 56
birth control
   overview 460–2
   vasectomy 454
   withdrawal, overview 464–6
"Birth Control Methods Fact Sheet"
   (OWH) 460n
bisphosphonate therapy, prostate
   cancer 314
bladder
   benign prostatic hyperplasia 422
   perineum 408
   prostate cancer 301
   urgency incontinence 357
bladder training, urgency
   incontinence 357
blood alcohol concentration (BAC)
   binge drinking 614
   impaired driving 258
blood alcohol levels, health risks 12
blood pressure
   abdominal aortic aneurysm 39
   alcohol health risks 12
   chronic kidney disease 227
   coronary heart disease 116
   erectile dysfunction 439
   heart attack 192
   heart failure 174
   sleep apnea 578
   stroke 328
blood tests
   balanitis 368
   cholesterol 45
   chronic kidney disease 223
   cirrhosis 146
   colorectal cancer 48
   coronary heart disease 187
   hepatitis 60
   kidney stones 346
   liver cancer 145
   muscular dystrophy 549
   pneumonia 221
   syphilis 504

blood thinners
  heart attack 200
  stroke 332
  see also anticoagulant
blotter (slang) 632
blow (slang) 631
BMI *see* body mass index
body dysmorphic disorder (BDD),
  overview 651–4
"Body Dysmorphic Disorder"
  (The Nemours Foundation/
  KidsHealth®) 651n
body image, overview 645–9
body mass index (BMI)
  screening tests for men 38
  cholesterol 71
  weight and health risk 82
  overview 84–8
  healthy eating for men 104
bone density test, osteoporosis
  screening 52
bone mineral density test,
  osteoporosis 570
booster doses, hepatitis B 489
Botox, urgency incontinence 359
BPH *see* benign prostatic hyperplasia
brain
  Alzheimer disease 127
  anabolic steroids 634
  bleeding 529
  gender difference 4
  perineal injury 408
  schizophrenia 606
  smoking 617
  stroke 325
BRCA1, breast self-examination 26
BRCA2
  breast self-examination 26
  male breast cancer 555
breast cancer
  men 554
  self-examination 26
breast self-examination, overview 26–8
"Breast Self-Examination"
  (Omnigraphics) 26n
breathing devices, sleep apnea 579
The British Columbia Eating
  Disorders Association (BCEDA),
  contact 671

bronchodilators, chronic obstructive
  pulmonary disease 155
bruit, stroke 330
buddy system, drowning 287
bullectomy, chronic obstructive
  pulmonary disease 157
bump (slang) 631
Bureau of Labor Statistics (BLS)
  publication
    fatal occupational
      injuries 275n

C

C-reactive protein (CRP)
  coronary heart disease 181
  physical activity 116
CABG *see* coronary artery bypass
  grafting
calcium oxalate stones
  kidney stones 346
  see also hypercalciuria
calories
  defined 662
  healthy eating for men 105
  healthy weight loss 92
  obesity 88
"Can an Aspirin a Day Help Prevent a
  Heart Attack?" (FDA) 199n
cancer
  alcohol use 14
  gender difference 8
  HIV 203
  human papillomavirus 492
  screening tests 48
  statistics 124
"Cancer among Men" (CDC) 124n
Cancer Care, contact 670
candida, balanitis 368
candy (slang) 631
carcinoma
  defined 662
  liver cancer 231
  male breast cancer 558
  penile cancer 295
  skin cancer 30
cardiomyopathy, heart failure 171
cardiopulmonary resuscitation,
  drowning 288

cardiovascular disease
  erectile dysfunction 440
  gender difference 8
  obesity 90
  screening tests for men 38
Cardiovascular Research Foundation
  (CRF), contact 672
Cardura (doxazosin)
  tabulated *426*
  urgency incontinence 358
carotid angiography, stroke 330
carotid artery, stroke 331
catheter
  percutaneous coronary
    intervention 195
  stroke complications 329
  urinary incontinence 361
CAT scan *see* computed axial
  tomography scan
cat valium (slang) 632
Caucasian, osteoporosis risk 569
CDC *see* Centers for Disease Control
  and Prevention
cefoxitin, epididymitis 390
ceftriaxone
  epididymitis 390
  syphilis 505
cell phones, distracted driving 251
Centers for Disease Control and
  Prevention (CDC)
  publications
      adult vaccine information 58n
      alcohol and public
        health 612n
      alcohol use and health 10n
      cancer 124n
      chlamydia 475n
      cholesterol 70n
      circumcision 364n
      colorectal cancer 161n
      coping with stress 75n
      diabetes 165n
      drowsy driving 254n
      epididymitis 386n
      genital herpes 480n
      gonorrhea 485n
      healthy weight 84n
      heart disease 14n
      hepatitis B 488n

Centers for Disease Control and
  Prevention (CDC)
  publications, *continued*
      home and recreational safety
        266n, 284n
      HPV and men 490n
      HPV vaccine for boys 61n
      impaired driving 257n
      influenza (flu) 63n, 216n
      liver cancer 229n
      lung cancer 239n
      neglected parasitic
        infections 507n
      older drivers 261n
      overweight and obesity 88n
      physical activity 112n
      poisonings prevention 280n
      pubic ("crab") lice 494n
      quitting smoking 625n
      sexually transmitted
        diseases 472n
      smoking and tobacco use 628n
      syphilis 501n
      viral hepatitis 134n
Center for Eating Disorders (CED),
  contact 671
cerebrovascular accident *see* stroke
chalk (slang) 632
chancres, syphilis 501
Chantix® 627
chemoembolization, liver cancer
  treatment 238
chemotherapy
  breast cancer 561
  described 309
  heart failure factor 171
  liver cancer 148, 237
  lung cancer 244
  male infertility causes 450
  penile cancer 300
  prostate cancer 314
  testicular cancer 33, 317
chickenpox vaccine *see* varicella
  vaccine
children
  Affordable Care Act 59
  chlamydia 476
  color blindness 520
  depression 590

children, *continued*
  domestic abuse 639
  drowning 284
  enough sleep 73
  fragile X syndrome 522
  heart disease 15
  hemophilia 534
  hernia repair 399
  influenza 216
  muscular dystrophy 549
  paraphimosis 382
  perineal injury 412
  poisoning 280
  pubic lice 495
  scabies 498
  sleep apnea 576
  stress 77
  vaccinations 58, 135
chlamydia
  balanitis 368
  defined 662
  epididymitis 388
  overview 475–80
"Chlamydia—CDC Fact Sheet
    (Detailed)" (CDC) 475n
cholangiocarcinoma
  defined 662
  see also liver cancer
cholesterol
  balanced diet 109
  cirrhosis 140
  defined 662
  high cholesterol prevention,
    overview 70–2
  obesity 90
  screening, overview 44–6
  statin 185
  see also heart disease; high-density
    lipoprotein (HDL) cholesterol;
    low-density lipoprotein (LDL)
    cholesterol
"Cholesterol" (CDC) 70n
Christmas disease *see* hemophilia
chronic conditions
  asthma 151
  cirrhosis 140
  epididymitis 386
  flu 217
  hepatitis B 136

chronic conditions, *continued*
  HIV infection 208
  kidney stones 345
  liver cancer 229
  penile cancer 370
  perineal injury 407, 413
  Peyronie disease 376
  prostatitis 429
  transient incontinence 354
chronic bronchitis *see* chronic
    obstructive pulmonary disease
chronic kidney disease (CKD),
    overview 223–7
"Chronic Kidney Disease (CKD)
    Basics" (NIDDK) 223n
chronic obstructive pulmonary disease
    (COPD)
  osteoporosis 566
  overview 149–59
  smoking 626
chronic perineal injury, depicted *411*
Cialis (tadalafil) 441
circumcision
  defined 298
  hemophilia 528
  liver cancer 230
  overview 364–6
  paraphimosis 382
  penile cancer 291
cirrhosis
  alcohol intoxication 616
  breast cancer in men 555
  hepatitis B 137
  liver cancer 230
  overview 140–8
"Cirrhosis" (NIDDK) 140n
"Civilian Fire Injuries in Residential
    Buildings (2012–2014)"
    (USFA) 269n
clinical trials
  adult primary liver cancer 235
  Alzheimer disease 131
  penile cancer 297
  prostate cancer 55
  screening tests 48
clonazepam (Klonopin) 436
clot-busting medication, stroke 331
clotrimazole 368

cocaine
  coronary artery spasm 191
  defined 663
  heart failure 171
  illegal drugs 630
  priapism 445
  substance abuse 19
cognitive function
  Alzheimer disease 127
  defined 115
  driving abilities 262
cognitive restructuring, defined 598
coitus interruptus *see* withdrawal
coke (slang) 631
collagenase (Xiaflex) 379
colon
  alcohol 12
  cancer 47
  depicted *162*
  screening 36
colonoscopy, defined 49
colorectal cancer
  overview 161–3
  screening, overview 47–51
  statistics 124
"Colorectal (Colon) Cancer" (CDC) 161n
Colorectal Cancer Control Program
  (CRCCP), contact 670
"Colorectal Cancer Screening
  (PDQ®)–Patient Version" (NCI) 47n
color vision deficiency,
  overview 514–20
computed axial tomography scan
  (CAT; CT)
  Alzheimer disease 131
  described 294
  lung cancer 242
  prostate cancer 308
  stroke 330
condoms
  birth control 461
  chlamydia 476
  defined 663
  dermatitis 368
  genital herpes 484
  overview 462–4
  premature ejaculation 444
  safer sex 467
  syphilis 506

congestive heart failure
  flu complications 217
  overview 170–8
constipation
  inguinal hernias 400
  perineal injury 412
  poly-X Klinefelter syndrome 539
  stroke complications 329
  transient incontinence 354
continuous positive airway pressure
  (CPAP)
  described 579
  sleep apnea 577
COPD *see* chronic obstructive
  pulmonary disease
"COPD" (NHLBI) 149n
"Coping with Stress" (CDC) 75n
coronary angiography
  coronary heart disease 184
  heart attack 194
  heart failure 173
coronary angioplasty, defined 195
coronary artery
  blood clots 181
  percutaneous coronary
    intervention 195
  plaque buildup 70, 116
  spasm 190
coronary artery bypass grafting
  (CABG)
  blood cholesterol level 185
  defined 196
coronary artery disease
  overview 179–88
  see also heart disease
coronary heart disease
  androgenetic alopecia 583
  heart attack 191
  heart failure 171
  physical activity 115
  obesity 90
  statistics 16
  see also coronary artery disease
"Coronary Heart Disease"
  (NHLBI) 179n
corpora cavernosa, defined 291
corpus spongiosum, defined 291
CPAP *see* continuous positive airway
  pressure

crabs *see* pubic lice
crack (slang) 631
crank (slang) 632
Crohn disease, colon cancer 48
crusted scabies, described 499
cryosurgery
  defined 298
  impotence 311
cryotherapy *see* cryosurgery
cryptorchidism
  defined 415
  sperm formation 450
  testicular cancer 34
crystal (slang) 632
CT scan *see* computed axial
  tomography scan
cystinuria, defined 345
cystoscopy
  described 435
  prostatitis 434

D

dabigatran (Pradaxa) 200
darifenacin (Enablex) 358
dementia
  Alzheimer disease 127
  excessive alcohol use 12
  syphilis 503
depression
  defined 663
  erectile dysfunction 440
  heart attack 198
  Klinefelter syndrome 539
  overview 588–93
  physical activity 115
  screenings 36
  suicide 336
  traumatic event 75
"Depression" (NIMH) 588n
Depression and Bipolar Support
  Alliance (DBSA), contact 672
desmopressin (DDAVP) 532
Detrol (tolterodine) 358
diabetes
  body mass index 82
  chronic kidney disease 223
  cirrhosis 145
  defined 663

diabetes, *continued*
  heart attack 192
  heart disease 15
  overview 165–8
  screenings 37
  types 166
diabetes mellitus *see* diabetes
dialysis
  chronic kidney disease 226
  cirrhosis 147
  defined 663
diastolic blood pressure *see* blood
  pressure
diet and nutrition
  constipation 414
  inguinal hernias 400
  kidney stones 350
  prostatitis 438
Dietary Guidelines for Americans
  drinking levels 11, 613
  healthy diet 89
dietary supplements
  depression 591
  lung cancer 241
  prostatitis 437
digestive system, colorectal cancer 47
digital rectal exam (DRE)
  prostate cancer 304
  screening tests 49
  urinary incontinence 356
Digoxin 175
dihydrotestosterone (DHT), hair
  loss 584
diphtheria, immunization 38
distracted driving, overview 248–54
"Distracted Driving at Work"
  (NIOSH) 248n
diuretic
  chronic kidney disease 225
  defined 663
  heart failure 175
  kidney stones 345
DNA Stool Test, defined 50
domestic abuse, overview 638–40
donepezil (Aricept®) 132
dopamine
  defined 663
  nicotine effect 6
doxazosin 358

drinking problem, healthcare
  provider 616
drowning
  excessive alcohol use 616
  statistics 284
drowsy driving, overview 254–7
"Drowsy Driving" (CDC) 254n
dual energy X-ray absorptiometry
  (DXA)
  body mass index 84
  defined 570
ductal carcinoma in situ, defined 554
dutasteride 359
dysthymia, defined 588

E

eating disorders
  weight loss 96
  see also body dysmorphic disorder
ecstasy, illegal drugs 445, 630
ECT see electroconvulsive therapy
edema
  cirrhosis 142
  defined 663
ejaculation
  chlamydia 475
  described 442
  gonorrhea 485
  prostatitis 432
  withdrawal 465
electrical nerve stimulation, urinary
  incontinence 359
electrocardiogram (EKG)
  coronary heart disease 184
  heart attack 194
  heart disease 15
  heart failure 175
  stroke 330
electroconvulsive therapy (ECT),
  depression 590
Eliquis (apixiban) 200
emphysema
  chronic obstructive pulmonary
    disease 157
  defined 663
  described 619
Enablex (darifenacin) 358
epididymitis, overview 386–90
"Epididymitis" (CDC) 386n

epididymo-orchitis see epididymitis
erectile dysfunction (ED)
  defined 620
  described 439
  male menopause 656
  perineal nerves 408
  Peyronie disease 375
  smoking 624
  see also sexual dysfunction
erection
  nerve-sparing surgery 307
  penile cancer 296
  phimosis 382
  priapism 444
  smoking 620
  vasectomy 456
  see also erectile dysfunction
erythroplasia of Queyrat see penile
  intraepithelial neoplasia
estrogen
  defined 8
  gynecomastia 563
  male breast cancer 26, 555
  prostate cancer 309
Eunice Kennedy Shriver National
  Institute of Child Health and
  Human Development (NICHD)
  contact 669
  publications
    causes of male infertility 449n
    fragile X syndrome 521n
    Klinefelter syndrome (KS) 535n
    muscular dystrophy 543n
    treatment options for male
      infertility 449n
    vasectomy 453n
excessive drinking, described 11
Exelon (rivastigmine) 132
exercise
  blood pressure 68
  cardiac rehabilitation 186
  healthy muscles 108
  heart disease 16
  osteoporosis 53
  pulmonary rehabilitation 156
  urgency incontinence 357
expedited partner therapy,
  chlamydia 479
exposure therapy, defined 598

F

"Facts about Color Blindness"
 (NEI) 514n
"Fact Sheets—Alcohol Use and Your
 Health" (CDC) 10n
"Fact Sheets—Excessive Alcohol
 Use and Risks to Men's Health"
 (CDC) 10n
falls
 excessive alcohol use 12
 overview 266–8
false-negative test result, defined 50
false-positive test result, defined 56
familial adenomatous polyposis (FAP),
 colorectal cancer 48, 162
family history
 chronic obstructive pulmonary
  disease 152
 cirrhosis 145
 coronary heart disease 186
 inguinal hernia 397
 Klinefelter syndrome 542
 lung cancer 241
 obesity 83
 prostate cancer 54
 Peyronie disease 378
 stroke 334
 testicular cancer 34, 316
 type 2 diabetes 166
fatalities
 construction 278
 drowsy driving 255
fecal occult blood test (FOBT)
 colorectal cancer 51
 described 49
fertility
 assistive reproductive
  technologies 452
 cryptorchidism 415
 prostate fluid 428
 retrograde ejaculation 446
 spermatocele 401
 varicocele 450
 vasectomy 457
fesoterodine (Toviaz) 358
finasteride (Proscar) 359
fire (slang) 632
fire-related injuries, overview 269–74

first line therapy, lindane 496
5-alpha reductase inhibitors, defined
 359, 425
Flomax (tamsulosin) 358
flu *see* influenza
flu shots
 chronic obstructive pulmonary
  disease 156
 vaccination 63
follow-up test
 cancer 56, 312, 324
 colorectal cancer 51
 recurrent penile cancer 300
foot care, diabetes 167
foreskin removal *see* circumcision
forget-me pill (slang) 632
fragile X syndrome, overview 521–5
"Fragile X Syndrome" (NICHD) 521n

G

G (slang) 631
galantamine, mental function 132
gallstone
 body mass index 82
 defined 663
 described 144
ganja (slang) 632
Gay Men's Health Crisis (GMHC),
 contact 673
"Gender Differences in Primary
 Substance of Abuse across Age
 Groups" (SAMSHA) 17n
gene
 color blindness 514
 defined 663
gene therapy, defined 663
genetic testing, described 549
genital herpes, overview 480–5
"Genital Herpes—CDC Fact Sheet
 (Detailed)" (CDC) 480n
genital warts
 defined 663
 HPV infections 491
Genetics Home Reference (GHR)
 publication
  androgenetic alopecia 583n
genitourinary bacteruria, acute
 epididymitis 388

Georgia Home Boy (slang) 631
germ cell tumor
  defined 663
  testicular cancer 315
"Get a Bone Density Test"
  (ODPHP) 52n
"Get Enough Sleep" (ODPHP) 72n
"Get the Facts to Feel and Look
  Better" (USDA) 104n
"Get Your Blood Pressure Checked"
  (ODPHP) 41n
"Get Your Cholesterol Checked"
  (ODPHP) 44n
GFR *see* glomerular filtration rate
Gleason score, prognosis 302
glomerular filtration rate (GFR),
  smoking 227
glucocorticoid medications
  muscular dystrophy 551
  osteoporosis 566
gonorrhea
  acute epididymitis 388
  overview 485–8
  sperm formation 450
"Gonorrhea—CDC Fact Sheet
  (Detailed Version)" (CDC) 485n
good cholesterol *see* high-density
  lipoprotein (HDL) cholesterol
gout, kidney stones 345
grass (slang) 632
gynecomastia
  Klinefelter syndrome 538
  male breast self-examination 27
  overview 563–4
"Gynecomastia" (The Nemours
  Foundation/KidsHealth®) 563n

H

HDL cholesterol *see* high-density
  lipoprotein (HDL) cholesterol
head injury, falls 266
"Health Effects" (NCI) 617n
"Healthy Muscles Matter"
  (NIAMS) 106n
"Healthy Weight" (CDC) 84n
heart attack
  heart diseases 15
  overview 189–99

heart attack, *continued*
  physical activity 116
  stressed heart 618
"Heart Attack" (NHLBI) 189n
heart disease
  described 14
  overview 169–201
  risk factors 590
  smoking 72
heart failure
  described 183
  high blood pressure 37
  overview 170–8
  sleep apnea 575
  spirometry test results 153
"Heart Failure" (NHLBI) 170n
Heart Rhythm Society (HRS),
  contact 672
heavy drinking *see* excessive drinking
hemochromatosis, liver cancer 230
hemophilia, overview 526–35
"Hemophilia" (NHLBI) 526n
hemorrhagic stroke
  defined 663
  described 328
hepatic encephalopathy, described 144
hepatitis A, described 134
hepatitis B
  described 135
  liver cancer 229
  overview 488–90
"Hepatitis B" (CDC) 488n
hepatitis C virus
  described 37
  liver cancer 230
Hepatitis Foundation International
  (HFI), contact 672
hepatocellular carcinoma, adult
  primary liver cancer 231
herb (slang) 632
heroin
  gender profiles 18
  gynecomastia 564
  illegal drugs 631
herpes simplex viruses (HSV), genital
  herpes 480
HHS *see* U.S. Department of Health
  and Human Services
high blood pressure *see* hypertension

"High Blood Pressure" (NIA) 68n
high-density lipoprotein (HDL)
  cholesterol, healthy diet 71
Hispanics, heart disease 16
HIV *see* human immunodeficiency
  virus
"HIV/AIDS" (OWH) 467n
HIV infection
  described 390
  genital herpes 482
  syphilis 504
"Home and Recreational Safety"
  (CDC) 266n, 284n
homicide
  excessive alcohol use 617
  overview 211–4
  short-term health risks 12
"Homicide" (Omnigraphics) 211n
hormone
  defined 663
  gynecomastia 564
  male menopause 656
  sperm formation 450
hormone therapy, described 309
horse (slang) 632
"How Much Physical Activity Do
  Adults Need?" (CDC) 112n
HPV *see* human papillomavirus
"HPV and Men—Fact Sheet" (CDC) 490n
"HPV Vaccine Is Recommended for
  Boys" (CDC) 61n
human immunodeficiency virus (HIV)
  defined 663
  see HIV infection
human papillomavirus (HPV)
  defined 664
  male circumcision 365
  oral cancer 28
  overview 490–4
hydrocele, overview 390–3
"Hydrocele" (Omnigraphics) 390n
hydrocelectomy, described 392
hypercalciuria, described 569
hyperparathyroidism, secondary
  osteoporosis 566
hypertension
  defined 664
  described 42
  obesity 90

hyperuricosuria, kidney stones 351
hypogonadism, described 567
Hytrin (terazosin), alpha-
  blockers 358

I

ICD *see* implantable cardioverter
  defibrillator
ice (slang) 632
"If You Need to Lose Weight"
  (OWH) 92n
imaging, defined 664
imipramine (Tofranil), tricyclic
  antidepressants 359
immune system
  autoimmune disorders 6
  biologic therapy 310
  defined 664
  HIV 203
  targeted therapy 562
immunization *see* vaccinations
immunosuppressant
  defined 664
  drug therapy 551
impaired driving, overview 257–61
"Impaired Driving: Get the Facts"
  (CDC) 257n
implantable cardioverter defibrillator
  (ICD), heart failure 176
impotence
  cryosurgery 311
  reproductive health 14
  transurethral resection 426
  see also erectile dysfunction
in vitro fertilization (IVF), male
  fertility 452
incontinence
  defined 664
  prostatectomy 426
indirect inguinal hernia
  depicted *394*
  described 394
infertility
  erectile dysfunction 620
  male menopause 656
  retrograde ejaculation 447
  sexual function 14
  testicular cancer 317

infiltrating ductal carcinoma, breast
cancer 554
influenza (flu)
chronic obstructive pulmonary
disease 151
nasal spray vaccine 64
overview 216–8
"Influenza (Flu)" (CDC) 63n
inguinal hernia, overview 393–400
"Inguinal Hernia" (NIDDK) 393n
inhalants, tabulated *632*
inhaled glucocorticosteroids, chronic
obstructive pulmonary disease 149
inhaled steroids, bronchodilators 155
inheritance pattern for hemophilia,
depicted *527*
injection drug use
defined 664
hepatitis B 488
insulin
diabetes 167
type 2 diabetes 145
insulin resistance
androgenetic alopecia 583
coronary heart disease 180
"Interested in Losing Weight?"
(USDA) 92n
intracerebral hemorrhage
defined 664
hemorrhagic stroke 327
invasive cancer
carcinoma in situ 558
colorectal cancer 162
defined 664
ischemia, defined 664
ischemic stroke, described 326
ivermectin, scabies 498

J

jaundice
cirrhosis 143
defined 664
hepatitis B 488
jogging
body image 648
healthy muscles 108
osteoporosis prevention 571
junk (slang) 632

K

K (slang) 632
Kegel exercises, described 358
kidney disease, smoking 227
kidney failure
diabetes 165
flu complications 218
hypertension 42
kidney stones, overview 344–51
"Kidney Stones in Adults"
(NIDDK) 344n
kidneys
cystine stones 346
depicted *224*
diabetes 37
Klinefelter syndrome,
overview 535–42
"Klinefelter Syndrome (KS)" (NICHD)
535n
"Know the Facts about Heart Disease"
(CDC) 14n

L

lactulose, hepatic
encephalopathy 147
laparoscopic hernia repair,
described 399
laparoscopy
adult primary liver cancer 233
hydrocelectomy 392
laser surgery, described 427
latent syphilis, over-the-counter
drugs 505
latex condoms
balanitis 368
trichomoniasis 508
see also condoms
laxative
hepatic encephalopathy 147
virtual colonoscopy 50
LDL cholesterol *see* low-density
lipoprotein cholesterol
leukoplakia, oral disease 629
Levitra (vardenafil), erectile
dysfunction 441
life expectancy, acquired
immunodeficiency syndrome 204

lifestyle changes
  dialysis 226
  erectile dysfunction 441
  stroke 331
lindane shampoo, pubic lice
  infestation 496
lipoprotein
  coronary heart disease 187
  defined 664
  high cholesterol 70
liquid ecstasy (slang) 631
liver cancer
  described 145
  hepatitis B 488
  overview 229–38
"Liver Cancer" (CDC) 229n
liver disorders *see* cirrhosis; hepatitis;
  liver cancer
liver failure, cirrhosis 148
lobe
  adult primary liver cancer 231
  defined 664
  prostate cancer 304
low-density lipoprotein (LDL)
  cholesterol
  defined 664
  healthy diet 71
LSD, tabulated *632*
lung cancer
  cancer 124
  described 37
  DNA 620
  overview 239–44
"Lung Cancer" (CDC) 239n
lung function tests, described 152
lungs with chronic obstructive
  pulmonary disease, depicted *150*
lung transplant, chronic obstructive
  pulmonary disease 157
lung volume reduction surgery, lung
  volume reduction surgery 157
lupus
  defined 664
  immunosuppressants 551
luteinizing hormone releasing
  hormone (LH-RH) agonists,
  hormone therapy 309
lymph nodes
  defined 664

lymph nodes, *continued*
  lung cancer 242
  testicular cancer 33
lymphadenectomy, prostate
  cancer 312

M

magnetic resonance imaging (MRI)
  adult primary liver cancer 231
  Alzheimer disease 131
  biopsy 435
  cirrhosis 146
  defined 665
  described 294
  imaging tests 146
  liver cancer 234
  penile cancer 294
  prostate cancer 303
  stroke 330
major depression, persistent
  depressive disorder 588
malathion, pubic lice infestation 496
"Male Breast Cancer Treatment
  (PDQ®)—Patient Version"
  (NCI) 554n
"Male Circumcision" (CDC) 364n
male condom, described 462
"Male Condom Fact Sheet"
  (OPA) 462n
male menopause, overview 655–7
"Male Menopause"
  (Omnigraphics) 655n
male pattern baldness,
  overview 583–5
male perineum, depicted *407*
male sling, surgery 360
marijuana
  gender profiles 18
  gynecomastia 564
  illegal drugs 630
measles, mumps, and rubella (MMR),
  described 60
medical test
  Alzheimer disease 131
  defined 665
  described 433
Medicare, abdominal aortic
  aneurysm 41

medications
  acquired immunodeficiency
    syndrome 206
  Alzheimer disease 132
  ascites 147
  benign prostatic hyperplasia 426
  cholesterol level 185
  chronic bacterial prostatitis 438
  cirrhosis 146
  depression 590
  drowsy driving 254
  erectile dysfunction 441
  fragile X syndrome 525
  gender differences 4
  hepatitis C 139
  herpes 484
  high blood pressure 68
  interactions 609
  kidney stones 351
  muscular dystrophy 551
  osteoporosis 570
  penile intraepithelial neoplasia 371
  Peyronie disease 379
  poisoning 281
  posttraumatic stress disorder 597
  premature ejaculation 444
  prostatitis 436
  pubic lice infestation 496
  quitting smoking 627
  retrograde ejaculation 446
  schizophrenia 607
  trichomoniasis 509
  urgency incontinence 358
melanoma, defined 665
memantine (Namenda), mental
  function 132
"Men and Heart Disease Fact Sheet"
  (CDC) 14n
"Men and Sexual Trauma"
  (VA) 641n
"Men and Women" (USDA) 104n
"Men: Stay Healthy at Any Age"
  (AHRQ) 36n
men who have sex with men (MSM)
  HIV infection 365
  HPV vaccines 493
metabolic syndrome
  coronary heart disease 181
  sleep apnea 575

metabolism
  cirrhosis 140
  defined 665
metastasis, cancer 557
meth (slang) 632
methamphetamine
  described 19
  illegal drugs 445
  see also amphetamines
Mirabegron (Myrbetriq), beta-3
  agonists 359
MMR *see* measles, mumps, and
  rubella
moderate drinking, described 11
monoclonal antibody
  defined 665
  hormone therapy 310
mortality
  health consequences 90
  overview 121–5
  scabies 498
"Mortality in the United States, 2014"
  (CDC) 122n
mosaicism, fragile X syndrome 523
mouthpieces, sleep apnea 578
multiple sclerosis (MS)
  autoimmune disorders 6
  erectile dysfunction 440
  urgency incontinence 353
  weakened immune system 621
muscle building, anabolic steroids 633
muscles of the arm, depicted *107*
muscular dystrophy, overview 543–51
"Muscular Dystrophy" (NICHD) 543n
mutation, defined 665
"Myths and Realities of
  Domestic Abuse against Men"
  (Omnigraphics) 638n

N

National Cancer Institute (NCI)
  contact 670
  publications
        adult primary liver cancer
          treatment 229n
        benefits of quitting 617n
        colorectal cancer screening 47n
        health effects 617n

National Cancer Institute (NCI)
publications, *continued*
    male breast cancer
      treatment 554n
    penile cancer treatment 291n
    prostate cancer screening 53n
    prostate cancer
      treatment 301n
    testicular cancer
      treatment 315n
    understanding prostate
      changes 422n
"National Census of Fatal
Occupational Injuries in 2014"
(BLS) 275n
National Council on Alcoholism and
Drug Dependence, Inc. (NCADD),
contact 670
National Eye Institute (NEI)
publication
    facts about color
      blindness 514n
National Heart, Lung, and Blood
Institute (NHLBI)
contact 672
publications
    aim for a healthy weight 82n
    benefits of physical
      activity 115n
    COPD 149n
    coronary heart disease 179n
    heart attack 189n
    heart failure 170n
    hemophilia 526n
    sleep apnea 573n
    stroke 325n
National Human Genome Research
Institute (NHGRI), contact 669
National Institute for Occupational
Safety and Health (NIOSH)
publication
    distracted driving 248n
National Institute of Arthritis and
Musculoskeletal and Skin Diseases
(NIAMS)
publications
    healthy muscles 106n
    osteoporosis in men 565n

National Institute of Diabetes and
Digestive and Kidney Diseases
(NIDDK)
contact 669
publications
    chronic kidney disease
      (CKD) 223n
    cirrhosis 140n
    inguinal hernia 393n
    kidney stones in adults 344n
    penile curvature (Peyronie
      disease) 374n
    perineal injury in males 407n
    prostatitis: inflammation of the
      prostate 428n
    urinary incontinence in
      men 351n
    weight management 97n
National Institute of Dental and
Craniofacial Research (NIDCR)
publication
    oral cancer exam 28n
National Institute of Mental Health
(NIMH)
contact 673
publications
    depression 588n
    posttraumatic stress
      disorder 593n
    schizophrenia 600n
National Institute on Aging (NIA)
publications
    Alzheimer disease 127n
    high blood pressure 68n
National Institute on Drug Abuse
(NIDA)
contact 671
publication
    anabolic steroids 633n
National Institutes of Health (NIH)
publication
    sex and gender 4n
National Kidney and Urologic
Diseases Information Clearinghouse
(NKUDIC), contact 673
NCI *see* National Cancer Institute
needle aspiration, treatment 392
needle biopsy, defined 665

"Neglected Parasitic Infections in the United States" (CDC) 507n
The Nemours Foundation/ KidsHealth®
  publications
    body image 645n
    drugs 630n
    body dysmorphic disorder 651n
    gynecomastia 563n
    pneumonia 219n
    testicular torsion 403n
    undescended testicles 414n
    varicocele 416n
neonatal pain rating system, male circumcision 365
neoplasm
  defined 665
  testicular cancer 33
nephrostomy tube, depicted *349*
nerve cells, Alzheimer disease 128
neurosyphilis, described 503
mild cognitive impairment (MCI), memory problems 128
NIA *see* National Institute on Aging
NIAID *see* National Institute of Allergy and Infectious Diseases
NIAMS *see* National Institute of Arthritis and Musculoskeletal and Skin Diseases
NICHD *see Eunice Kennedy Shriver* National Institute of Child Health and Human Development
nicotine, dopamine release 6
NIDA *see* National Institute on Drug Abuse
NIDDK *see* National Institute of Diabetes and Digestive and Kidney Diseases
nitroglycerin pill, emergency medical care 190
nocturnal erection test, erectile dysfunction 441
nonalcoholic fatty liver disease (NAFLD), cirrhosis 142
non-melanoma skin cancer, potential skin cancers 30
nonseminoma
  defined 665
  testicular germ cell tumors 315

Norwegian scabies *see* crusted scabies

O

obesity
  androgenetic alopecia 583
  body mass index 82
  heart disease 17
  urinary incontinence 352
obstruction
  alpha-blockers 358
  defined 665
  open prostatectomy 427
occupational injuries, overview 275–80
Occupational Safety and Health Administration (OSHA), contact 670
ocular syphilis, neurosyphilis 503
Office of Disease Prevention and Health Promotion (ODPHP)
  publications
    cholesterol 44n
    sleep 72n
    blood pressure 41n
    abdominal aortic aneurysm 39n
    bone density test 52n
Office of Population Affairs (OPA)
  publication
    condom 462n
Office on Women's Health (OWH)
  publications
    birth control methods 460n
    HIV/AIDS 467n
    lose weight 92n
ofloxacin, epididymitis 389
"Older Adult Drivers" (CDC) 261n
older adults
  Alzheimer disease 127
  depression 590
  impaired driving 281
  physical activity 112
oligospermia, infertility 450
Omnigraphics
  publications
    aggressive driving 246n
    balanitis 367n
    breast self-examination 26n
    domestic abuse against men 638n

Omnigraphics
  publications, *continued*
    homicide 211n
    hydrocele 390n
    male menopause 655n
    penile intraepithelial
      neoplasia 370n
    penile trauma 372n
    phimosis and paraphimosis 381n
    sexual dysfunction 439n
    skin cancer self-
      examination 30n
    spermatocele 401n
    testicular self-examination 33n
    withdrawal 464n
    women's longevity 7n
oncologist
  defined 665
  lung cancer 244
open hernia repair, described 398
opioid
  anabolic steroids 635
  defined 665
opportunistic infection
  defined 665
  HIV 203
oral cancer, risk 28
"Oral Cancer: Causes and Symptoms
  and the Oral Cancer Exam"
  (NIDCR) 28n
"The Oral Cancer Exam" (NIDCR) 28n
oral cancer self-examination,
  overview 28–30
oral sex, syphilis 501
orchiectomy, defined 406
osteoarthritis, obesity 90
osteoporosis, metabolic bone
  diseases 144
"Osteoporosis in Men" (NIAMS) 565n
osteoporosis screening, overview 52–3
outpatient surgery
  defined 665
  vasectomy 456
overflow incontinence, urine spills 354
overweight *see* obesity
"Overweight and Obesity" (CDC) 88n
oxybutynin (Oxytrol),
  antimuscarinics 358
oxygen therapy, described 156

P

pacemaker, myotonic MD 551
  heart failure 175
  muscular dystrophy 551
Pacific Islanders, diabetes 166
Paget disease of the nipple, male
  breast cancer 554
pancreas
  cirrhosis 143
  defined 665
  hemochromatosis 232
  insulin 165
  virtual colonoscopy 51
pap test, defined 665
paraphimosis, described 382
Parkinson disease, depression 590
paroxetine, antidepressant
  medications 444
PE *see* premature ejaculation
penectomy, surgery 298
penile anatomy, depicted *292*
penile cancer, overview 291–300
"Penile Cancer Treatment (PDQ®)–
  Patient Version" (NCI) 291n
"Penile Curvature (Peyronie's
  Disease)" (NIDDK) 374n
penile intraepithelial neoplasia,
  overview 370–1
penile trauma, overview 372–4
"Penile Trauma"
  (Omnigraphics) 372n
penis
  chlamydia 475
  depicted *292*
  Klinefelter syndrome 537
percutaneous ethanol injection, adult
  primary liver cancer 237
percutaneous nephrolithotomy
  depicted *348*
  kidney stones 347
perineal injury, overview 407–14
"Perineal Injury in Males"
  (NIDDK) 407n
perineal urethroplasty, perineal
  injury 409
permethrin, lice-killing lotion 496
PET scan *see* positron emission
  tomography

Peyronie disease
  erectile dysfunction 440
  overview 374–81
phimosis, described 381
"Phimosis and Paraphimosis"
  (Omnigraphics) 381n
physical activity, muscular
  dystrophy 550
physical examination
  chlamydia 476
  male menopause 656
  perineal injury 412
piperonyl butoxide, lice-killing
  lotion 496
plaque, defined 666
pneumonia
  immunization 38
  muscular dystrophy 550
  overview 219–21
"Pneumonia" (The Nemours
  Foundation/KidsHealth®) 219n
poisoning, smokeless tobacco 630
polyps, colon cancer 48
polysomnogram, sleep studies 577
polyurethane condoms, male
  condom 462
portable monitor, described 578
portal hypertension, described 143
positron emission tomography (PET)
  scan, defined 666
posttraumatic stress disorder (PTSD)
  overview 593–600
  sexual assault 641
"Posttraumatic Stress Disorder"
  (NIMH) 593n
potassium permanganate,
  balanitis 369
Pradaxa (dabigatran), blood
  thinners 200
prednisone, muscular dystrophy 551
prehypertension, blood pressure 42
premature ejaculation (PE), male
  sexual dysfunction 439
presumptive therapy, acute
  epididymitis 388
priapism
  described 444
  persistent partial erection 410
proctitis, chlamydia 475

prognosis, defined 666
propecia, tabulated *426*
Proscar (finasteride)
  5-alpha reductase inhibitors 359
  see also propecia
prostate, depicted *429*
prostate cancer
  benign prostatic hyperplasia 422
  risk factors 54
  testosterone levels 568
prostate cancer gene 3 (PCA3) test,
  described 55
prostate cancer screening,
  overview 53–6
"Prostate Cancer Screening (PDQ®)–
  Patient Version" (NCI) 53n
"Prostate Cancer Treatment (PDQ®)–
  Patient Version" (NCI) 301n
prostate-specific antigen (PSA) test,
  cancer 303
prostatectomy, recurrent prostate
  cancer 314
prostatitis, overview 428–38
Prostatitis Foundation (PF),
  contact 673
"Prostatitis: Inflammation of the
  Prostate" (NIDDK) 428n
pruritus, scabies 498
psychosis
  defined 666
  schizophrenia 603
  see also depression
psychotherapy, described 598
PTSD *see* posttraumatic stress
  disorder
"PTSD Study: Men Versus Women"
  (VA) 21n
"Pubic "Crab" Lice" (CDC) 494n
pubic lice
  defined 666
  overview 494–8
pulmonary rehabilitation,
  described 156
pulmonologist, lung cancer 244
pyrethrins 496

Q

"Quitting Smoking" (CDC) 625n

R

radiation
  defined 666
  male breast cancer 26, 555
radiation therapy
  chest 241
  described 298
  prostate cancer 56
radical prostatectomy, inguinal
  hernia 307
radiofrequency ablation, ablation
  therapy 236
Razadyne (galantamine), Alzheimer
  disease 132
Recurrent Adult Primary Liver
  Cancer, treatment 238
rectum hepatic encephalopathy 147
rectum
  colorectal cancer 161
  depicted *162*
  hepatic encephalopathy 147
recurrence
  defined 666
  penile intraepithelial neoplasia 371
recurrent prostate cancer
reefer (slang) 632
relapse
  defined 666
  psychosocial treatments 609
renal tubular acidosis, kidney
  stones 345
resection, defined 666
retrograde ejaculation, male sexual
  dysfunction 439
risky sexual behavior, drinking 617
rivaroxaban (Xarelto), blood
  thinners 200
retrograde ejaculation, described 446
roach (slang) 632
robo (slang) 632
rock (slang) 631
Rohypnol, tabulated *632*
roofies (slang) 632

S

safe sex, overview 467–9
Sanctura (trospium chloride),
  antimuscarinics 358

Sarcoptes scabiei 498
SCA *see* sudden cardiac arrest
scabies
  defined 666
  overview 498–500
schizophrenia, overview 600–610
"Schizophrenia" (NIMH) 600n
sclerotherapy, hydrocele
  treatment 392
screening tests
  abdominal aortic aneurysm 39
  blood pressure 41
  cholesterol 44
  color blindness 520
  colorectal cancer 47
  liver cancer 148
  lung cancer 242
  osteoporosis 52
  overview 36–8
  prostate cancer 53, 306
scrotum
  chronic epididymitis 386
  defined 666
  granuloma 455
  hydrocele 390
  inguinal hernia symptom 396
  prostatitis symptom 430
  retractile testes 415
  spermatocele 401
  testicular self-examination (TSE) 34
  testicular torsion 404
  undescended testicle 414
  varicocele 417, 450
seasonal flu *see* influenza
secondary syphilis, symptoms 502
secondhand smoke
  COPD risk factor 151
  described 240
self-examinations
  breast cancer 26
  oral cancer 28
  skin cancer 30
  spermatocele 402
  testicular cancer 33
semen
  defined 666
  ejaculation 442
  5-alpha reductase inhibitors side
    effect 425

semen, *continued*
  hepatitis B 136, 488
  HIV transmission 204
  prostate 428
  retrograde ejaculation 446
  vasectomy 453
semen analysis, described 436
seminal fluid 453
seminal vesicles, prostate cancer 305
sentinel lymph node biopsy
  breast cancer 559
  described 294
serotonin
  body dysmorphic disorder 652
  defined 666
  premature ejaculation cause 442
  steroid abuse 634
sertraline, premature ejaculation
  treatment 444
serum tumor marker test
  adult primary liver cancer 233
  testicular cancer 316
"Sex and Gender" (NIH) 4n
sexual assault
  alcohol health risk 12
  alcohol/drug abuse risk 469
  overview 641–3
  posttraumatic stress disorder risk
    factor 596
sexual dysfunction
  overview 439–47
  penile trauma consequence 372
  prostatitis complication 432
"Sexual Dysfunction"
  (Omnigraphics) 439n
sexual function
  alcohol effect 14
  benign prostatic hyperplasia
    (BPH) 54
  hormonal therapy 309
  male circumcision 365
  perineal injury 413
Sexuality Information and Education
  Council of the United States
  (SIECUS), contact 673
sexually transmitted disease (STD)
  defined 666
  excessive alcohol use consequence 14
  HIV in uncircumcised men 364

sexually transmitted disease (STD),
  continued
  withdrawal risk 465
  overview 471–509
"Sexually Transmitted Diseases"
  (CDC) 472n
"Sexually Transmitted Diseases
  Treatment Guidelines" (CDC) 498n
shingles
  immunizations 38
  older adults 59
side effects
  alpha-blockers 425
  anabolic steroids 634
  antipsychotic medications 607
  CPAP 580
  electroconvulsive therapy 592
  5-alpha reductase inhibitors 425
  hormone therapy 309
  HPV vaccine 62
  prednisone 551
  synthetic hormone 657
  TURP 426
sigmoidoscopy, described 49
sildenafil (Viagra), ED treatment 441
skin cancer self-examination,
  overview 30–2
"Skin Cancer Self-Examination"
  (Omnigraphics) 30n
sleep apnea
  CHD risk factor 182
  drowsy driving 256
  inadequate sleep factors 75
  obesity consequences 90
  overview 573–581
"Sleep Apnea" (NHLBI) 573n
sleep disorders
  drowsy driving risks 254
  inadequate sleep factors 75
  male menopause symptoms 656
sleep studies 577
smokeless tobacco, overview 628–30
smoker's cough, COPD symptom 151
smoking
  AAA risk factor 39
  COPD cause 149
  effect on dopamine 5
  heart disease risk factor 15, 45, 72
  high blood pressure risk 69

smoking, *continued*
  lung cancer 37
  obesity risk factor 83
  oral cancer 28
  osteoporosis risk 53
  reactions to stress 76
  unhealthy HDL cholesterol level 46
"Smoking and Tobacco Use" (CDC) 628n
smoking cessation, bupropion 604
snow (slang) 631
solifenacin (VESIcare),
  antimuscarinics 358
special K (slang) 632
speeding 246
spermatic cord
  testicles 315
  testicular cancer stage 318
  epididymitis 387
  inguinal hernia 394
  testicular torsion 403
  varicocele diagnosis 418
spermatocele, overview 401–3
"Spermatocele" (Omnigraphics) 401n
spermatocelectomy 402
spermicide
  birth control methods, tabulated *462*
  contraceptives 468
  defined 666
  dermatitis 368
spirometry
  depicted *153*
  described 153
splenomegaly
  imaging tests 146
  portal hypertension complication 144
sprain
  described 108
  prevention 110
stages
  adult primary liver cancer 234
  BCLC staging system 235
  breast cancer 557
  defined 666
  heart failure treatment 174
  penile cancer 295
  prostate cancer 304
  syphilis 502
  testicular cancer 318
standard drink, described 11, 260

statin
  cholesterol treatment 185
  heart attack treatment 195
statistics
  cancer 124
  civilian fire injuries 269
  distracted driving 251
  drinking levels 13
  erectile dysfunction 439
  fragile X syndrome 523
  genital herpes 480
  homicide 211
  Klinefelter syndrome 536
  life expectancy 7
  mortality 122
  occupational injuries 275
  substance abuse 17
  suicide 335
STD *see* sexually transmitted disease
stem cell transplant 323
stent, percutaneous coronary
  intervention 195
steroids
  balanitis 368
  chronic obstructive pulmonary
    disease 155
  glucocorticoid medication 567
  Peyronie disease treatments 379
  phimosis 382
  see also anabolic steroids
strangulated hernia, inguinal
  hernias 396
strength training
  better body image 648
  *Physical Activity Guidelines for
    Americans* 89
stress
  adequate sleep 73
  CHD risk factor 182
  depression risk factors 590
  driving 254
  ED-related conditions 440
  high blood pressure prevention 44
  male menopause 656
  PE risk factors 443
  Peyronie disease complications 377
  smoking 625
  stroke 334
stress incontinence, described 353

stress management, overview 75–9
stress test
  coronary heart disease 184
  heart disease 15
  heart failure 173
stroke
  anabolic steroids 634
  aspirin 199
  defined 666
  high cholesterol 37, 44, 70
  obesity 90
  overview 325–34
  sleep apnea 575
  smokeless tobacco 629
  smoking 69
  statin 185
  urgency incontinence 353
"Stroke" (NHLBI) 325n
subarachnoid hemorrhage
  defined 666
  see also stroke
substance abuse
  gender differences, overview 17–20
  PTSD-correlated conditions 595
  schizophrenia 604
  sexual trauma 642
  suicide 335
  teens with Klinefelter syndrome 539
Substance Abuse and Mental Health
  Services Administration (SAMHSA)
  contact 671
  publication
      suicide prevention 335n
sudden cardiac arrest (SCA),
  arrhythmia 184
suicide
  alcohol abuse risk 12, 617
  anabolic steroids 635
  body dysmorphic disorder 654
  depression symptoms 589
  overview 335–9
  prostate cancer 56
  schizophrenia 604
"Suicide Prevention" (SAMHSA) 335n
Suicide Prevention Resource Center
  (SPRC), contact 674
support groups
  chronic obstructive pulmonary
      disease 159

support groups, *continued*
  domestic violence 640
  heart attack 198
  posttraumatic stress disorder 597
  smoking 154
surgery
  aneurysm clipping 332
  bariatric surgery 101
  benign prostatic hyperplasia 426
  breast cancer 561
  coronary heart disease 186
  heart failure 175
  hemorrhagic stroke 332
  hydrocelectomy 392
  infertility 451
  inguinal hernia 396
  lung cancer 244
  male circumcision 364
  muscular dystrophy 551
  orchiectomy 309
  orchiopexy 416
  penile cancer 297
  penile fracture 373
  penile intraepithelial neoplasia 371
  perineal surgery 409
  perineal urethroplasty 409
  Peyronie disease 380
  priapism 445
  prostate cancer 307
  prostatectomy 409
  retrograde ejaculation 446
  sleep apnea 580
  spermatocelectomy 402
  standard cancer treatment types 236
  testicular torsion 405
  torn/bleeding aneurysm 40
  urgency incontinence 360
  vasectomy 458
syphilis, overview 501–6
"Syphilis-CDC Fact Sheet (Detailed)"
  (CDC) 501n
systolic blood pressure 68

T

tadalafil (Cialis), ED treatment 441
"Talk to Your Doctor about Abdominal
  Aortic Aneurysm" (ODPHP) 39n
tamsulosin, urgency incontinence 358

targeted therapy
  breast cancer 562
  adult primary liver cancer 237
  standard treatment types 236
  lung cancer 244
  monoclonal antibody therapy 562
  prostate cancer 310
tattoos, hepatitis B 489
terazosin (Hytrin), urgency
  incontinence 358
testes *see* testicles
testicles (testes)
  congenital hydroceles 391
  cryptorchidism 34, 415
  defined 666
  described 315
  hormone therapy 309
  hydrocele 390
  inguinal hernias 394
  retractile testes 415
  sperm formation 450
  testicular exam 418
  testicular torsion 403
  testosterone 655
  undescended testicle 414
  varicocele 417
  vasectomy 454
testicular asymmetry 34
testicular cancer
  testicular self-examination 33
  overview 315–24
"Testicular Cancer Treatment
  (PDQ®)–Patient Version"
  (NCI) 315n
testicular self-examination,
  overview 33–4
"Testicular Self-Examination"
  (Omnigraphics) 315n
testicular torsion, overview 403–6
"Testicular Torsion" (The Nemours
  Foundation/KidsHealth®) 403n
testosterone
  anabolic steroids 633
  5-alpha reductase inhibitors 425
  hormone therapy 309
  hypogonadism 568
  Klinefelter syndrome 537
  male menopause 655
  secondary osteoporosis 566

tetanus, recommended
  vaccinations 58
thrombosis, defined 667
TIA *see* transient ischemic attack
"Tips to Prevent Poisonings"
  (CDC) 280n
tobacco use
  colorectal cancer 152
  tobacco/nicotine dependence 625
Tofranil (imipramine), urgency
  incontinence 359
tolterodine (Detrol), urgency
  incontinence 359
total cholesterol 46
transient ischemic attack (TIA)
  defined 667
  described 329
transmission
  defined 667
  genital herpes 481
  HIV 205
  syphilis 506
transplantation
  heart 176
  kidney 226
  liver 148
  lung 157
  pancreas 168
  stem cell 323
transrectal ultrasound
  described 435
  prostate cancer 302
transurethral incision of the prostate
  (TUIP) 426
transurethral microwave
  thermotherapy (TUMT) 427
transurethral needle ablation
  (TUNA) 427
transurethral resection of the prostate
  (TURP) 426
Trichomonas vaginalis 507
trichomoniasis, defined 667
triglycerides
  defined 667
  overview 507–9
triple C (slang) 632
trospium (Sanctura), urgency
  incontinence 358

tunica albuginea
  penis fracture 373
  Peyronie disease 374

U

ugly duckling sign, described 32
ulcer
  defined 667
  smoking 618
ulcerative colitis *see* Crohn disease
ultrasound
  abdominal aortic aneurysm 36
  cryosurgery 311
  defined 667
  described 413
  liver cancer 145
"Understanding Prostate Changes"
  (NCI) 422n
undescended testicle,
  overview 414–6
"Undescended Testicles"
  (The Nemours Foundation/
  KidsHealth®) 414n
United Network for Organ Sharing
  (UNOS), contact 672
unprotected sex, hepatitis B
  vaccine 489
ureteroscopic stone removal,
  depicted *348*
ureteroscopy, described 347
urethra
  prostate cancer 53
  sexual problems 408
  ureteroscopy 347
uric acid stones *see* hyperuricosuria
urinalysis
  defined 667
  described 434
  kidney stones 346
  retrograde ejaculation 446
urinary incontinence,
  overview 351–60
"Urinary Incontinence in Men"
  (NIDDK) 351n
urinary tract
  defined 667
  epididymitis 386
  stress incontinence 353

urine flow
  diagnostic tests 356
  kidney stones 347
  pelvic floor muscle 358
urodynamic testing, diagnostic
  tests 356
uroflowmetry
  diagnostic tests 356
  urodynamic tests 435
urolithiasis, kidney stone 344
Uroxatral (alfuzosin), alpha-
  blockers 358
U.S. Department of Agriculture
  (USDA)
  publications
    feel and look better 104n
    lose weight 92n
    men and women 104n
U.S. Department of Health and
  Human Services (HHS)
  contact 670
  publications
    condoms 462n
    HIV/AIDS 203n
U.S. Department of Veterans Affairs
  (VA)
  publications
    men and sexual trauma 641n
    PTSD 21n
U.S. Fire Administration (USFA)
  publication
    civilian fire injuries 269n
U.S. Food and Drug Administration
  (FDA)
  contact 670
  publication
    aspirin and heart attack 199n
"Using Condoms" (HHS) 462n

V

"Vaccine Information for Adults"
  (CDC) 58n
vaccines
  defined 667
  overview 58–66
vacuum devices, medical therapies 380
vardenafil (Levitra), erectile
  dysfunction 441

varicella, described 60
varicocele, overview 416–9
"Varicocele" (The Nemours
  Foundation/KidsHealth®) 416n
varicocelectomy, varicocele 419
vas deferens
  testicular cancers 315
  vasectomy failure 455
vasectomy, overview 453–7
"Vasectomy: Condition Information"
  (NICHD) 453n
ventricular fibrillation, heart
  attack 190
verapamil, nonsurgical
  treatments 379
Viagra (sildenafil), oral
  medications 441
viral hepatitis *see* hepatitis
"Viral Hepatitis" (CDC) 134n
virus
  defined 667
  HIV treatment 206
vitamin D supplement,
  osteoporosis 570

W

waist circumference, described 83
walking pneumonia,
  contagiousness 220
warfarin, blood thinners 200
watchful waiting, described 306
water-related accidents,
  overview 284–9
weight control
  defined 667
  weight-loss program 98
weight loss
  body mass index 93
  overview 97–101

weight management, weight loss
  plan 93
"Weight Management" (NIDDK) 97n
Western blot, genital herpes 483
"What Are the Causes of Male
  Infertility?" (NICHD) 449n
"What Is HIV/AIDS?" (HHS) 203n
"What Treatment Options Are
  Available for Male Infertility?"
  (NICHD) 449n
"What You Need to Know about
  Drugs" (The Nemours Foundation/
  KidsHealth®) 630n
whooping cough
  immunizations 38
  pneumonia 220
  Tdap vaccine 58
"Why Women Live Longer than Men"
  (Omnigraphics) 4n
withdrawal, overview 464–6
"Withdrawal" (Omnigraphics) 464n

X

Xarelto (rivaroxaban), blood
  thinners 200

Y

yawning, drowsy driving 255
yeast infection, balanitis 368
yoga, physical activity 115

Z

zero tolerance laws, impaired
  driving 260
zoledronate 310
zoster vaccine, shingles 59
Zyban® 627
Zyloprim 351